UCSF-VA
JOHNS HOPKINS-CDC

Human Sacrifice, Genocide, Child Porn

MANDATED REPORT
On the Socialization of Violence and Abuse to
DOJ/OIG and the Social Body

PRIMUM NON NOCERCE

First Do No Harm

Dr. Richard L. Matteoli
CALIFORNIA PENAL CODES
FEDERAL CODE 42 AND WIC.

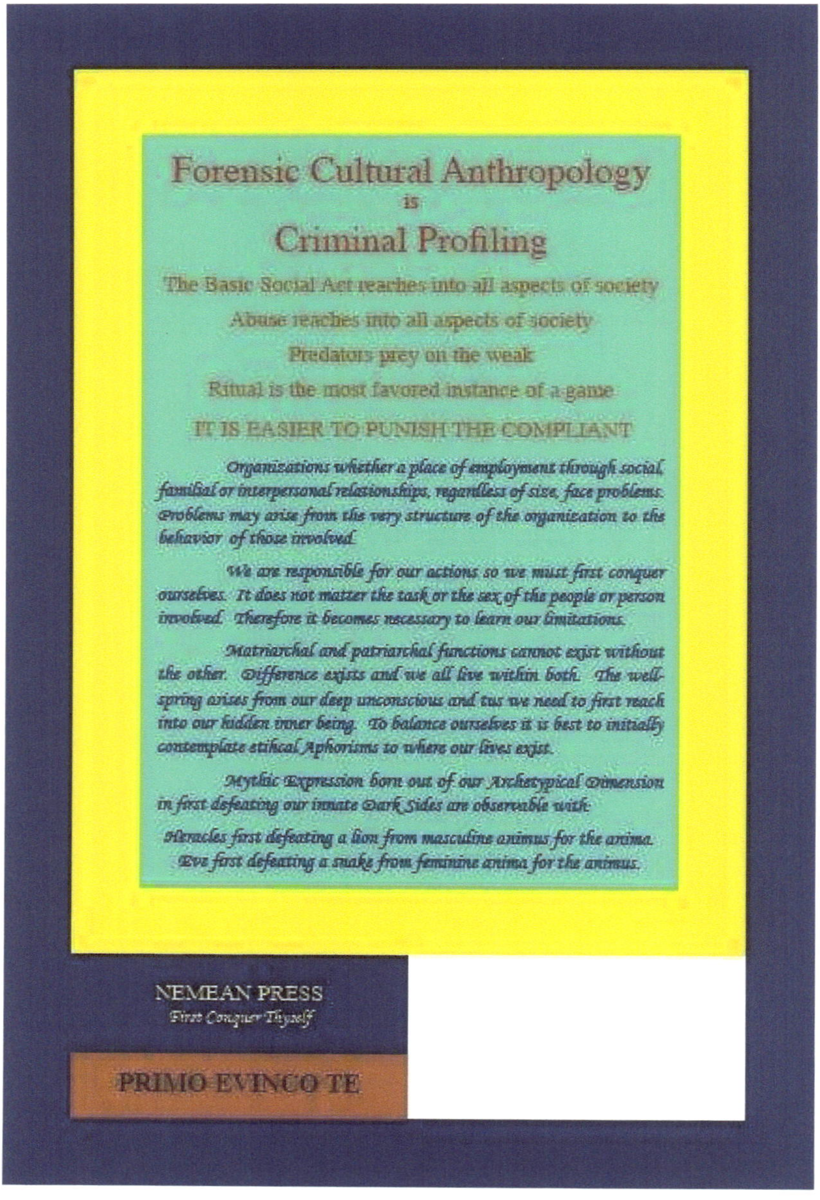

Forensic Cultural Anthropology

is

Criminal Profiling

The Basic Social Act reaches into all aspects of society

Abuse reaches into all aspects of society

Predators prey on the weak

Ritual is the most favored instance of a game

IT IS EASIER TO PUNISH THE COMPLIANT

Organizations whether a place of employment through social, familial or interpersonal relationships, regardless of sise, face problems. Problems may arise from the very structure of the organization to the behavior of those involved.

We are responsible for our actions so we must first conquer ourselves. It does not matter the task or the sex of the people or person involved. Therefore it becomes necessary to learn our limitations.

Matriarchal and patriarchal functions cannot exist without the other. Difference exists and we all live within both. The well-spring arises from our deep unconscious and tus we need to first reach into our hidden inner being. To balance ourselves it is best to initially contemplate etihcal Aphorisms to where our lives exist.

Mythic Expression born out of our Archetypical Dimension in first defeating our innate Dark Sides are observable with:

Heracles first defeating a lion from masculine animus for the anima.
Eve first defeating a snake from feminine anima for the animus.

NEMEAN PRESS
First Conquer Thyself

PRIMO EVINCO TE

UCSF-VA
Johns Hopkins-CDC
Human Sacrifice, Genocide, Child Porn

MANDATED REPORT
On the Socialization of Violence and Abuse to DOJ/OIG and the Social Body

INTRODUCTION
REFERENCE LIBRARY Conversational Study Guide
TITLE Leads to Mythic Expression
DOUBLE TITLES and PHOTO to Archetypical Dimension

Dr. Richard L. Matteoli

California Penal Codes
Federal Code 42 and wic.

First Conquer Thyself:
Nemean Press
Monterey, CA 93940
USA

Richard L. Matteoli

Primo Evinco Te

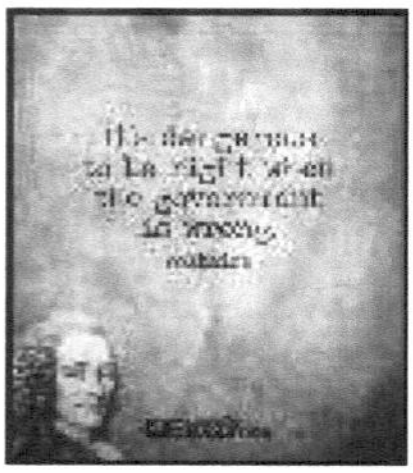

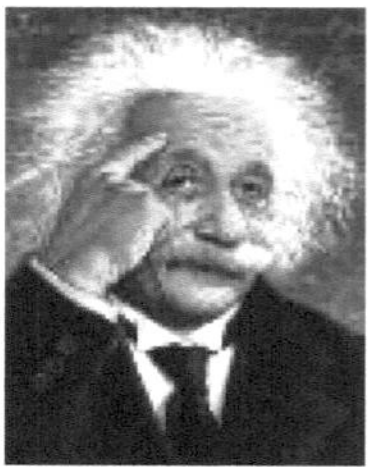

I: UCSF Medical School to VA to CDC: BDSM Child Pornography Sites and Practice of Two Aspects of Human Sacrifice Turned Genocidal
ISBN: 978-1-943347-14-8

Acknowledgment: *John J. Whitworth.*

From ***Mandated Reports***, in part to the Social Body, regarding the socialization of violence and abuse. Confidentiality limits though. Per *required*: In part, Individual State Penal Codes as well as Federal Codes wic. 15630-15632 and 42 U.S. Code Section § 13031 in Reporting Suspicions. Reports are made and sent to appropriate authorities for their decision to proceed. Being a Social Issue, the Social Body is a valid appropriate authority.

Images courtesy Google and used in the **Mandated Reports** as well as appropriate images from those Reports also inserted when structurally usable.

Mandated Report VA to CDC - Matteoli

Because of the expansiveness of this subject the following is sufficient for initial use by both individuals and Law Enforcement Investigations.

For government employees this Mandated Report will aid in Self-Correction and WHISTLEBLOWER PROTECTION.

Read copyright section allowing free use EXCEPT FOR PROFIT.

This Report is Legally Mandated. Discuss as you will.
Prove me correct or incorrect. That is your job.
There is a Military connotation with the subject regarding life-long Sub-clinical PTSD that is easily EXACERBATED to Clinical Significance; AFFECTING BOTH Self and Society, Nationally and Internationally.
Severity depends on many factors.
NOT DISCUSSABLE HERE

Do so in an appropriate, respectful and responsible manner.

The text is too expensive because of size, cost of color paper and printing. It cannot be priced less due to Publisher Rules and Regulations.

Print two sided and place in a binder if you care to have a hard copy.

When making any type of Complaint you may store on a disc with all other pertinent information to send to proper authorities with the written Complaint(s).

If you send to an authority that knows a more appropriate authority, they will forward.

Upon reaching THE proper authority, they will create as many copies as they require and store a copy for their records.

MANDATED REPORT

Full Report Sent Separate
SOCIAL GENOCIDE OF ANIMUS SERVANCY

MENS REA, SIGNATURE'S DESIRE, MODUS OPERANDI

MENS REA: Dominant Personalities Functional Scenario under DESTROYER-PROSTITUTE Child Archetypes in THANTOS

SIGNATURE'S DESIRE: Wealth, Power, Control, Authority, Domination, Selfishness, Unchangeable THANTOS = The Ritual

MODUS OPERANDI: THANTOS Behavior with a series of steps using TRANSFERENCE in COLLECTIVE TRANSMISSION taking advantage of Victim's Inverted Self-Regard (per: Henry A. Flynt) for Due Process and Blaming the Victim that the Victim or aide is the person to be feared:

1): PERPETRATOR: Initial existence of Neurotic Anxiety created from the Fear of Illicit Behavior being Discovered by Victim-Society.

2): Upon Ideation, whether true or false, of Discovery is Transferred Psychosis.

3): Perception and Flow Transference of Aggression occurs and increases until abated.

4): In turn in the Victim is a Transference Neurosis to Transferred Anxiety, if unabated exacerbations expand depending on Victim.

5): Then through the CON Approach through Internal Authoritative Justification procedures, a veiling is created in blaming the victim and those who aid the victim.

6): RESULT: correlates to all Bovine and Human Sacrifices, actual or attenuated, in Mythic Expression through the Archetypical Dimension.

7): WHY? Dissociation of Victim's Humanity in Malignant Narcissism.

SUSPICIONS

Hobbs Act; RICO Act, Feres Doctrine, Collusion Tucker Act; Federal Tort; Color of Law/Authority; Honest Services; Endangerment; Patient Abandonment; Malice Aforethought; Violations of Contract Intent by United States with Service Member; Breach of Duty; Hate Crime; Civil Conspiracy; Domesticated Violence; Elder Abuse Financial and Physical; Incompetence; Willful and Wanton Disregard of Patient Well Being; Deliberate Indifference; Gross Indifference; Deliberate Difference; Extortive Exercise power, control and authority; Dual Responsibility with Conflict of Interest; Fraud: Constructive, in Factum and Misrepresentation; Transference of Aggression; Quid Pro Quo; Infliction Emotional Distress;: Actual and Constructive; Punitive Personality Disorder; Malignant Narcissism; Doubling per Robert Lifton; Lack of Inverted Self Regard per Henry Flint; Attribution per Darley and Latane in Diffusion of Responsibility; Dishonest Gaming per Eric Berne in Transactional Analysis; Babelian Imperative; Fear Conditioning; Libel Personal and Professional Character; Lack of Supervision including: Hiring, Training, Control of Employees; Denial Equal Protection and due Process; Affective Bribery; Dismissive Cognition and/or Cognitive Dissonance; Malignant Hero Syndrome both Medical and Procedural; Violation of State and Federal Disability Acts including: age, race, national origin and religion; Misdirection in Diagnosis; Refusal to Diagnose; Practicing Below the International Usual and Customary Standards of Care; Hostile Environment; Coercion; Patient Molestation; Mens Rea in both Commission and Omission; Questionable Staff Relationships; Questionable Construction, Maintenance and Management of Patient Records; Dissociation of Service Member Humanity; Harassment; Administrative and Clinical Patient Maltreatment; Affective: Cycle of Betrayal, Abuse, Power and Control; Violence per Signature's Desire; Decreasing Patient Value within the Legal Triangle; Culture Bound and/or Culture Specific Syndromes in Shared Psychotic Disorder in Delusion; Retaliation in Social Transference; Factitious Disorder with: Munchausen by Proxy including: Transgenerational; Collective Transmission; Social Agency with Direct Agency; and For Profit; Antisocial Personality Disorder; Sociopathy; Psychopathy; Team Predation; Phased Genocidal Behavior; Assault with a Deadly Weapon (Improper Assault use of meds with prescription and a Battery if taken –Commission-omission unless agreed upon). Interference proper doctor-patient relationship; Homicide all categories depending; Phased Genocidal Activity with Cultural Imperialism: In Part.

Mandated Report VA to CDC - Matteoli

If I can stop one heart from breaking,
I shall not live in vain:
If I can ease one life from aching,
Or cool one pain,
Or help one fainting robin
Unto his nest again,
I shall not live in vain.
Emily Dickinson

Perhaps the sentiments contained in the following pages
are not yet sufficiently fashionable to procure them general favor.
A long habit of not thinking a thing wrong
gives it a superficial appearance of being right
and raises at first a formidable outcry in defense of custom.
Time makes more converts than reason.
Thomas Paine

The woman becomes the vehicle of nature.
The man becomes the vehicle of society, the social order, the social purpose.
The woman is life. The man is the servant of life…
Life has overtaken her. Woman is what it is all about,
the giving of birth and the giving of nourishment.
Without him she would become overwhelmed.
Joseph Campbell, *The Power of Myth*

Abuse occurs when one person controls or subjugates another through humiliation, fear, intimidation, and physical or verbal abuse.
People do not have to use their fists to abuse one another.
Aaron

He found himself envying those under the maternal embrace of the organization.

Marie Louise von Franz in Jung's: Man and his Symbols.

I should have left him alone. But he irritated me…
Stay away from me or I'll kill you.
Marie. *Innocent Blood.*

Be my victim. My altar awaits your sacrifice.
***Candyman.* Candyman 3**

Pitiful earth brains… It amuses me to watch your puny efforts.
Naya. *Devil Girl from Mars*

WHEN DOES THE SERVANT BECOME A SLAVE?
Matteoli

TABLE OF CONTENTS

MONTELEONE

GUIDELINE TEXT FOR MANDATED REPORTERS

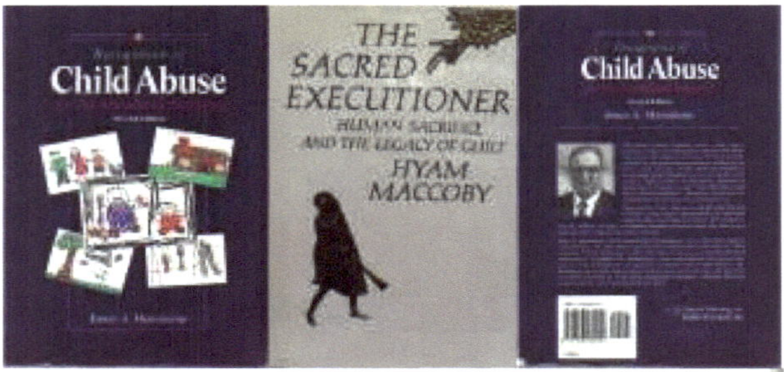
Child Abuse
THE SACRED EXECUTIONER
HYAM MACCOBY
Child Abuse

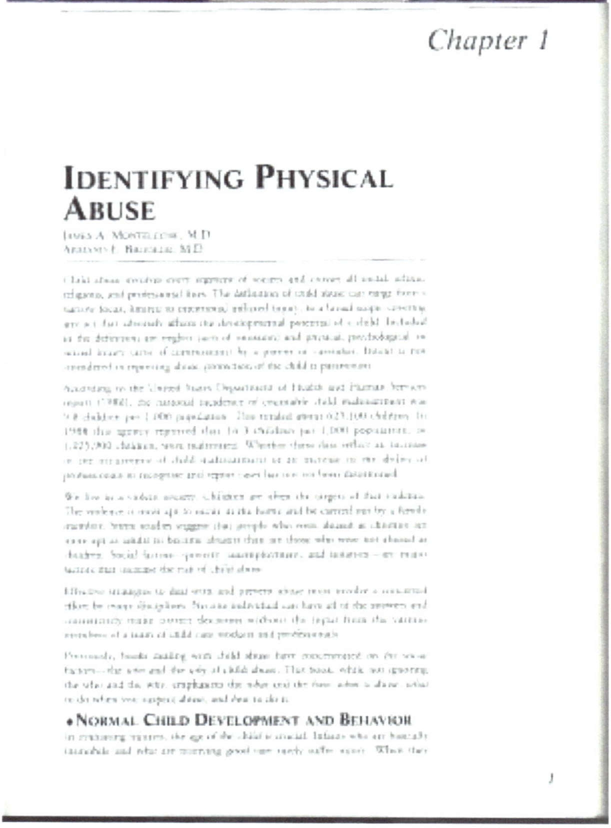

Chapter 1

IDENTIFYING PHYSICAL ABUSE

James A. Monteleone, M.D.
[illegible], M.D.

[illegible]

NORMAL CHILD DEVELOPMENT AND BEHAVIOR

[illegible]

Mandated Report VA to CDC - Matteoli

Read Picture Line as a Sentence

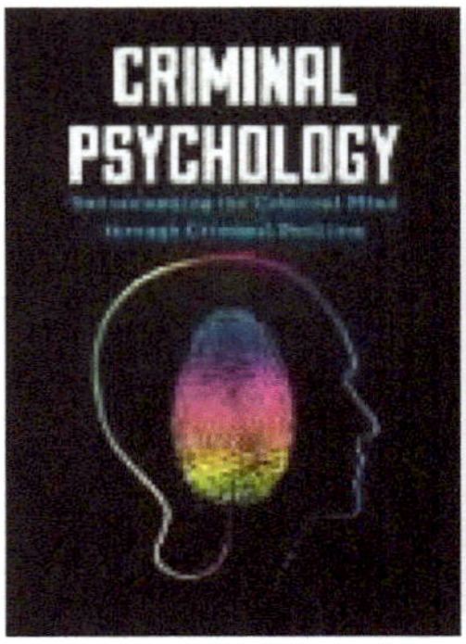

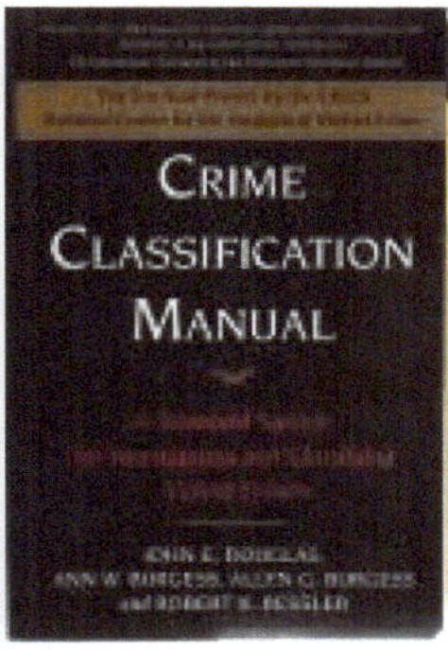

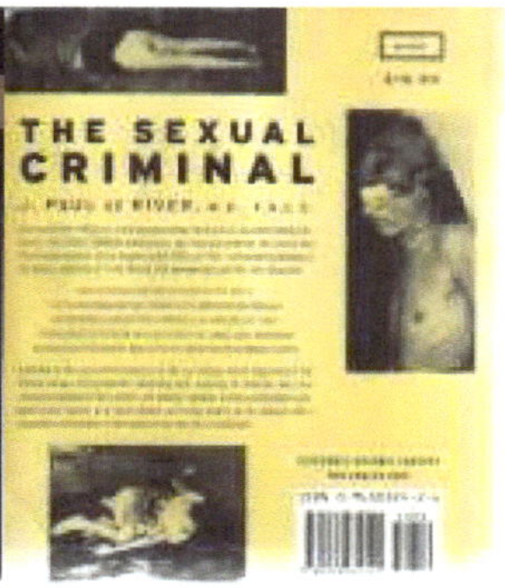

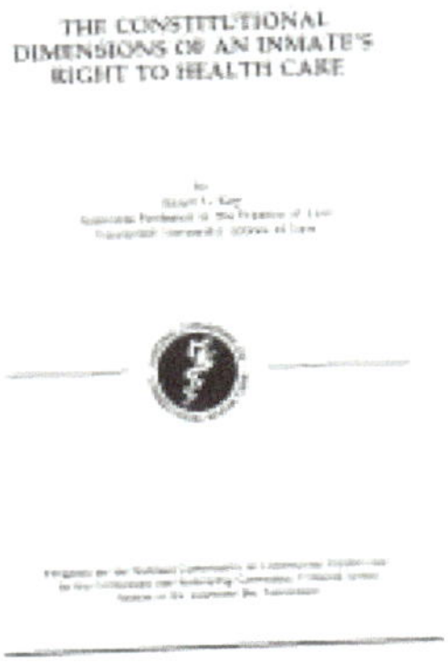

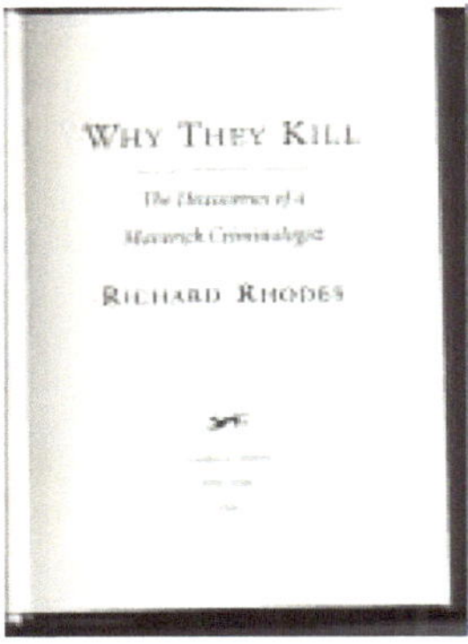

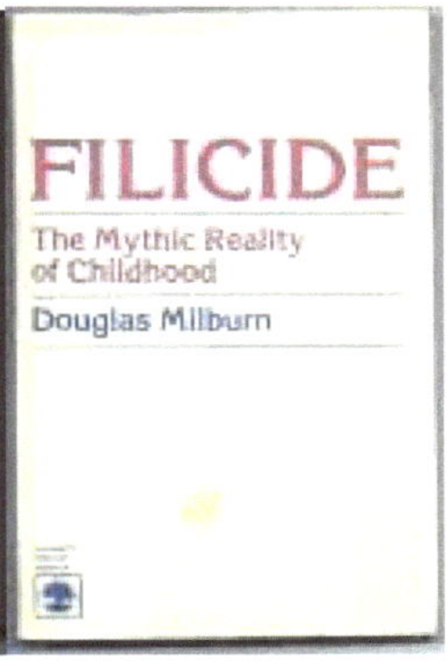

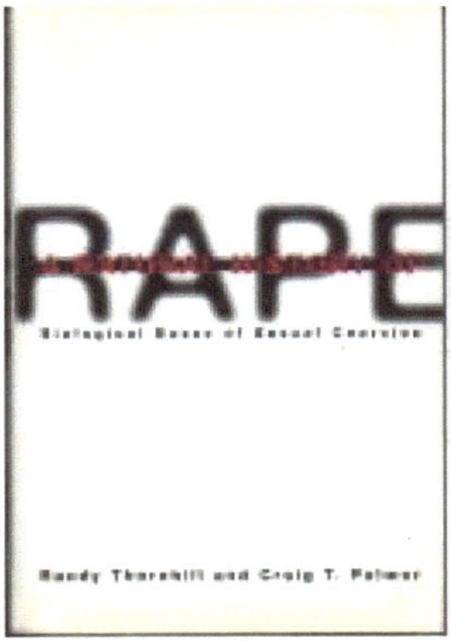

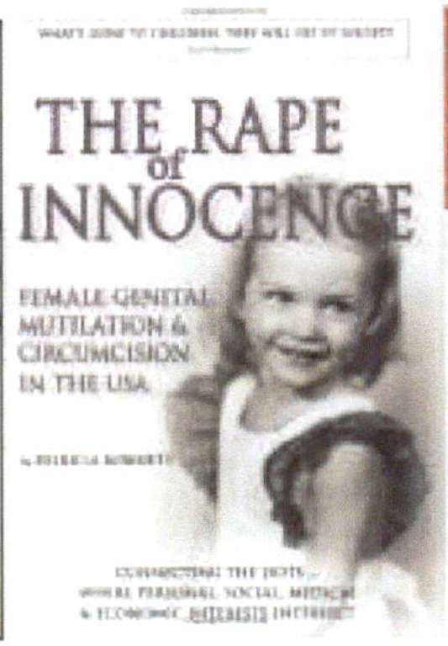

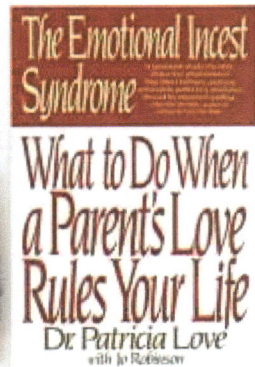

Mandated Report VA to CDC - Matteoli

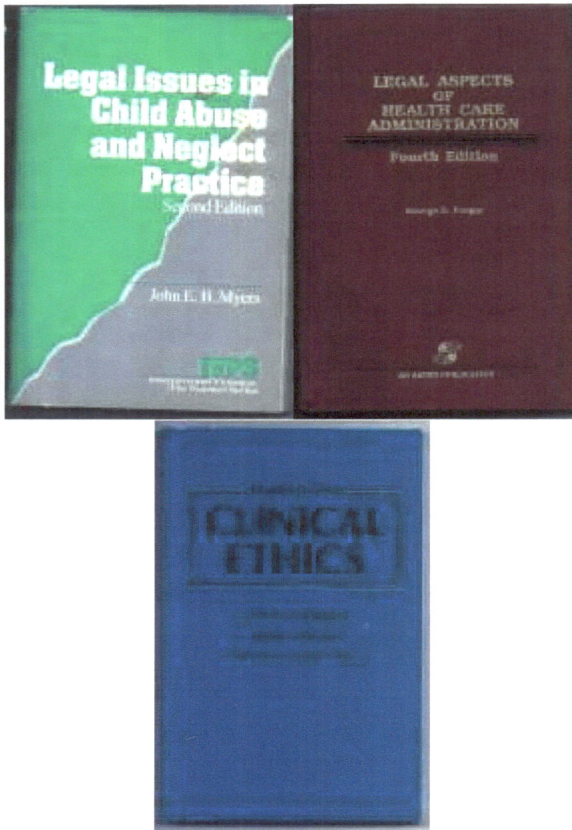

Thantos, the **Death Wish**, is stronger than the Pleasure Principle
History-Fantasy-Reality-Intertwine-**Myth-Archetype-Present**
The **Totemic Analogy** replaced the
Metaphor in One-God Theology

Preliminary Mandated Reports sent to DOJ/OIG and VA
Personal Counseling given as best possible
Ethics Course **Submitted** to VA Appeals and Resolution Boards
From this was another Retaliation Attempt by the VA

Mandated Report VA to CDC - Matteoli

PRELIMINARY FINDINGS

1): There is a criminal sub-culture that has resulted in Loss of Life within the VA. RESOLUTION: Immediate Law Enforcement.

2): Per HOBBS and RICO Federal Government Bonuses are against the law and considered a form of Bribery and Racketeering. RESOLUTION: The bonus system needs immediate termination and restitution made via an individual monthly repayment plan.

3): Pharmaceuticals are not properly used, including such ancillary requirements as liver monitoring for Tuberculosis Prophylaxis. RESOLUTION: A): Directive that Material Safety Data Sheets (MSDS) in the Physician's Desk Reference by followed with CODICILE for testing efficacy of concerns per doctor-patient agreement. B): Each Region establish a Collegial in-house pharmaceutical Review/Q&A/Hotline.

4): Clinic notes obfuscating for impropriety is inappropriate, especially with regard to illicit Red Flagging and refusal to deliver appropriate Consideration clinically and financially to the Veteran from implied Intent of Contract made by Veteran with the United States government. RESOLUTION: Institute proper SOAP NOTEing.

5): Improper Diagnostic Test for PATHOLOGY using 4000Hz scale for Hearing Loss and Tinnitus. RESOLUTION: A): ALL Denials be reviewed and retesting if required. B): Only Disability Claims need testing to proper 8000Hz and specific determination made.

6): Current All-or-Nothing Disability Decisions are too adversarial. RESOLUTION: Alter to Shared Responsibility procedures.

7): DoD purges Medical Records more-so than VA. RESOLUTION: A): Restructure VA. B): Consolidate with DoD. C): Allow Tricare Family Plan for Veterans from which the choice of plan be determined by the Veteran with payment by veteran, depending on individual case with Shared Responsibility scale.

CONTINUING

Elementary Criminology

(Child) abuse involves every segment of society and crosses all social, religious, and professional lines. The definition of (child) abuse can range from a narrow focus, limited to intentional inflicted injury, to a broad scope, covering any act that adversely affects the developmental potential of a (child). Included in the definition are neglect (acts of commission) and physical, psychological, or sexual injury (acts of commission) by a parent or caretaker. Intent is not considered in reporting abuse, protection of the child is paramount. *Monteleone.*

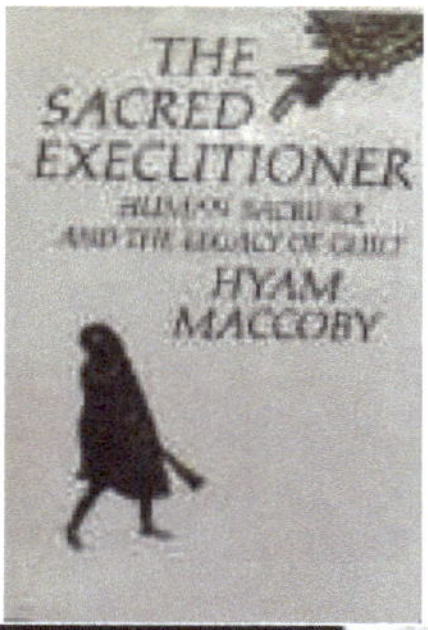

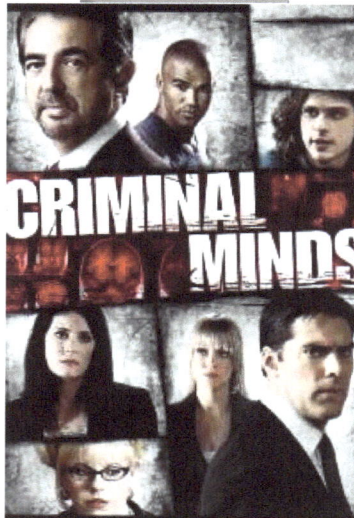

Mandated Report VA to CDC - Matteoli

Read Picture Line as a Sentence

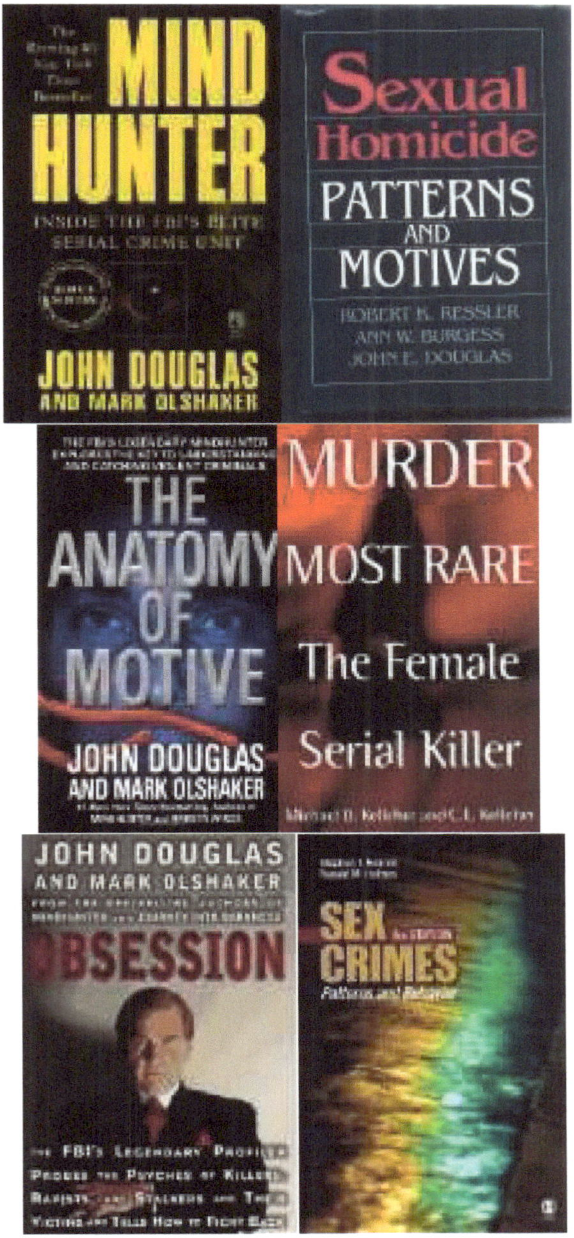

Mandated Report VA to CDC - Matteoli

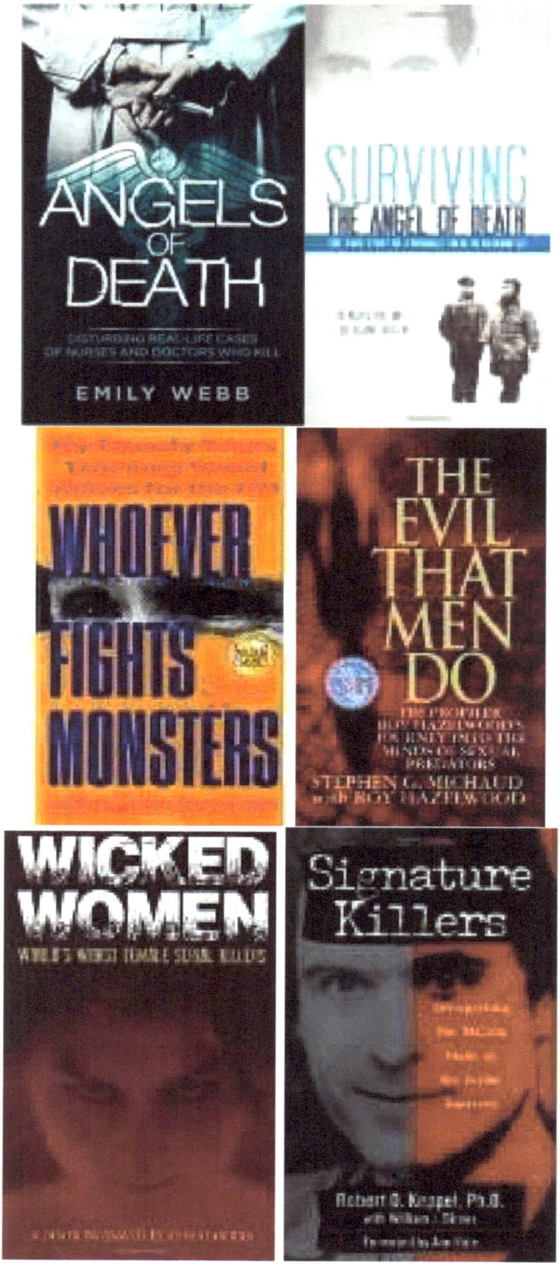

JOURNEY INTO DARKNESS
JOHN DOUGLAS
AND MARK OLSHAKER

I HAVE LIVED IN THE MONSTER
Inside the minds of the world's most notorious serial killers
ROBERT K. RESSLER
AND TOM SHACHTMAN

SOCIOPATH
PAUL SORENSEN

THE PSYCHOPATH

Suffer the Child
JUDITH SPENCER

THE CASES THAT HAUNT US
JOHN DOUGLAS
MARK OLSHAKER

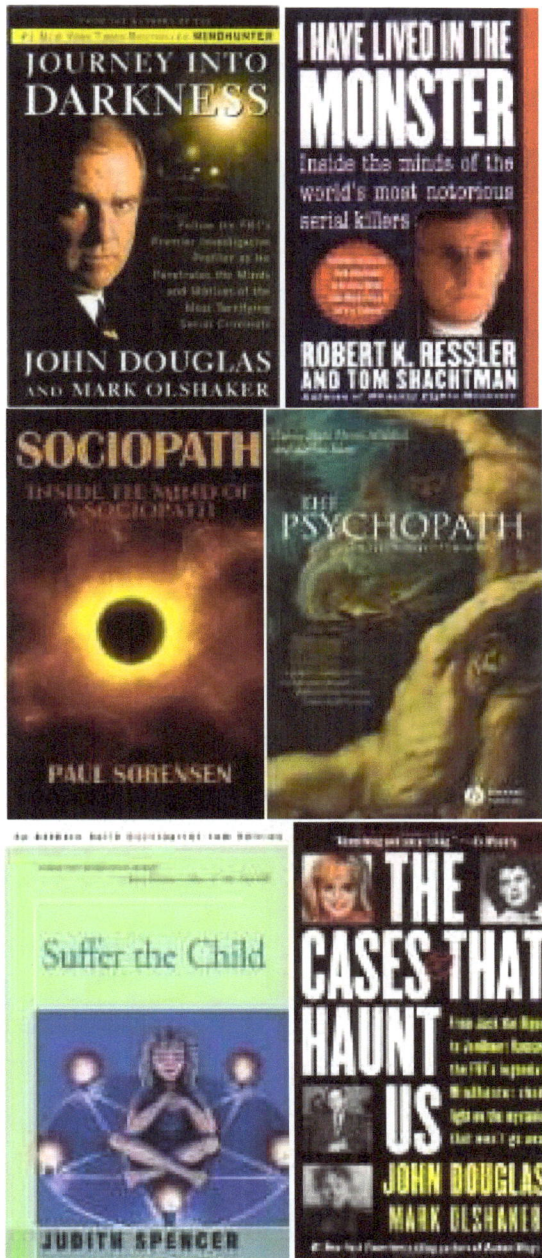

BEHAVIOR REFLECTS PERSONALITY

John Douglas with Mark Olshaker

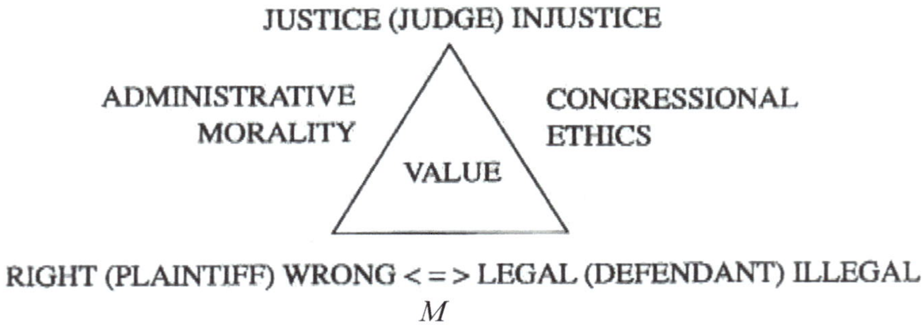
JUSTICE (JUDGE) INJUSTICE
ADMINISTRATIVE MORALITY
CONGRESSIONAL ETHICS
VALUE
RIGHT (PLAINTIFF) WRONG < = > LEGAL (DEFENDANT) ILLEGAL
M

LACK OF EMPATHY

Dissociation: The inability to perceive the humanity of another *syn*: disunion, separation, division, dividing, parting, split, splitting, sundering, break, rupture, rift, divorce, cleavage

TRANSFENCE OF AGGRESSION

Transference: the deliberate displacement of one's unresolved conflicts, dependencies and aggressions onto a substitute object

MODUS OPERANDI AND SIGNATURE

John Douglas with Mark Olshaker: "In part:"
Mind Hunter: Inside the FBI's Elite Serial Crime Unit, p.252

Modus Operandi: "- MO – is learned behavior. It's what the perpetrator does to commit the crime. It's dynamic – that is, it can change." Change is refinement for safety and security.

Signature = Ritual: "Signature, a term I [Douglas] coined to distinguish it from MO, is what the perpetrator has to do to fulfill himself. It is static; it does not change." Signature is the psychological drive. Dismemberment is a Signature and Ritual.

Mandated Report VA to CDC - Matteoli

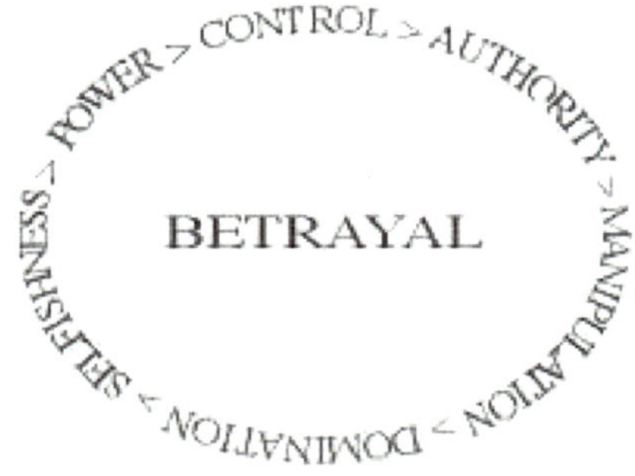
POWER > CONTROL > AUTHORITY > MANIPULATION > DOMINATION > SELFISHNESS >
BETRAYAL

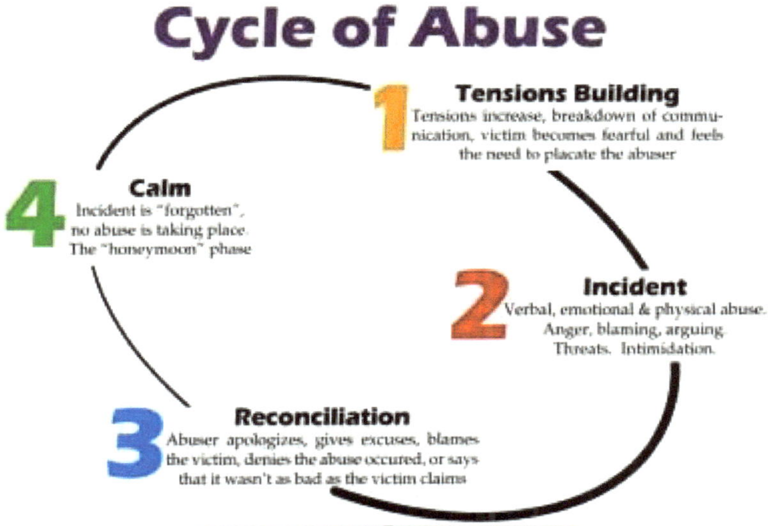
Cycle of Abuse
1 Tensions Building
Tensions increase, breakdown of communication, victim becomes fearful and feels the need to placate the abuser
2 Incident
Verbal, emotional & physical abuse. Anger, blaming, arguing. Threats. Intimidation.
3 Reconciliation
Abuser apologizes, gives excuses, blames the victim, denies the abuse occured, or says that it wasn't as bad as the victim claims
4 Calm
Incident is "forgotten", no abuse is taking place. The "honeymoon" phase

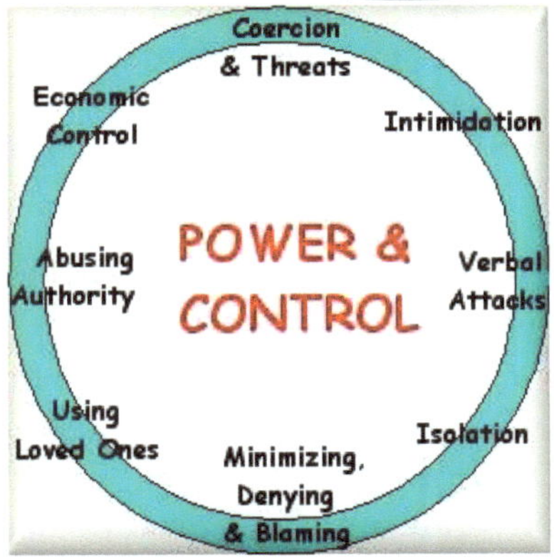
Coercion & Threats
Intimidation
Verbal Attacks
Isolation
Minimizing, Denying & Blaming
Using Loved Ones
Abusing Authority
Economic Control
POWER & CONTROL

SERIAL KILLERS [PREDATORS] ARE USUALLY CREATURES OF HABIT; THEY FIND A METHOD OF DESTRUCTION THAT WORK AND STICK TO IT.
Colin Evans, *The Casebook of Forensic Detection*

CRIMINAL APPROACH

CON: The Con is used to gain the victim's confidence. They act friendly and have a calm attitude. Often they wear uniforms. They are confident, organized, patient and meticulous. The Con approach increases over time as the serial predator becomes confident and organized. The Con uses a **Service Personality** used to disarm potential victims.

BLITZ: The Blitz is brutally violent. Suddenness is not the defining factor. The Blitz approach describes the attack itself. Total time with the act may vary. It is commonly used by the **Anger Retaliatory** type of predator.

SURPRISE: The victim is chosen and a trap is set. They usually attack from the behind. Threats are made if the victim does not cooperate. This approach is often used by the **Power Reassurance** perpetrator

PASSIVE INITIATION

PASSIVE INITIATION is having another person commit an act without the initiator's direct involvement. *Delegation* is common with females and some males. At 5' 2" Charles Manson is not an imposing physical figure.

VICTIMOLOGY

VICTIMOLOGY is the study of victim traits as: lifestyle, employment, background, finances, daily routines, likes and dislikes. Victimology aids law enforcement understanding why specific victims are targets. It enables investigators pinpoint persons who might be at risk, narrows the perpetrator's profile and allows proactive measures to draw out the perpetrator .and protect potential victims.

ABUSER-ABUSED CYCLE OF EMOTIONS

Nothing new happens in the world, for everything is but the repetition of the same primordial archetypes.
Mircea Eliade. *Myth of the Eternal Return.*

It's deja-vu all over again. Yogi Berra.

Abuser-Abused (Perpetrator-Victim) Cycles include individual emotions, actions and reactions as well as existing in cultural systems where such cycles exist.

Repetition Compulsion & Generational Abuse

Perpetrator ← → Victim
Betrayals

Distress Arises from an initial Betrayal	*Disfranchisement* Loss of privilege from immunity
Torment Increases with remembrance	*Self-esteem* Is lowered
Anger Evolves in displeasure	*Guilt* Is the mantle taken into the Self
Hate Is a result created	*Shame* Guilt's response in relation to others
Hostility Becomes activated	*Ignominy* Is the Self disgraced, debased
Aggression Follows from frustration	*Disgrace* Becomes the place of existence
Violence Onto another is perpetrated	*Humiliation* Is the living existence
Rage Is uncontrolled violence	*Envy* Of others formulates
Wrath Is a violent fit of rage	*Resentment* Of others is envy solidified
Abuse Is enacted to completion	*Desperation* Attempt to reconcile existence
Justification Is hypothesized to formality	*Hopelessness* despair in reality of unchanging

Victim ← → Perpetrator
Betrayals

ORGANIZED *V.* DISORGANIZED OFFENDERS

ORGANIZED offenders are often anal retentive personalities, which isd broadly defined as orderliness, stubbornness, a compulsion for control with an interest in collecting, possessing and retaining objects and a tendency toward obsessive-compulsive disorders.

DISORGANIZED offenders are more often anal expulsive personalities, which is broadly defined as exhibiting cruelty, emotional outbursts, disorganization, rebelliousness, carelessness, as well as artistic ability, generosity and self-confidence.

PERSONALITY TYPES

VISIONARY: The Con is used to gain the victim's confidence. They act friendly and have a calm attitude. Often they wear uniforms. They are confident, organized, patient and meticulous. The Con approach increases over time as the serial predator becomes confident and organized.

MISSION-ORIENTED: The Blitz is brutally violent. Suddenness is not the defining factor. The Blitz approach describes the attack itself. Total time with the act may vary. It is commonly used by the **Anger Retaliatory** type of predator.

HEDONISTIC: The Con is used to gain the victim's confidence. They act friendly and have a calm attitude. Often they wear uniforms. They are confident, organized, patient and meticulous. The Con approach increases over time as the serial predator becomes confident and organized.

POWER/CONTROL: The Con is used to gain the victim's confidence. They act friendly and have a calm attitude. Often they wear uniforms. They are confident, organized, patient and meticulous. The Con approach increases over time as the serial predator becomes confident and organized.

AXIS MUNDI

The **Axis Mundi** (also cosmic axis, world axis, world pillar and center of the world) in beliefs and philosophies is the world center, or the connection between Heaven and Earth. As the Celestial Pole and Geographic Pole, it expresses a point of connection between sky and earth where the four compass points meet. The Axis Mundi is the communication point between lower and higher realms where one may travel to and from.

The Axis Mundi is used in both the religious and secular found worldwide in shamanistic and animist belief systems, current major world religions. It is the Concept of the Center in which life revolves.

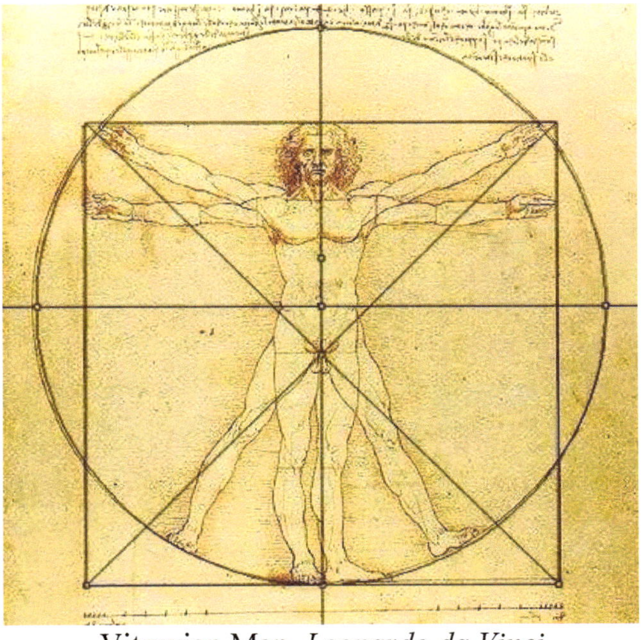

Vitruvian Man, *Leonardo da Vinci*
The Genitals are the Axis Mundi of the human body
Attacks on persons of the opposite sex often represent a genitalization of the victim's body in Transference.

ARCHETYPES

Archetypes are highly developed elements from the Collective Unconscious. Being unconscious, the existence of archetypes can only be deduced indirectly from examining behavior, art, images, myths, religions or dreams as the psychic counterpart of instinct.

CHILD ARCHETYPES

About Caroline Myss • Products • Ca

Home » Free Resources » Sacred Contracts and Your Archetypes » Appendix: The Four Archetypes of Survival

Appendix: The Four Archetypes of Survival

The Child, Victim, Prostitute, and Saboteur are all deeply involved in your most pressing challenges related to survival. Each one represents different issues, fears, and vulnerabilities that you need to confront and overcome as part of your Sacred Contract. In doing so, you come to see these four archetypes as your most trusted allies, which can represent spiritual as well as material strengths. They can become your guardians and will preserve your integrity, refusing to let you negotiate it away in the name of survival. Keep in mind that, like all archetypes, their energies are essentially neutral, despite the negative connotations of their names. (Although the Child itself sounds positive, variants such as the Wounded, Needy, or Orphan Child have a similar negative tonality.)

The outline of your Sacred Contract may have been agreed on before your birth, yet the way in which you respond to the challenges presented to you, and how you choose to interact with the people with whom you have Contracts, is fully up to you. If your choices are made unconsciously and you act defensively and fearfully, you may not learn and grow as you should. The more conscious you can remain about the archetypal patterns influencing your behavior, the more likely that your choices, and lessons, will be positive. Now let's take a brief look at each of the four survival archetypes and see how you can learn from them.

https://www.myss.com/free-resources/sacred-contracts-and-your-archetypes/appendix-the-f... 8/5/2015

The Child

The mature personality of the Child archetype nurtures that part of us that yearns to be lighthearted and innocent, expecting the wonders of tomorrow, regardless of age. This part of our nature contributes greatly to our ability to sense playfulness in our lives, balancing the seriousness of adult responsibilities. The balanced Child is a delight to be around because the energy that flows from this part of our personality is positively infectious and brings out the best in others, as well as in us.

The Child also establishes our perceptions of life, safety, nurture, loyalty, and family. Its many aspects include the Wounded Child, Abandoned or Orphan Child, Dependent, Innocent, Nature, and Divine Child. These energies may emerge in response to different situations in which you find yourself, yet the core issue of all the Child archetypes is dependency vs. responsibility: when to take responsibility, when to have a healthy dependency, when to stand up to the group, and when to embrace communal life. Each of the variants of the Child archetype is characterized by certain tendencies, including shadow tendencies.

Wounded Child

The Wounded Child archetype holds the memories of abuse, neglect, and other traumas that we have endured during childhood. This is the Child pattern most people relate to, particularly since it has become the focus of therapy since the 1960s. Many people blame the relationship with their parents that created their Wounded Child, for instance, for all their subsequent dysfunctional relationships. On the positive side, the painful experiences of the Wounded Child often awaken a deep sense of compassion and a desire to help other Wounded Children. From a spiritual perspective, a wounded childhood cracks open the learning path of forgiveness.

The shadow aspect may manifest as an abiding sense of self-pity, a tendency to blame our parents for any current shortcomings and to resist moving on through forgiveness. It may also lead us to seek out parental figures in all difficult situations rather than relying on our own resourcefulness.

Orphan Child

From Little Orphan Annie to Cinderella, the Orphan Child in most well known children's stories reflects the lives of people who feel from birth as if they are not a part of their family, including the family psyche or tribal spirit. But because orphans are not allowed into the family circle, they have to develop independence early on. The absence of family influences, attitudes, and traditions inspires or compels the Orphan Child to construct an inner reality based on personal judgment and experience.

The shadow aspect manifests when Orphans never recover from feelings of abandonment, and the scar tissue from family rejection stifles their maturation, often causing them to seek surrogate family structures to experience tribal union. Therapeutic support groups become shadow tribes or families for an Orphan Child who knows deep down that healing these wounds requires moving on to adulthood. For that reason, establishing mature relationships remains a challenge.

Magical/Innocent Child

The Magical Child sees the potential for sacred beauty in all things, and embodies qualities of wisdom and courage in the face of difficult circumstances. One example is Anne Frank, who wrote in her diary that in spite of all the horror surrounding her family while hiding from Nazis in an attic, she still believed that humanity was basically good. This archetype is also gifted with the power of imagination and the belief that everything is possible.

The shadow energy of the Magical Child manifests as the absence of the possibility of miracles and of the transformation of evil to good. Attitudes of pessimism and depression, particularly when exploring dreams, often emerge from an injured Magical Child whose dreams were "once upon a time" thought foolish by cynical adults. The shadow may also manifest as a belief that energy and action are not required, allowing one to retreat into fantasy.

Nature Child

This archetype inspires deep, intimate bonding with natural forces, and has a particular affinity for friendships with animals. Although the Nature Child has tender, emotional qualities, it can also have an inner toughness and ability to survive–the resilience of Nature herself. Nature Children can develop advanced skills of communicating with animals, and in stories reflecting this archetype an animal often comes to the rescue of its child companion. Many veterinarians and animal rights activists resonate with this archetype because they have felt a conscious rapport with animals since childhood. Other adults describe being in communication with nature spirits and learning to work in harmony with them in maintaining the order of nature.

The shadow aspect of the Nature Child manifests in a tendency to abuse animals and people and the environment.

A love of animals is not sufficient to qualify for this archetype, however. A life-long pattern of relating to animals in an intimate and caring way, to the extent that your psyche and spirit need these bonds as a crucial part of your own well-being, is your best clue.

Puer/Puella Eternis (Eternal Boy/Girl)

This archetype guides us to remain eternally young in body, mind, and spirit, and not to let age stop us from enjoying life. The shadow Eternal Child often manifests as an inability to grow up and embrace the responsible life of an adult. Like Peter Pan, the Eternal Boy resists ending a cycle of life in which he is free to live outside the boundaries of conventional adulthood. The shadow Puella Eternis can manifest in women as extreme dependence on those who take charge of their physical security. She cannot be relied on nor can she accept the aging process. Although few people delight in the end of their youth, the Eternal Child is sometimes left floundering and ungrounded between the stages of life, because of not having laid a foundation for a functioning adulthood.

Dependent Child

The Needy or Dependent Child carries a heavy feeling inside that nothing is ever enough, and is always seeking to replace something lost in childhood – although exactly wha never clear. As with the Wounded Child, this leads to bouts of depression, only more severe. The Dependent Child tends to be focused on his own needs, often unable to see the needs of others. As with all apparently negative archetypes, you can learn to recognize its emergence and use it as a guide to alert you when you are in danger of falling into needy, self-absorbed attitudes and behavior.

Divine Child

The Divine Child is closely related to both the Innocent and Magical Child, but is distinguished from them by its redemptive mission. It is associated with innocence, purity, and redemption, god-like qualities that suggest that the Child enjoys a special union with the Divine itself. Few people are inclined to choose the Divine Child as their dominant Child archetype, however, because they have difficulty acknowledging that they could live continually in divine innocence. And yet, divinity is also a reference point of your inner spirit that you can turn to when you are in a conscious process of choice. You may also assume that anything divine cannot have a shadow aspect, but that's not realistic. The shadow of this archetype manifests as an inability to defend itself against negative forces. Even the mythic gods and most spiritual masters — including Jesus, who is the template of the Divine Child for the Christian tradition — simultaneously expressed anger and divine strength when confronting those who claimed to represent heaven while manifesting injustice, arrogance, or other negative qualities (think of Jesus' wrath at the money-changers in the Temple). Assess your involvement with this archetype by asking whether you see life through the eyes of a benevolent, trusting God/Goddess, or whether you tend to respond initially with fear of being hurt or with a desire to hurt others first.

The Victim

Don't be misled by the name of this archetype. When properly recognized, the Victim can alert you to the possibility that you are about to let yourself be victimized, whether through passivity or inappropriate actions. It can also help you recognize your own tendency to victimize others for personal gain. We need to develop this clarity of insight, however, and that means learning the nature and intensity of the Victim within.

In its shadow manifestation, the Victim tells you that you are always taken advantage of and it's never your fault. We may like to play the Victim at times because of the positive feedback we get in the form of sympathy or pity. Our goal is always to learn how to recognize these inappropriate attitudes in ourselves or others, and to act accordingly. We are not meant to be victimized in life, but to learn how to handle challenges and outrun our fears.

In establishing contact with your own inner Victim, ask yourself:

- Do I blame others for the circumstances of my life?
- Do I spend time in the pit of self-pity?
- Do I envy others who always seem to get what they want out of life?
- Do I feel victimized by others when situations don't work out the way I wanted them to?
- Do I tend to feel more powerless than powerful?

The Saboteur

This may be the most difficult of all the archetypes to understand, because its name is associated with betrayal. Yet the purpose of this archetype is not to sabotage you, but to help you learn the many ways in which you undermine yourself. How often do you set new plans in motion, only to end up standing in your own way because of the fears that undermine those optimistic plans. Or you begin a new relationship and then destroy it because you begin to imagine a painful outcome. You begin a working relationship with another person and find yourself once again in a power struggle that could be settled peacefully — but you fall into the same destructive pattern because you fear the other person.

The Saboteur's fears and issues are all related to low self-esteem that causes you to make choices that block your own empowerment and success. As with the Victim and Prostitute, you need to face this powerful archetype that we all possess and make it an ally. When you do, you will find that it calls your attention to situations in which you are in danger of being sabotaged, or of sabotaging yourself. Once you are comfortable with the Saboteur, you learn to hear and heed these warnings, saving yourself untold grief from making the same mistakes over and over. Ignore it, and the shadow Saboteur will manifest in the form of self-destructive behavior or the desire to undermine others.

To learn how to become aware of the action of the Saboteur within, ask yourself these questions:

- What fears have the most authority over me? List three.
- What happens when a fear overtakes me? Does it make me silent?
- Do I allow people to speak for me?
- Do I agree to some things out of fear that I otherwise would not agree to?
- Have I let creative opportunities pass me by?
- How conscious am I in the moment that I am sabotaging myself?
- Am I able to recognize the Saboteur in others?
- Would I be able to offer others advice about how to challenge one's Saboteur? If so, what would it be?

The Prostitute

None of us thinks kindly of the term 'prostitute,' and yet from this archetype we learn the great gift of never again having to compromise our body, mind, or spirit. You may have already reached the point in which the Prostitute has become a mature part of yourself that circles you with a strong vibrational field that says, "Not for sale."

The Prostitute archetype engages lessons in the sale or negotiation of one's integrity or spirit due to fears of physical survival or for financial gain. It activates the aspects of the unconscious that are related to seduction and control, whereby you are as capable of buying a controlling interest in another person as you are of selling your own power. Prostitution should be understood as the selling or selling out of your talents, ideas, and any other expression of the self. The core learning of the Prostitute relates to the need to birth and refine self-esteem and self-respect.

We prostitute ourselves when we sell our bodies or minds for money or when we compromise our morals and ethics for financial gain. That may include remaining in a marriage or job that endangers our well being for reasons of financial security.

In identifying this archetype, ask yourself:

- Have I ever sold out to people or organizations that I did not truly believe in?
- Have I ever remained in a situation that offered me financial protection because of a desire for financial security?
- Have I ever put another person in the position of compromising him- or herself in order to gain power over that individual?
- Have I ever 'bought' another person's loyalty, support, or even silence, in order to have my way?

From another perspective:

- Have I ever offered to help another who was weakened by his or her Prostitute archetype?
- Do I judge others because they find themselves continually compromising themselves?
- Do I think of them as weak and myself as a better person?

And from yet another perspective:

- Have I ever felt myself being pulled into a circumstance that would require me to sell out my ethics, but then found myself strong enough to say "no"?

Once you have answered these questions, you may proceed to determining the rest of the 12 archetypes that make up your personal support team.

DEATH CULT RITUAL

The Basic Social Act

The Basic Social Act reaches into all aspects of life and society

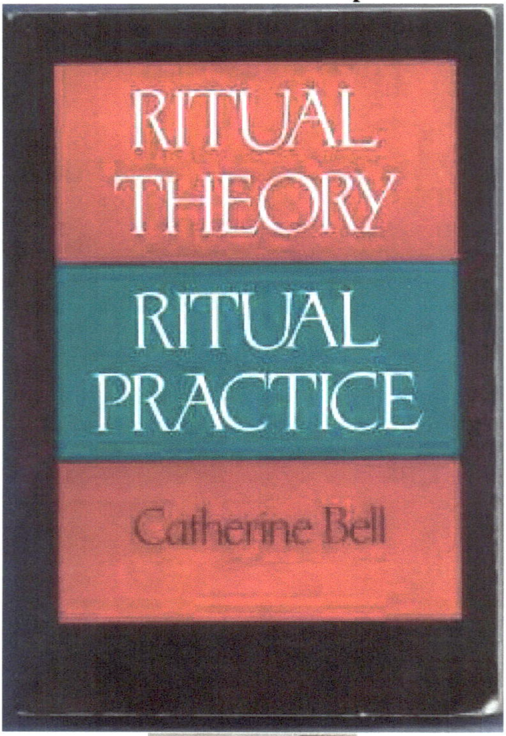

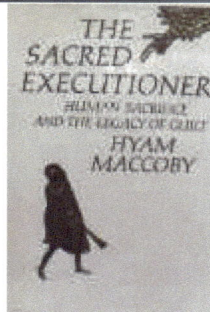

Read Picture Line as a Sentence

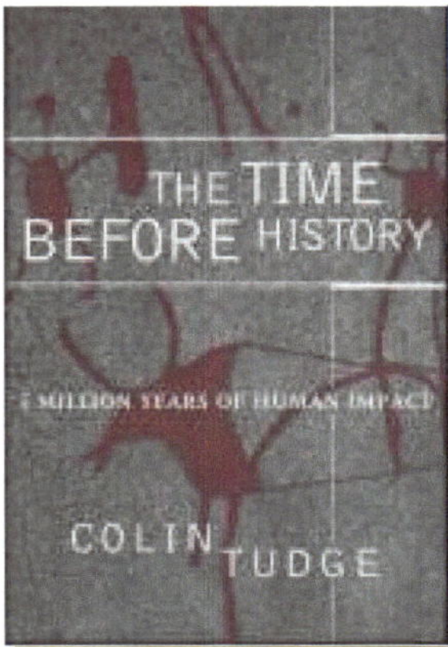

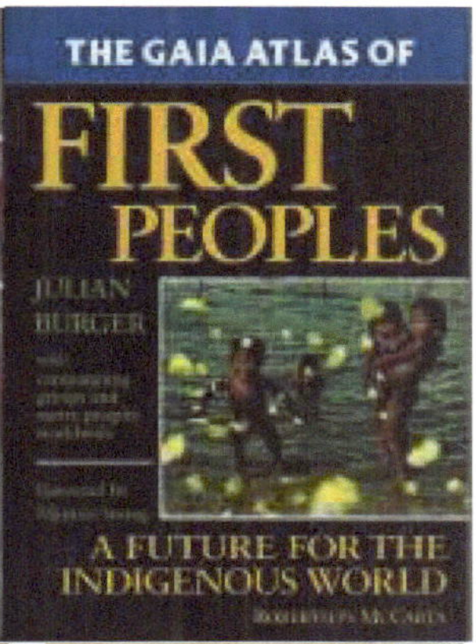

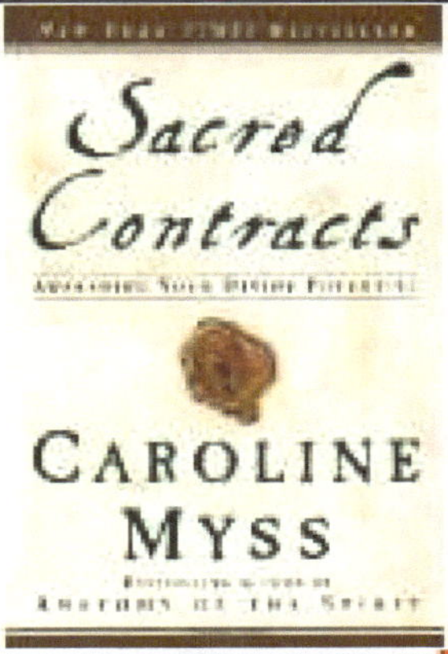

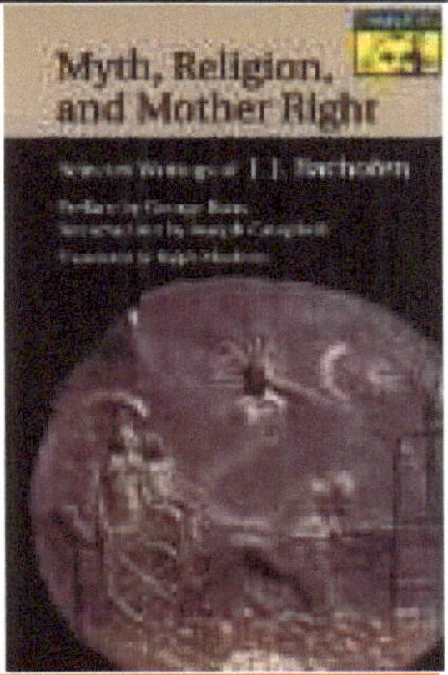

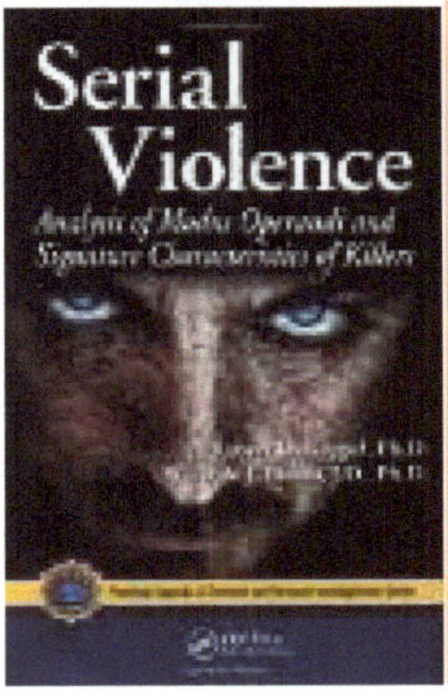

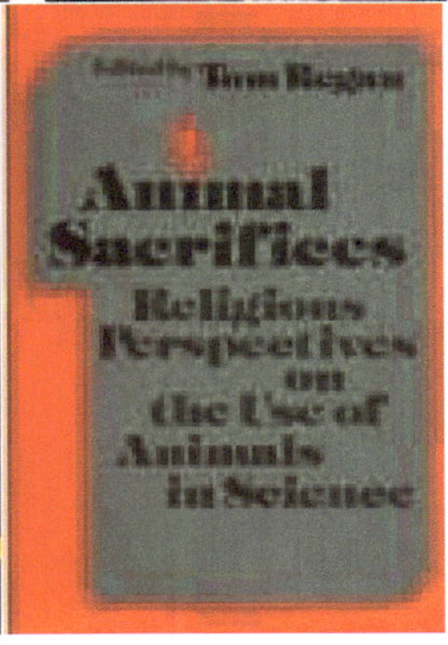

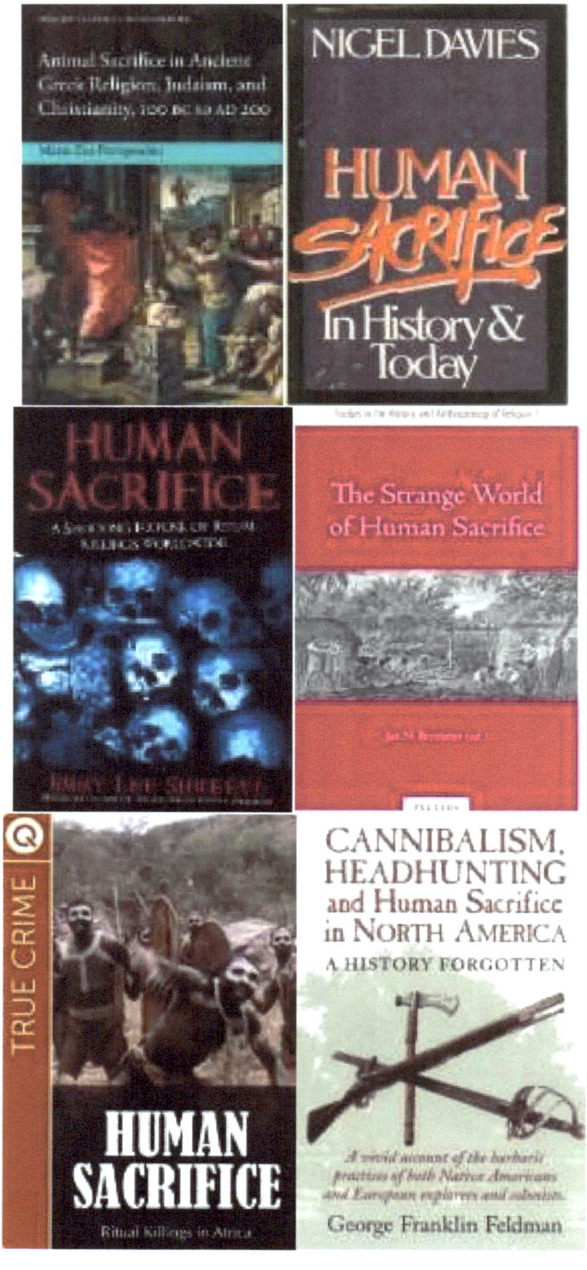
Animal Sacrifice in Ancient Greek Religion, Judaism, and Christianity, 100 BC to AD 200
NIGEL DAVIES
HUMAN SACRIFICE
In History & Today
HUMAN SACRIFICE
The Strange World of Human Sacrifice
TRUE CRIME
HUMAN SACRIFICE
Ritual Killings in Africa
CANNIBALISM, HEADHUNTING and Human Sacrifice in NORTH AMERICA
A HISTORY FORGOTTEN
A vivid account of the barbaric practices of both Native Americans and European explorers and colonists.
George Franklin Feldman

DISCOVERY OF LOST WORLDS
Edited by Joseph J. Thorndike, Jr.

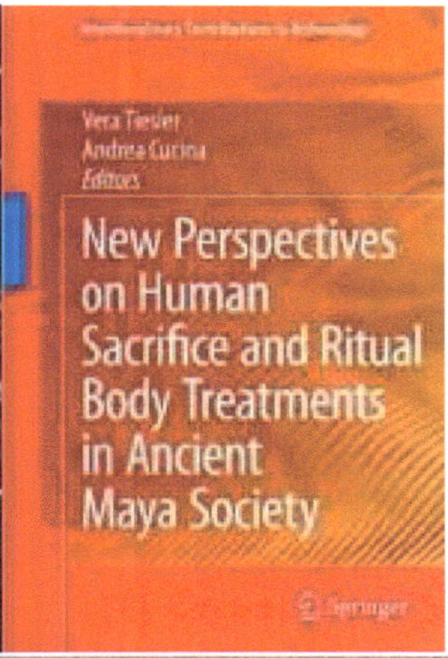
Vera Tiesler
Andrea Cucina
Editors
New Perspectives on Human Sacrifice and Ritual Body Treatments in Ancient Maya Society
Springer

THE ARYAN CHRIST
THE SECRET LIFE OF CARL JUNG
RICHARD NOLL

DYING FOR THE GODS

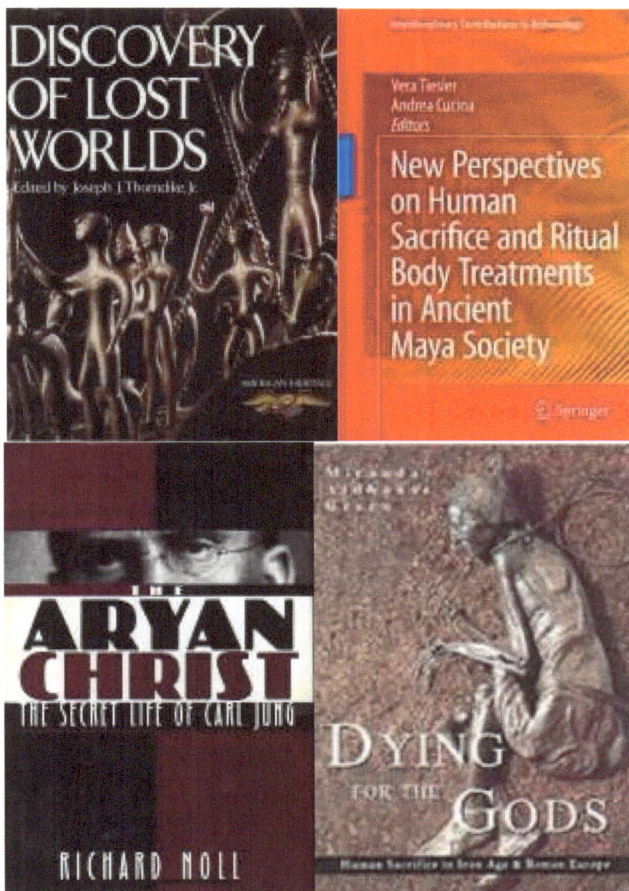

MOTHER NATURE DETERMINES RITUAL

SELF DEIFICATION

Quoting Bell

(Rituals) demonstrate that collective effervescences do not so much unite the community as strengthen the socially more dominant group through a **mobilization of bias**… Ritual is circular.

Hence, ritualization is central to culture as the means to **dominate** nature and the natural violence within human beings. Although ritual (=culture) is the necessary repression of this violence (=nature), **culture is still dependent upon the energy of aggression** as well as its restraint…

The orchestrated construction of **power** and **authority** in ritual, which is deeply evocative of the basic division of the social order, engage the social body in the objectification of opposites and deployment of schemes that effectively reproduce the **divisions of the social order**...

In this process such schemes become socially instinctive automatisms of the body and implicit strategies for **shifting power relationships** among symbols…

Culture uses ritual to **control** by means of **sets of assumptions** about the way things are and should be.

The Objectified and Manipulated Veteran

Ritual never defines anything except the terms of the **expedient relationships** that ritualization itself establishes among things, thereby **manipulating their relationships**…

What is distinctive about ritual is not what it says or symbolizes, but that first and foremost it **does things**: ritual is always a matter of the performance of gestures and the **manipulation of objects**.

To approach cultural rituals as rooted in **purely psychological conflicts** is to see ritual as an **oppression** inherently necessary to society, which is defined in turn as the **repression of the individual**...

Ritual structure is totally repressive, instead of channeling violence, the order of ritual completely denies it.

Ritual emerges as the means for a provisional synthesis of some form of **original opposition**...
Such dispositions are, in turn, further differentiated into two kinds: **moods and motivations**.

Ultimately, the struggle between the individual psyche and society is never seen as simply out there in the social arena, but within each person as well. The formulation of ritual often appears to involve a **distancing within actors of their private and social identities**...

Socialization cannot be anything less than the acquisition of schemes that can potentially **restructure and renuance both self and society**.

Ritual mastery is itself a capacity for, and relationship of, **relative domination**...

Binary oppositions almost always involve asymmetrical relations of **dominance** and **subordination** by which they generate hierarchically organized relationships...

Fairly standard understandings involve the positive notion of ***influence*** on the one hand and the negative notion of ***force*** on the other.

As institutions of **specialists take on the formulation of reality**, there is a decreased need for personal or collective rituals to assume that function.

As institutions of **specialists** take on the formulation of reality, there is a decreased need for personal or collective rituals to assume that function.

Ultimately, when the strategies of ritualization are **dominated by a special group**, recognized as official experts, the definition of reality that they objectify works primarily **to retain the status and authority of the experts themselves**.

Specific relations of **domination** and **subordination** are generated and orchestrated by the participants themselves simply by participating.

It is this type of **control** that must be understood. These bodies of knowledge act simultaneously to secure a particular form of **authority**.

Saying "NO" to the Destroyer-Prostitute Child Archetypes
The only real alternative to negotiated compliance is either **total resistance or asocial self-exclusion**.

MYTHIC EXPRESSION of the ARCHETYPICAL DIMENSION

Myths and rites referring to the mythological age, when the great mythological event took place that brought both **death** and **reproduction** into play and fixed the density of life-in-time through a chain reaction of significantly interlocked **transformations**, belong rather to the world system of **planters** than to the shamanistically dominated hunting sphere. Whenever such myths are found in a hunting society, **acculturation from some horticultural center can be supposed.**

Joseph Campbell, *Primitive Mythology: The Masks of God*

MASLOW'S HIERARCHY OF NEEDS

Unlike most, Maslow studied motivation in *normal* and *exemplary people* as well as *top students*. The process is lineal up-down between steps and more horizontal, relationship-wise, within each step.
The process is lineal where a step must be reasonably met before proceeding to the next. Regression occurs when a stage becomes compromised and descent returns to the compromised stage. Descent can be rapid.

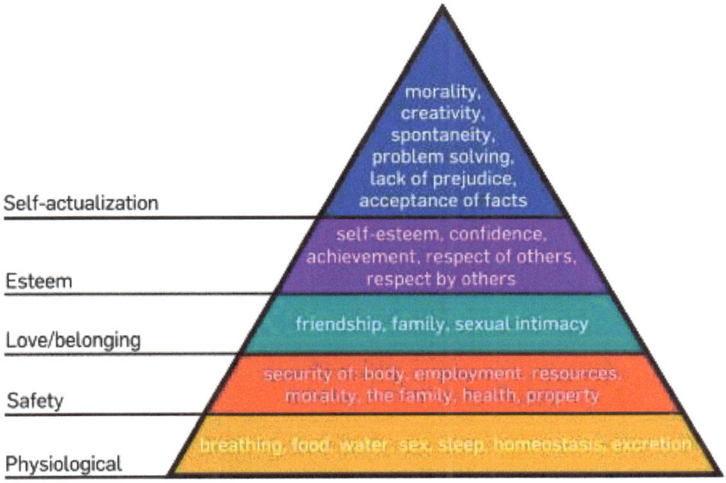

The problem with Self-actualization is it needs ***repetition*** *to maintain a perceived success and can, in negativity, become an excuse.*

REPETITION COMPULSION ARISES OUT OF THANTOS

Repetition Compulsion: is a psychological phenomenon in which a person repeats a traumatic event or its circumstances over and over again. This includes reenacting the event or putting oneself in situations where the event is likely to happen again.

COMIXIO RELIGIONIS

THE MIXING OF RELIGIONS

Ecumenism within the **Jungian Mana Family** observable in **Myth**.

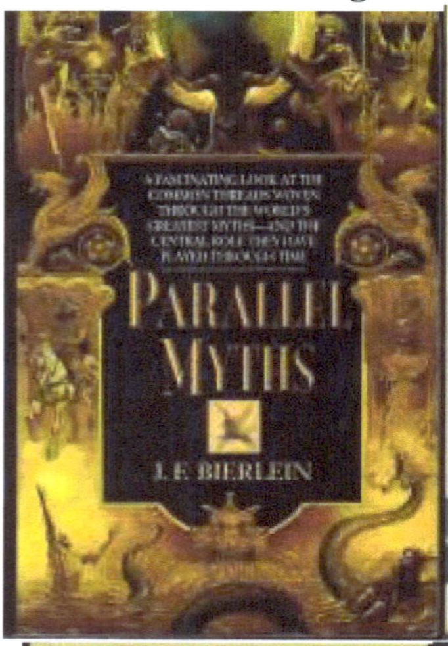

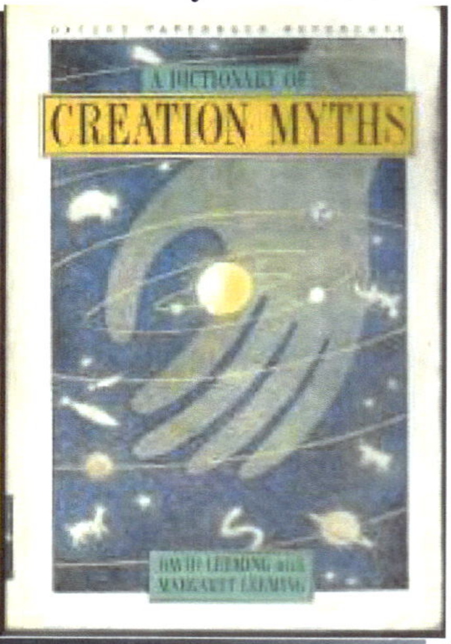

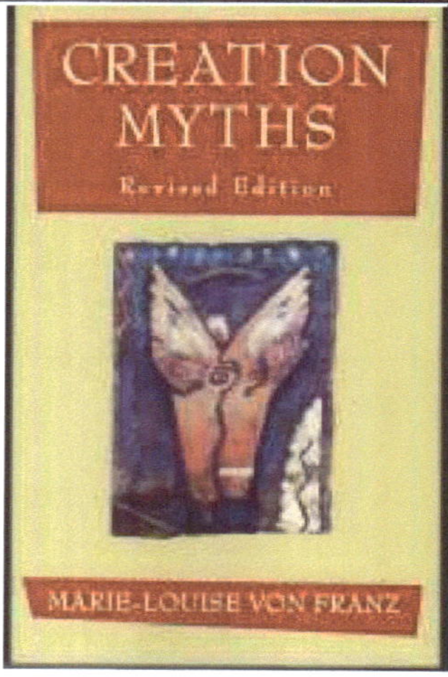

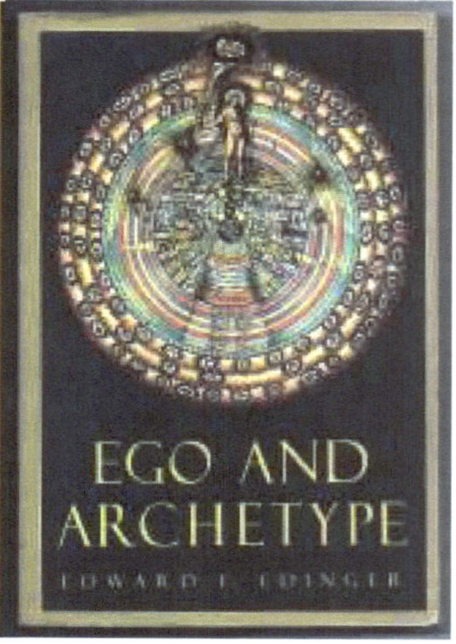

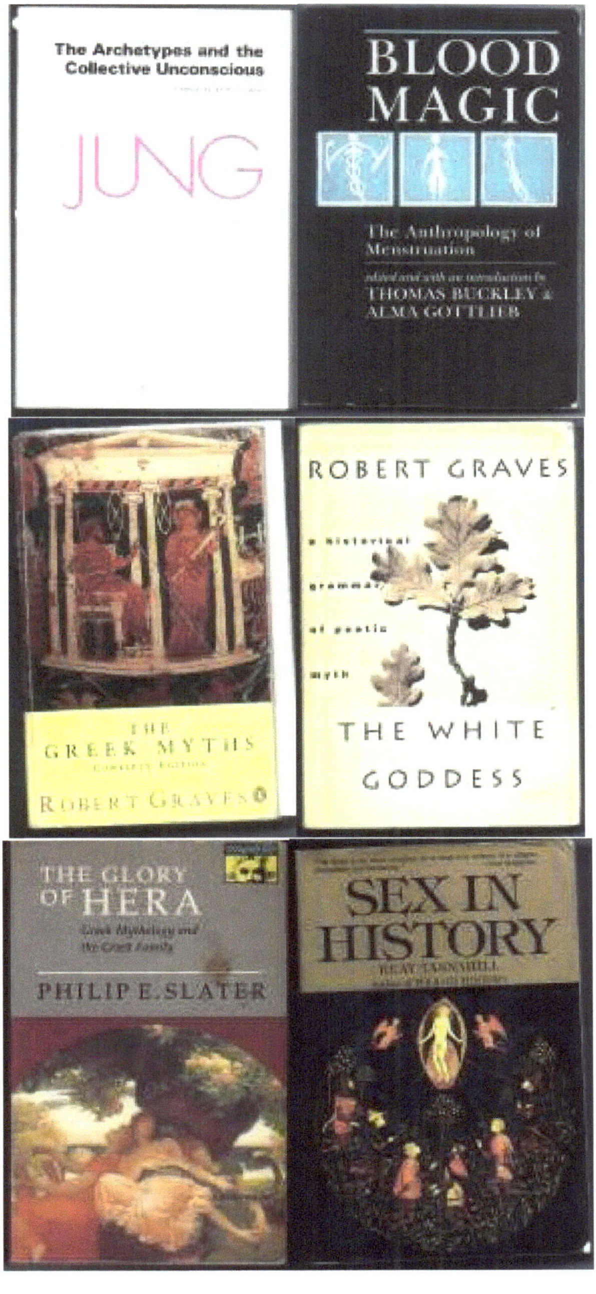
The Archetypes and the
Collective Unconscious
JUNG
BLOOD
MAGIC
The Anthropology of
Menstruation
THOMAS BUCKLEY &
ALMA GOTTLIEB
THE
GREEK MYTHS
ROBERT GRAVES
a historical
grammar
of poetic
myth
THE WHITE
GODDESS
THE GLORY
OF HERA
Greek Mythology and
the Greek Family
PHILIP E. SLATER
SEX IN
HISTORY
REAY TANNAHILL

Read Picture Line as a Sentence

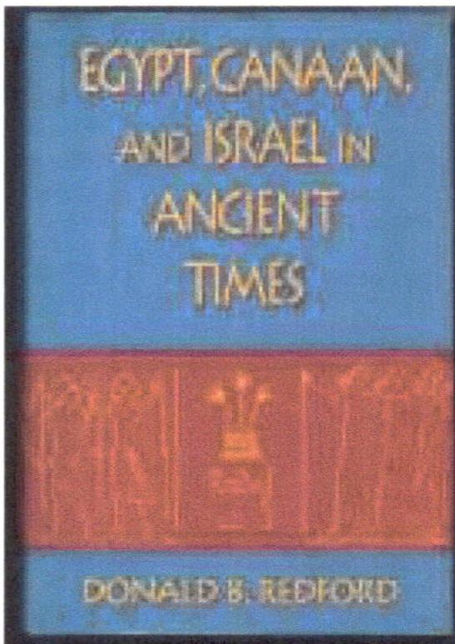

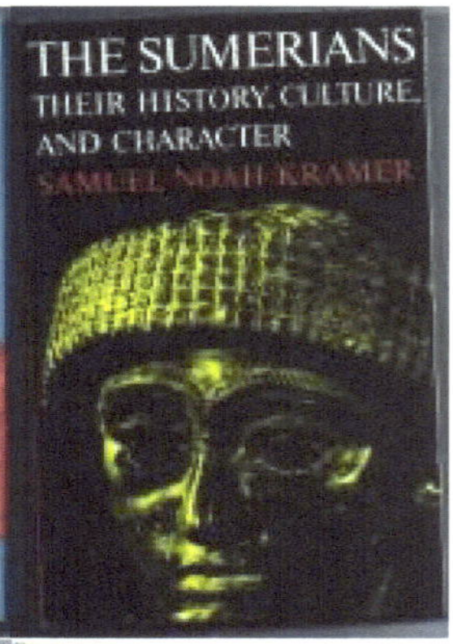

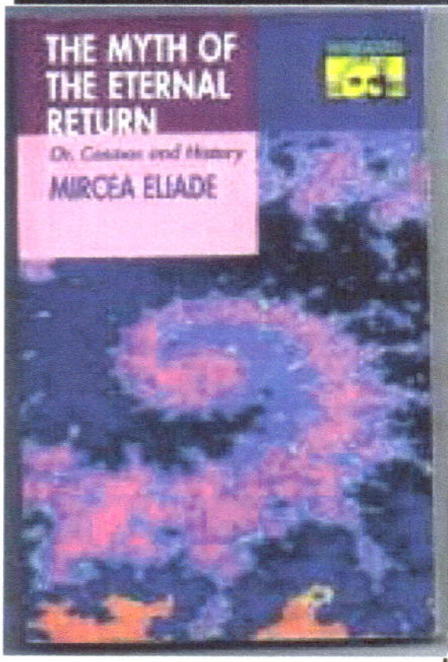

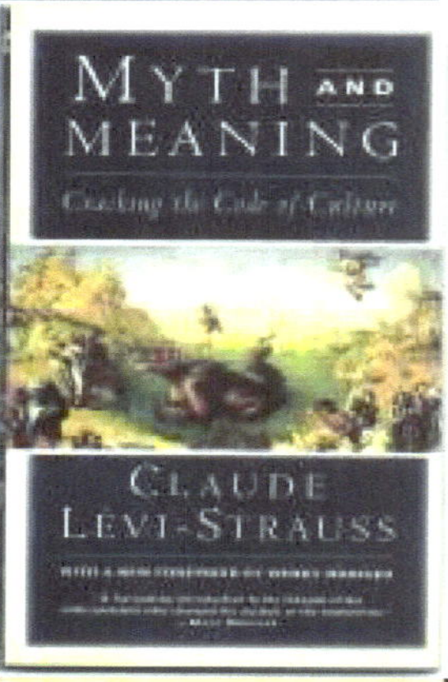

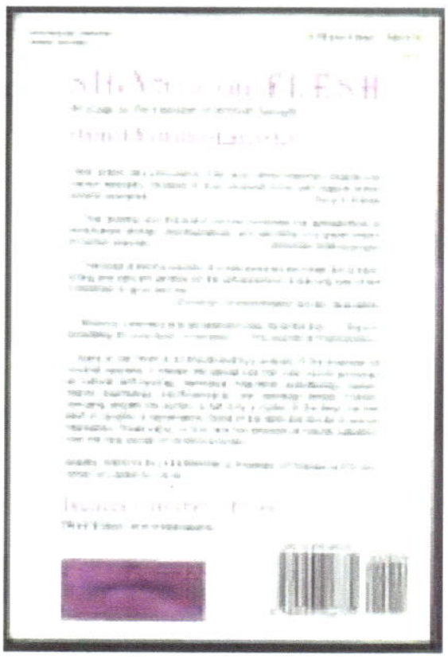

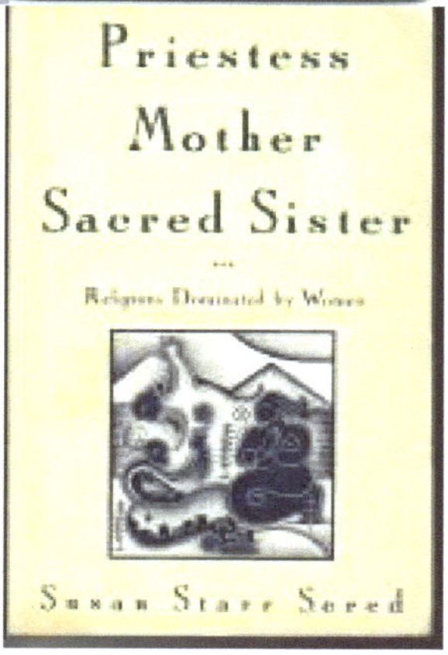

JOSEPH CAMPBELL
CREATIVE
MYTHOLOGY
JOSEPH CAMPBELL
ORIENTAL
MYTHOLOGY
THE MASKS OF GOD
JOSEPH CAMPBELL
PRIMITIVE
MYTHOLOGY
THE MASKS OF GOD
On Death and Dying
What the dying have to teach doctors, nurses, clergy, and their own families
Elisabeth Kübler-Ross, M.D.

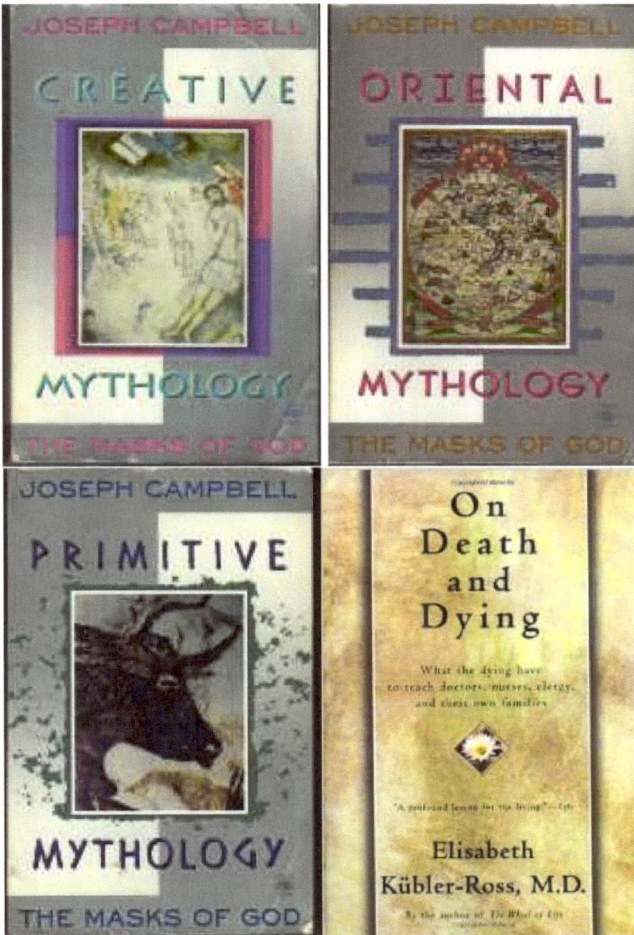

MOTHER NATURE DETERMINES THEO-RELIGIOUS SOCIAL EXISTENCE TO WHICH THE MASCULINE SERVES

BIOLOGY DICTATES

Women have 40% more nerves connecting brain hemispheres
The ANIMA perceives the whole - Existence
The ANIMUS perceives the separations - Function

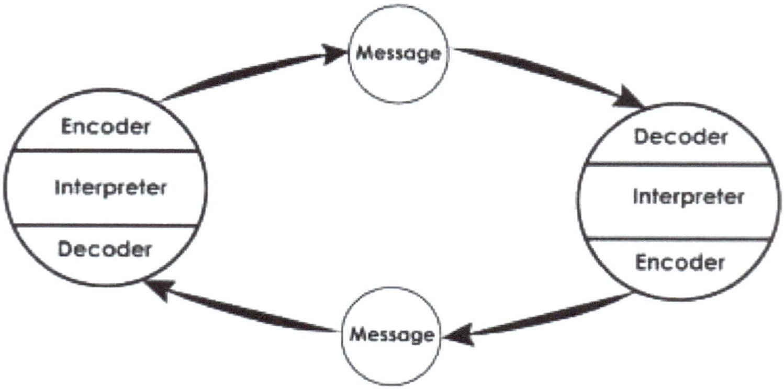

COMMUNICATIVE THEOLOGY

The feminine is OF nature.
The masculine is THROUGH nature
Spirituality is; Theology Explains; Religion Practices

COMMUNICATIVE THEOLOGY is the polarized psychosexual process of development and understanding of the realm of the Spiritual from the feminine horizontal communication in the circular and/with/or masculine vertical communication in the linear, *syn*: communico theologia

COMMONIS THEOLOGIA is the basic dogmatic expression of innate spirituality from which all variations stem usu. using the Collective Unconscious within the Jungian Mana Family. *syn*: common theology

FEMININE THEOLOGY (ANIMA) is spirituality addressed through horizontal circular communication and encompasses the Life/Dearh/Life Cycle most often using Maiden-Mother-Wise Woman, *syn*: femineus theologia

ANIMA-FEMININIZED DOMINANT FORM OF COMMUNICATION AND SOCIAL STRUCTURE
CIRCULAR

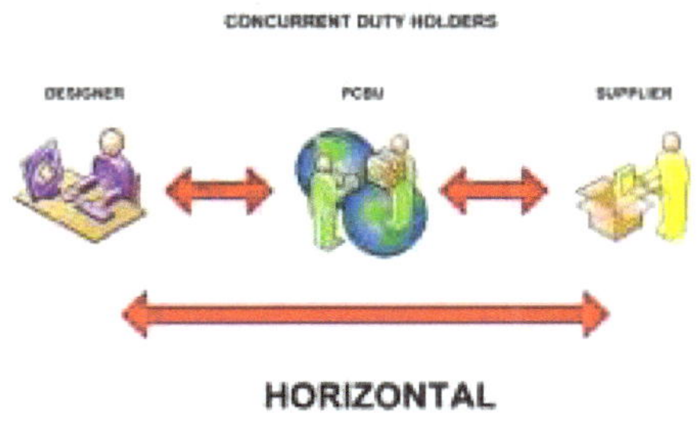

MASCULINE THEOLOGY (ANIMUS) is spirituality addressed through vertical linear communication and encompasses the Build/Destroy/Build Cycle most often using Sword-Scepter-Staff. *syn*: masculus theologia

ANIMUS-MASCULINIZED DOMINANT FORM OF COMMUNICATION AND SOCIAL STRUCTURE
LINEAR

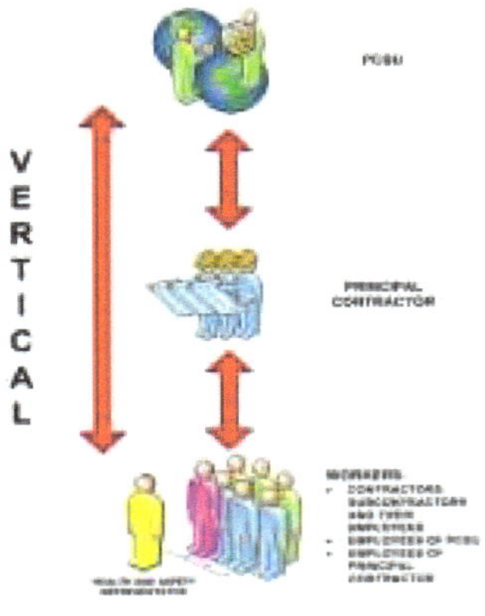

TOTEMIC ANALOGY

Semantics
Within One-God Theology
Eliminating the Metaphor

A HIDDEN LANGUAGE OF CONFLICT AND RESOLUTION

TOTEMIC ANALOGY: the use of non-metaphorical totemic symbolism in the form of a simile to explain parts of nature to nature: to spirituality, or to the conditions of humanity as they relate to one another.

SOCIOARITHMETICS: the use of arithmetic as a Totemic Analogy to explain social and spiritual dynamics: *syn*: numeric, *ant*: linguistic metaphoric Greek Isopsephy, Jewish Gematria

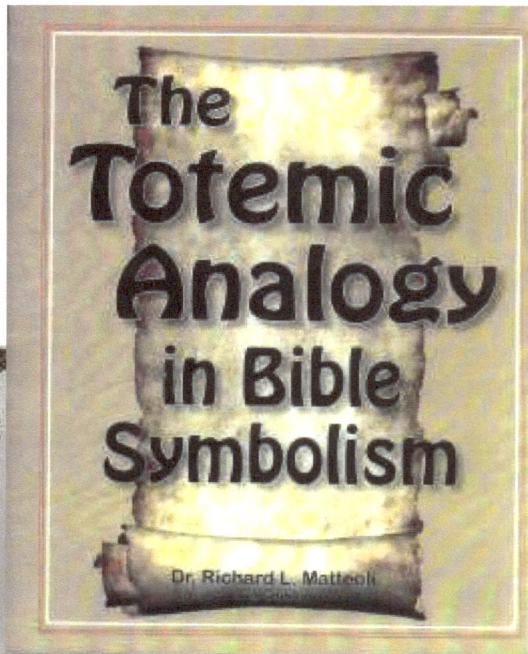

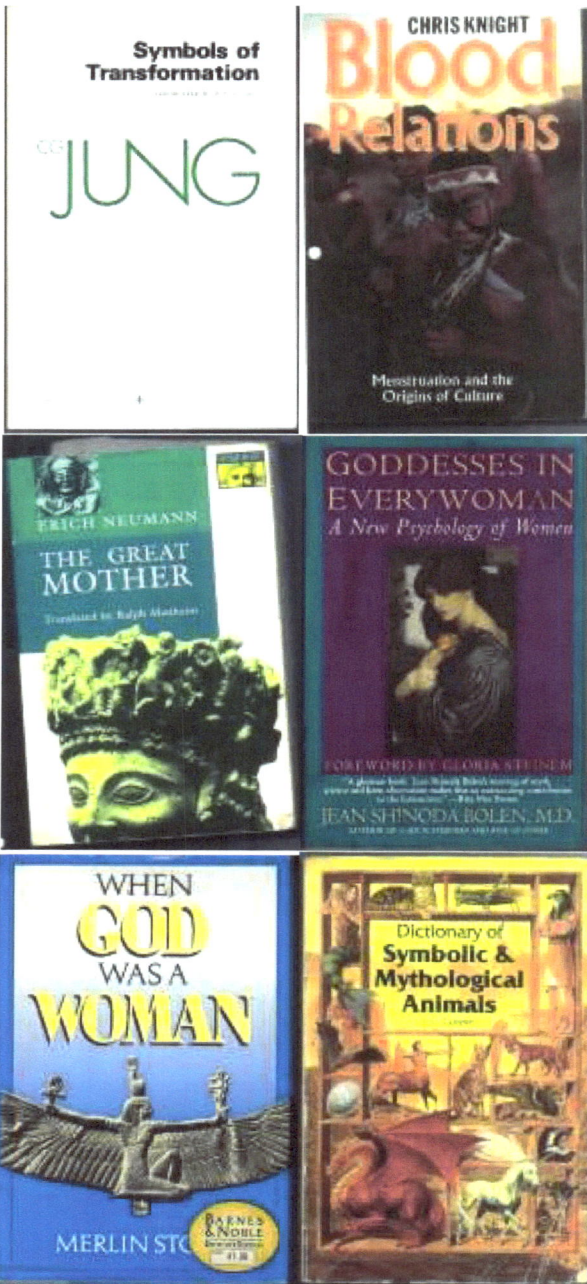

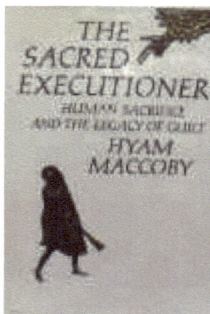

Mandated Report VA to CDC - Matteoli

Read Picture Line as a Sentence

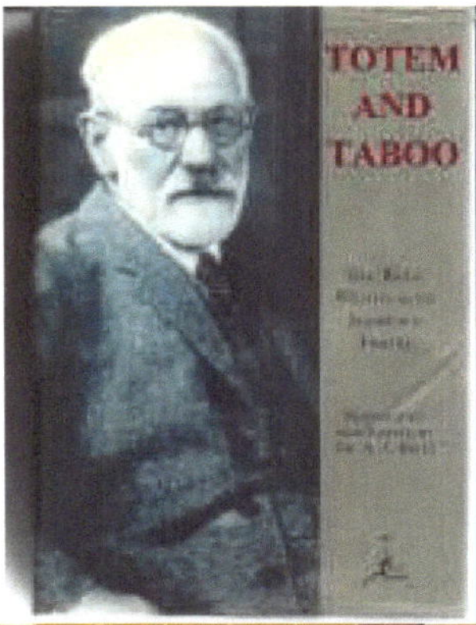

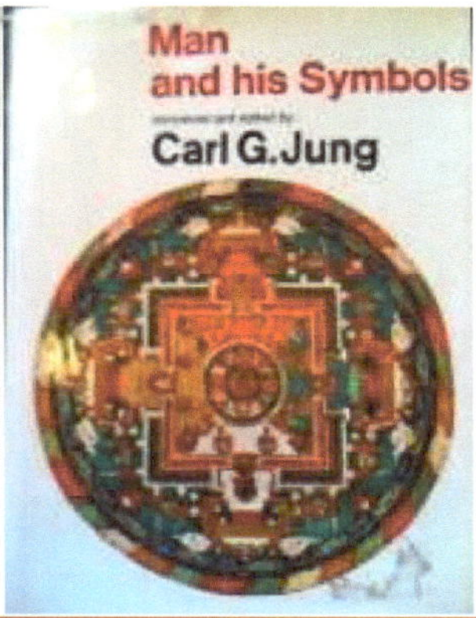

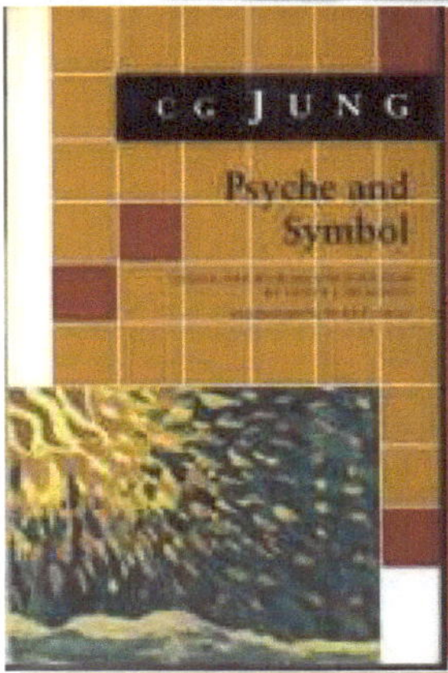

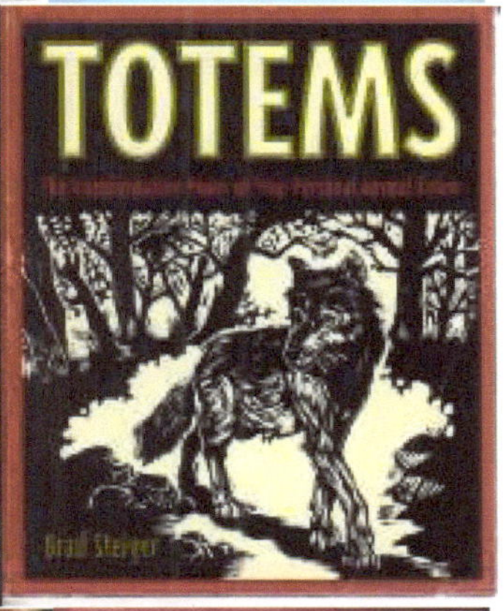

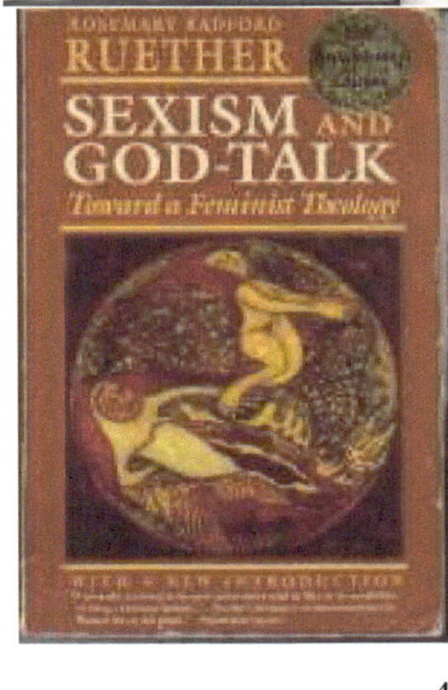

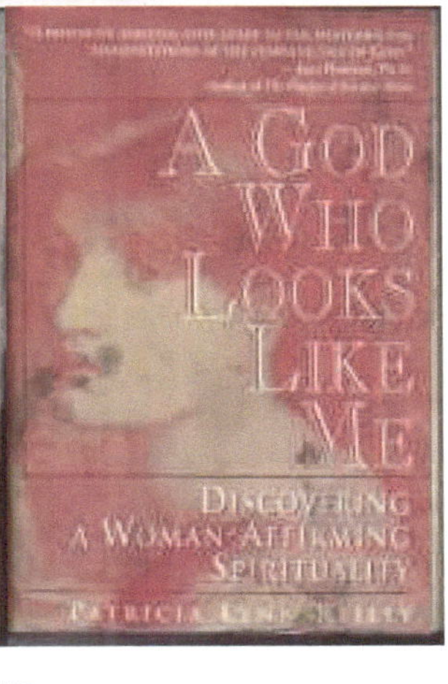

Mandated Report VA to CDC - Matteoli

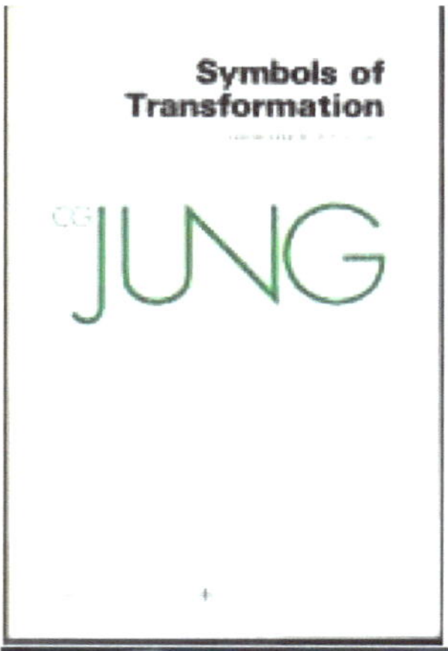
Symbols of
Transformation
C.G.
JUNG

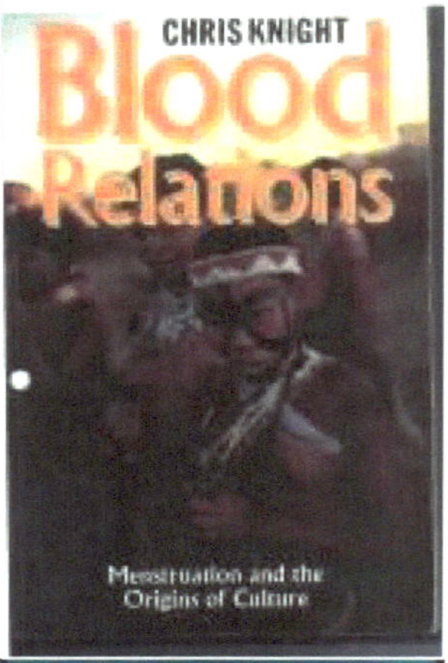
CHRIS KNIGHT
Blood
Relations
Menstruation and the
Origins of Culture

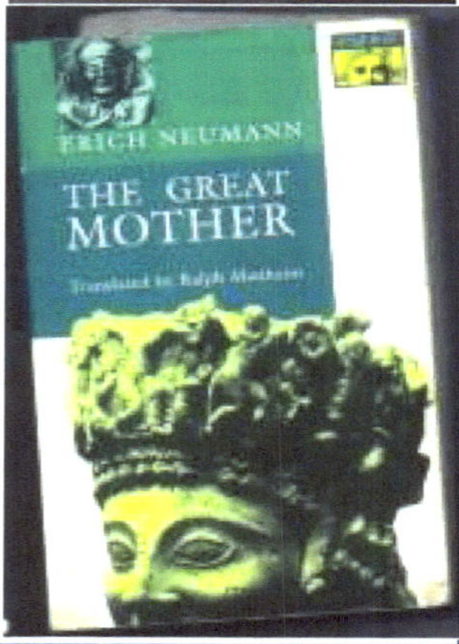
ERICH NEUMANN
THE GREAT
MOTHER

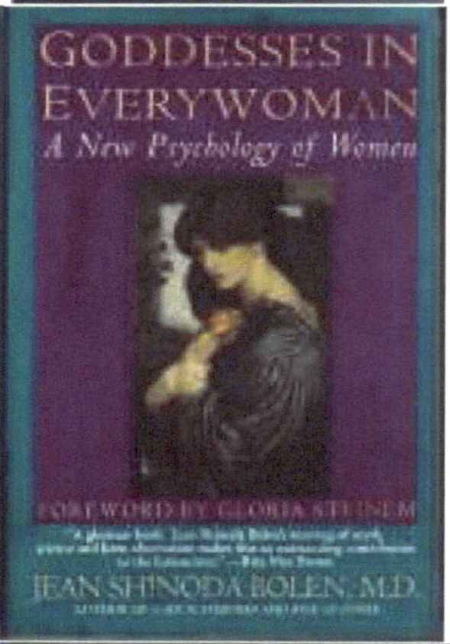
GODDESSES IN
EVERYWOMAN
A New Psychology of Women
FOREWORD BY GLORIA STEINEM
JEAN SHINODA BOLEN, M.D.

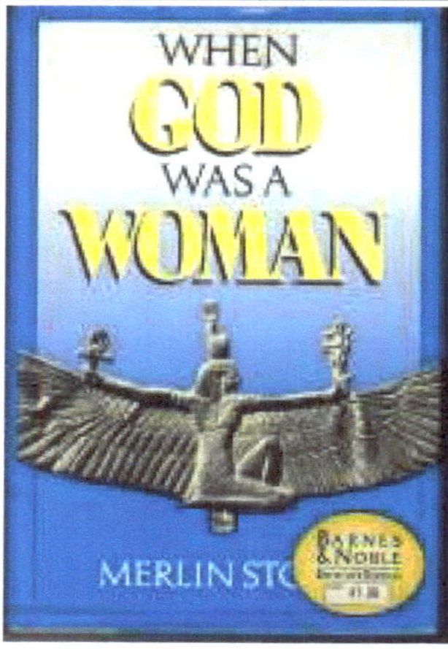
WHEN
GOD
WAS A
WOMAN
MERLIN STO
BARNES
& NOBLE

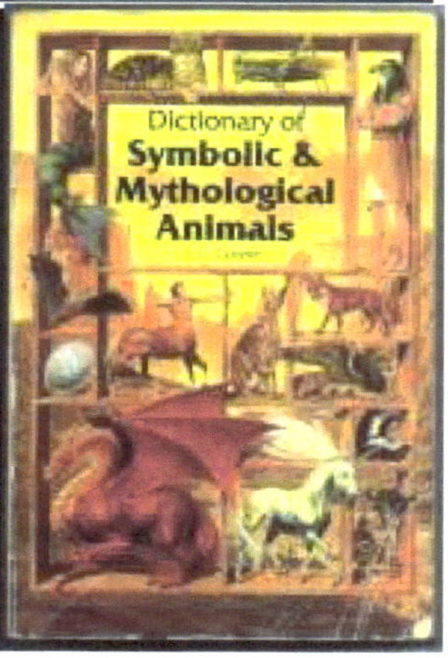
Dictionary of
Symbolic &
Mythological
Animals

MOTHER NATURE DETERMINES THEO-RELIGIOUS COMMUNICATION

TOTEM: A totem is a natural object or animal believed by a particular society to have spiritual significance and adopted by it as an emblem.

Words themselves also have totemic meaning

I asked him to give me an example of a metaphor.

He said: *So and so runs very fast. People say he runs **like** a deer.*

I said: *That's not a metaphor; the metaphor is: So and so **is** a deer.*

That's a lie. He said.

That's a metaphor. I said.

Even the categories of being and non-being - - those are categories of thought. I mean it is as simple as that. So it depends on how much you want to think about it. Whether it's putting you in touch with the mystery that's the ground of your own being.

If it isn't... Well, it's a lie.

JOSEPH CAMPBELL: A Biographical Portrait: THE HERO'S JOURNEY

Obviously, the metaphysical concepts of the archaic world were not formulated in theoretical language; but the symbol, the myth, the rite, express on different planes and through the means proper to them, a complex system that can be regarded as constituting metaphysics...

It is useless to search archaic languages for the terms so laboriously created by the great philosophic traditions: there is every likelihood that such words as ***being***, nonbeing, **real**, **becoming**, **illusionary**, are not to be found in the language of the Australians or of the ancient Mesopotamians. But if the word is lacking, the *thing*, is present; only it is *said* – that is, revealed in a coherent fashion – through *symbols* and *myth*.

Mircea Eliade, *The Myth of the Eternal Return*

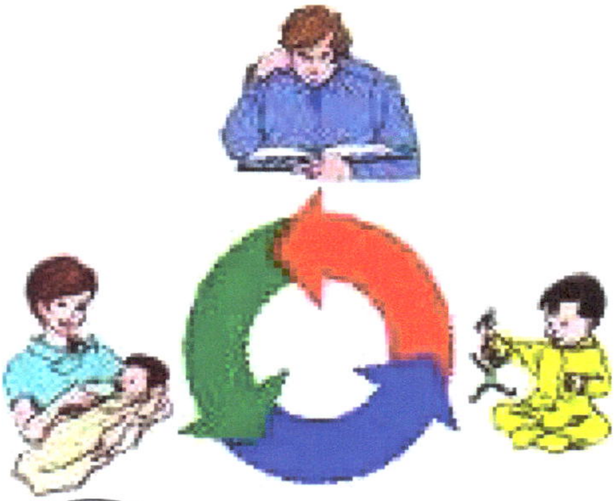

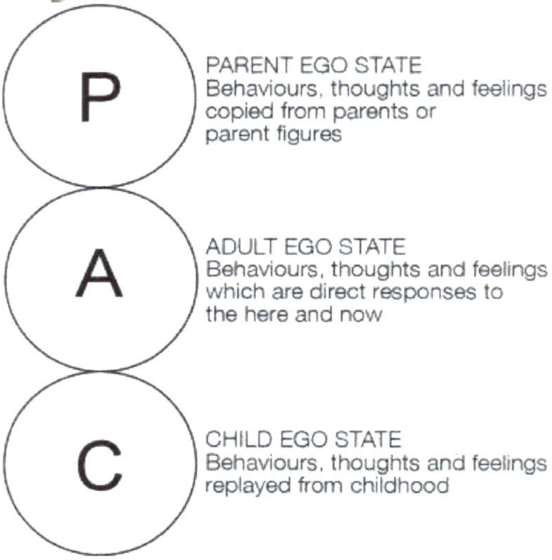
P
PARENT EGO STATE
Behaviours, thoughts and feelings copied from parents or parent figures
A
ADULT EGO STATE
Behaviours, thoughts and feelings which are direct responses to the here and now
C
CHILD EGO STATE
Behaviours, thoughts and feelings replayed from childhood

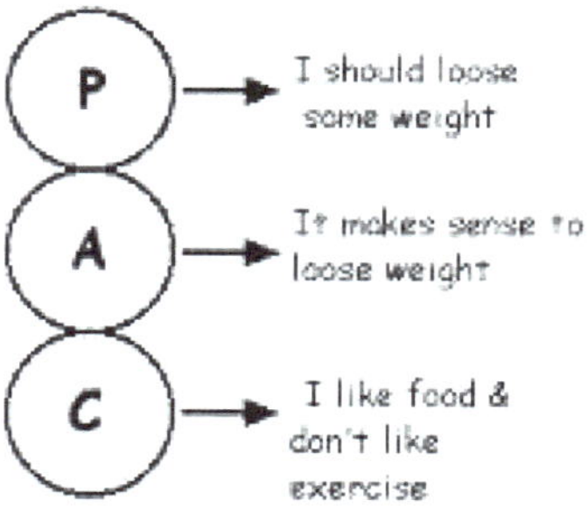
P
I should loose some weight
A
It makes sense to loose weight
C
I like food & don't like exercise

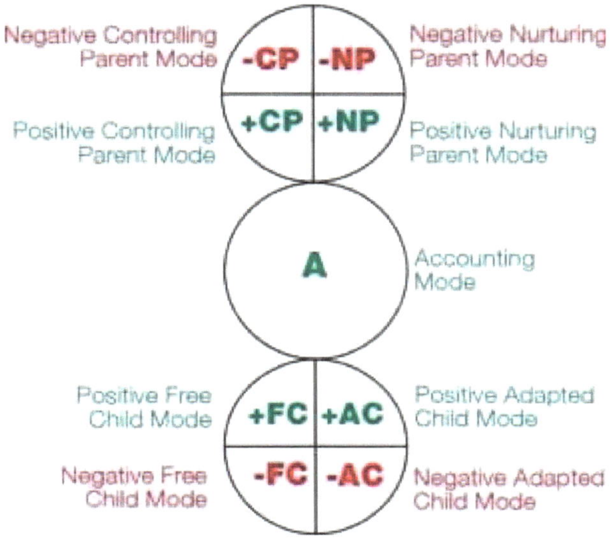
Negative Controlling Parent Mode
-CP
-NP
Negative Nurturing Parent Mode
Positive Controlling Parent Mode
+CP
+NP
Positive Nurturing Parent Mode
A
Accounting Mode
Positive Free Child Mode
+FC
+AC
Positive Adapted Child Mode
Negative Free Child Mode
-FC
-AC
Negative Adapted Child Mode

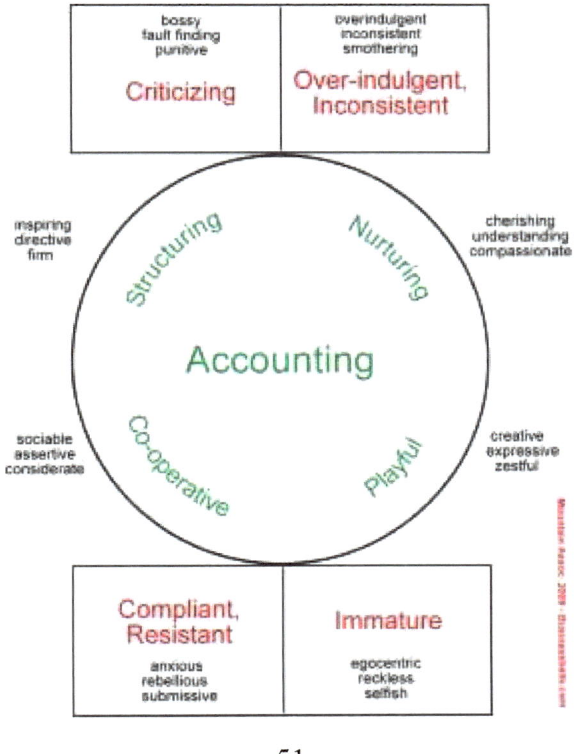
bossy
fault finding
punitive
Criticizing
overindulgent
inconsistent
smothering
Over-indulgent, Inconsistent
inspiring
directive
firm
Structuring
Nurturing
cherishing
understanding
compassionate
Accounting
sociable
assertive
considerate
Co-operative
Playful
creative
expressive
zestful
Compliant, Resistant
anxious
rebellious
submissive
Immature
egocentric
reckless
selfish

COMMUNICATIVE PROGRESSION TOWARD DISHONESTY

TRANSACTIONAL ANALYSIS

Eric Berne's discusses *communication* that segments into three ego 'negotiating' *ego* elements, Parent, Adult and Child, (PAC). Parent and Child communication is mediated through the Adult. Berne's categories are similar but not identical with Freud's psychology as: Parent/ego, Adult/superego, and Child/id. From Berne's *Games People Play*, Harper, 1967, pp. 29, 35-36, 36-37, 41, 48 and 24.

CHILD: The manner and intent of reaction is the same as it would be for a very little boy or girl

PARENT: To dominate and control children, parents assume certain postures, gestures, vocabulary, feelings, etc.

ADULT: This is the mature, autonomous, objective state that appraises situations and states thought processes, perceived problems and conclusions in a non-prejudicial manner.

NORMAL: Adults flirting and sex are engaging in Child-Child Interaction.

TRANSACTION: The unit of social intercourse is called a *transaction.* If two or more people encounter each other in social aggregation, sooner or later one of them will speak, or give some other indication of acknowledging the presence of others. This is called 'transactional stimulus.' Another person will say or do something which in some way related to this stimulus, and that is called 'transactional response.' Simple transactional analysis is concerned with diagnosing which ego state implemented the transactional stimulus, and which one executed the response. The simplest transaction are those in which both stimulus and response arise from the Adults of the parties concerned. The agent, estimating the data before him that a scalpel is now the instrument of choice, holds out his hand. The respondent appraises this gesture correctly, estimates the forces and distances involved, and places the handle of the scalpel exactly where the surgeon expects it. Next in simplicity are Child-Parent *transactions*. The fevered child asks for a glass of water, and the nurturing mother brings it. Both these *transactions* are 'complementary;' that is, the response is appropriate and expected and follows the natural order of healthy human relationships.

PROCEDURE: A *procedure* is series of simple complementary Adult transactions directed toward the manipulation of reality... *Procedures* are based on data processing and probability estimates concerning the 'material' of reality, and reach their highest development in professional techniques... Two variables are used in evaluating *procedures*: A procedure is said to be 'efficient' when the agent makes the best possible use of the data and experience available to him, regardless of any deficiencies that may exist in his knowledge. If the Parent or the Child interferes with the Adult's data processing, the procedure becomes 'contaminated' and will be less efficient. The 'effectiveness' of a procedure is judged by the actual results. The efficiency is a psychological criterion and effectiveness is a material one.

RITUAL: A *ritual* is a stereotyped series of simple complementary transactions programmed by external forces. An *informal ritual*, such as social leave-taking, may be subject to considerable local variations in details, although the basic form remains the same. A *formal ritual*, such as a Roman Catholic mass, offers much less option... Many formal rituals started off as heavily contaminated through fairly efficient procedures, but as time passed and circumstances changed, they lost all procedural validity while still retaining their usefulness as acts of faith. Transactionally, they represent guilt-relieving or reward-seeking compliances with Parental demands. They offer a safe, reassuring (apotropaic), and often an enjoyable method of structuring time.

PASTIMES: This may be defined as a series of semi-ritualistic, simple, complementary transactions arranged around a single field of material, whose primary object is to structure of time. The beginning and the end of the interval are typically signaled by procedures or rituals. The transactions are adaptively programmed so that each party will obtain the maximum gains or advantages during the interval. The better his adaptation, the more he will get out of it.

GAME: A *Game* is an ongoing series of complementary ulterior transactions progressing to a well-defined, predictable outcome. Descriptively it is a recurring set of transactions, often repetitious, superficially plausible, with a snare, or "gimmick." Games are clearly differentiated from procedures, rituals and pastimes by two chief characteristics: (1) their ulterior quality and (2) the payoff. Procedures may be successful, rituals effective, and pastimes profitable, but all of them are by definition candid, and ending may be sensational, but it is not dramatic. Every *Game*, on the other hand, is basically dishonest, and the outcome has a dramatic, as distinct from exciting quality.

NEGATING CONFLICT RESOLUTION

Destroyer and Prostitute Child Archetypes

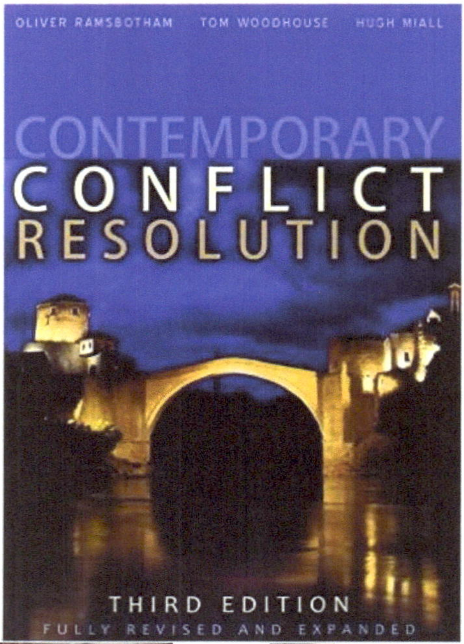

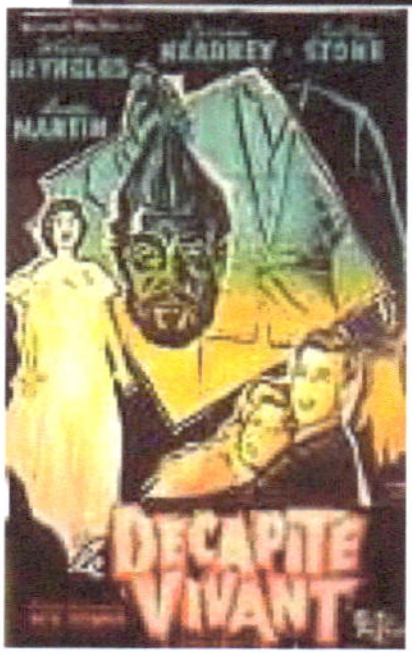

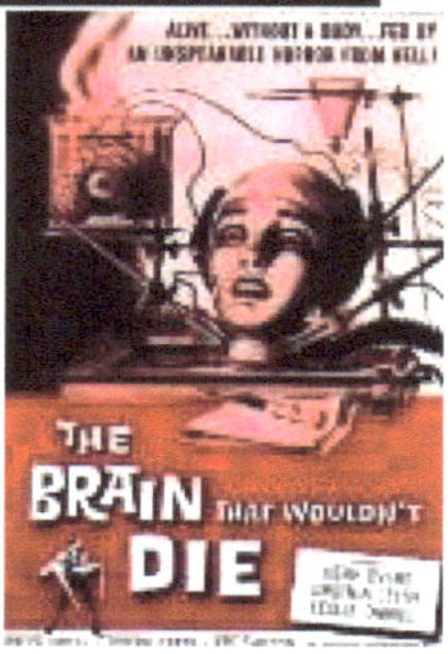

The Thing That Couldn't-Wouldn't Die

We have found the enemy and he is us.
Comic Strip. *Pogo*.

CYCLIC RESURRECTION

GENETICS

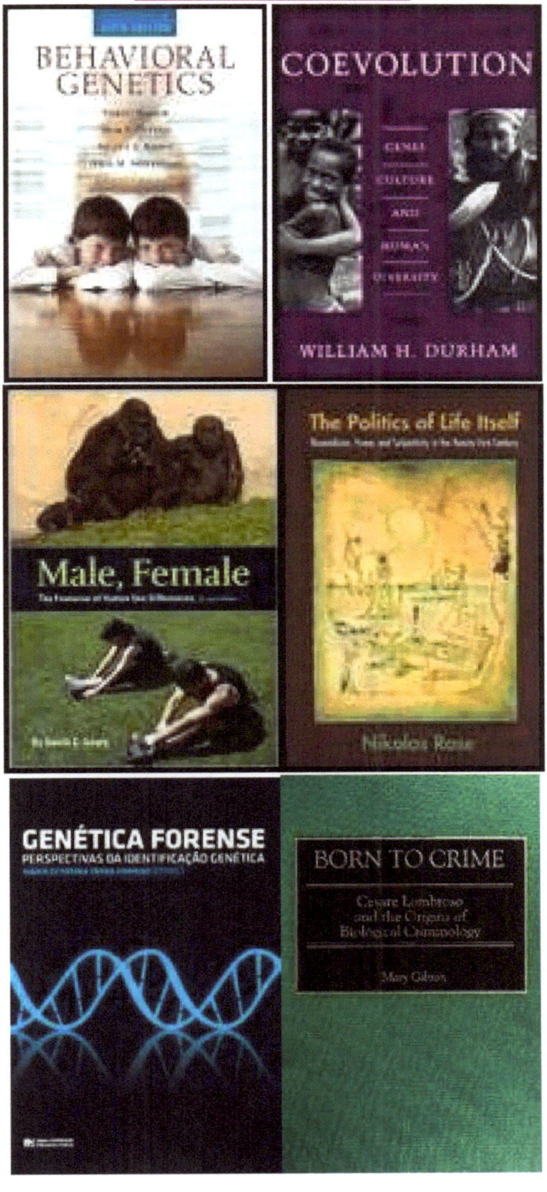

Mandated Report VA to CDC - Matteoli

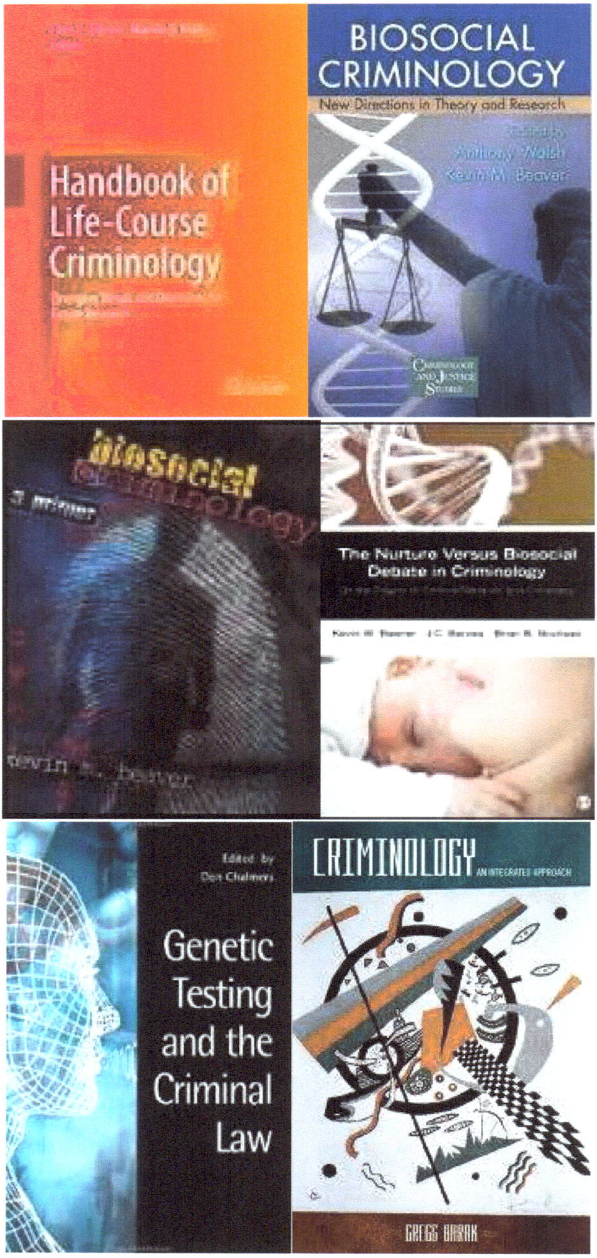

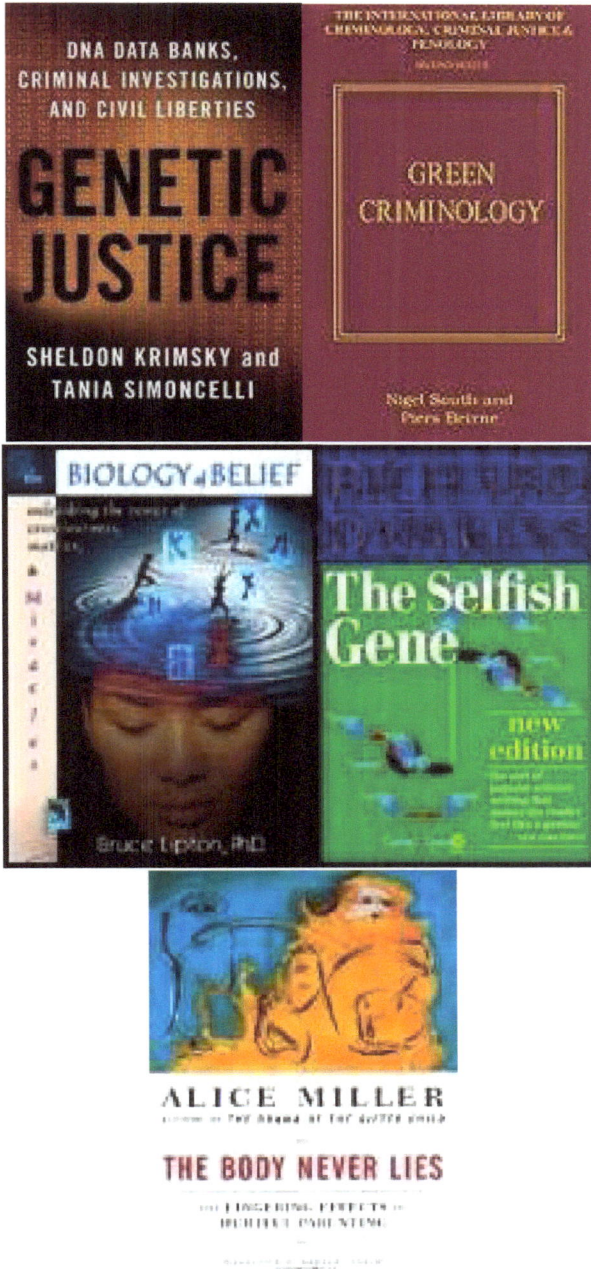

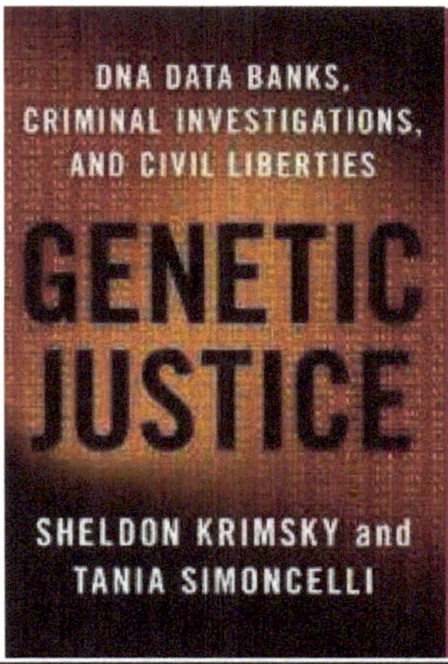
DNA DATA BANKS,
CRIMINAL INVESTIGATIONS,
AND CIVIL LIBERTIES
GENETIC
JUSTICE
SHELDON KRIMSKY and
TANIA SIMONCELLI

GREEN
CRIMINOLOGY
Nigel South and
Piers Beirne

BIOLOGY of BELIEF
Bruce Lipton, PhD

The Selfish
Gene
new
edition

ALICE MILLER
THE BODY NEVER LIES

GENOCIDE
Self-Deification

VA Secular in Medical Environment

COMMON HUMANITY IS EXPRESSED IN BLOOD AND FLESH

Genocide eventually turns in on itself.

CDR Robert Harger, USN, (Ret.), SEAL

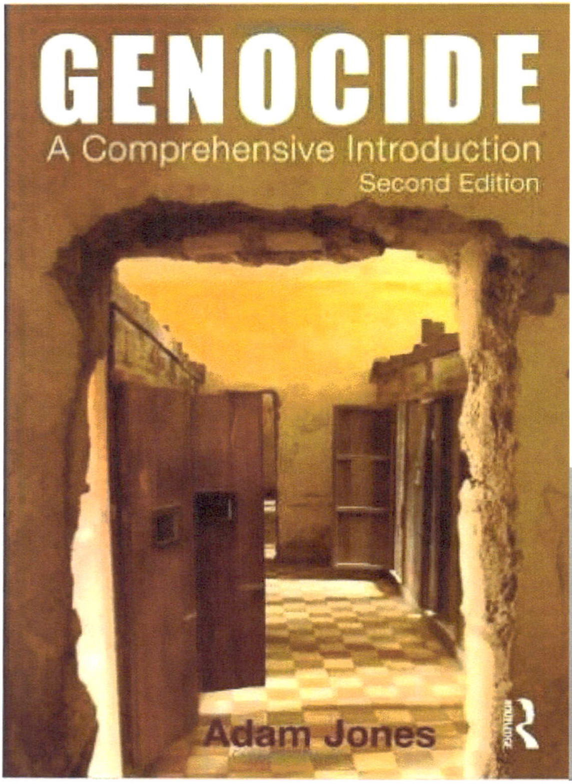

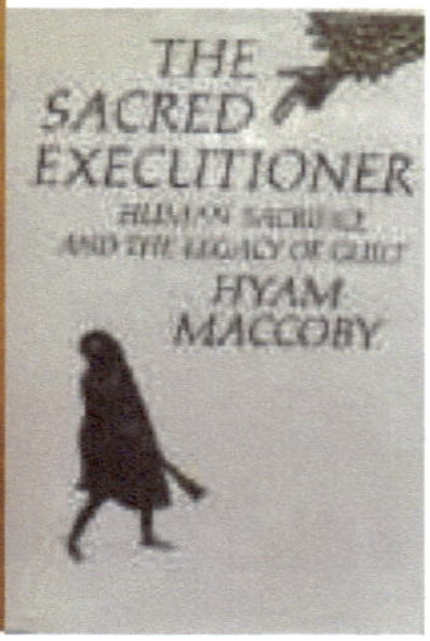

Read Picture Line as a Sentence

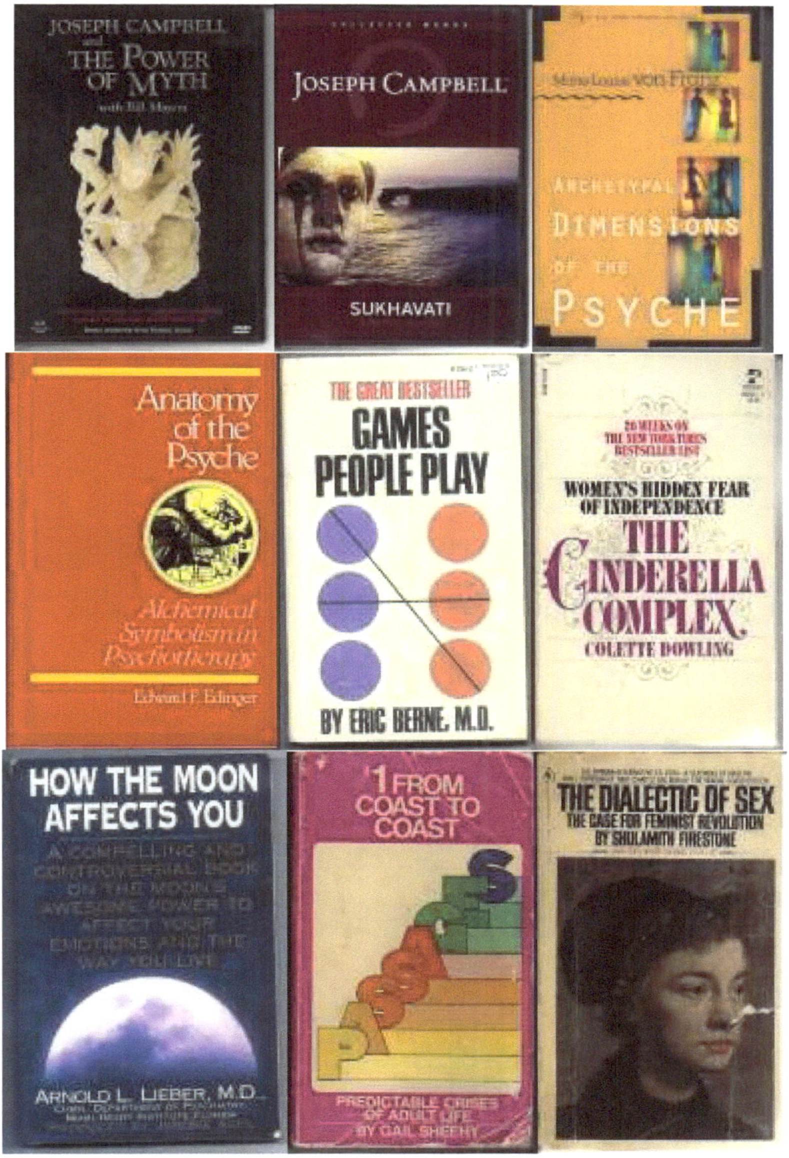

CONTINUING

ADDITIONAL REFERENCES WITHIN THE MYTHIC EXPRESSION AND ARCHETYPICAL DIMENSION

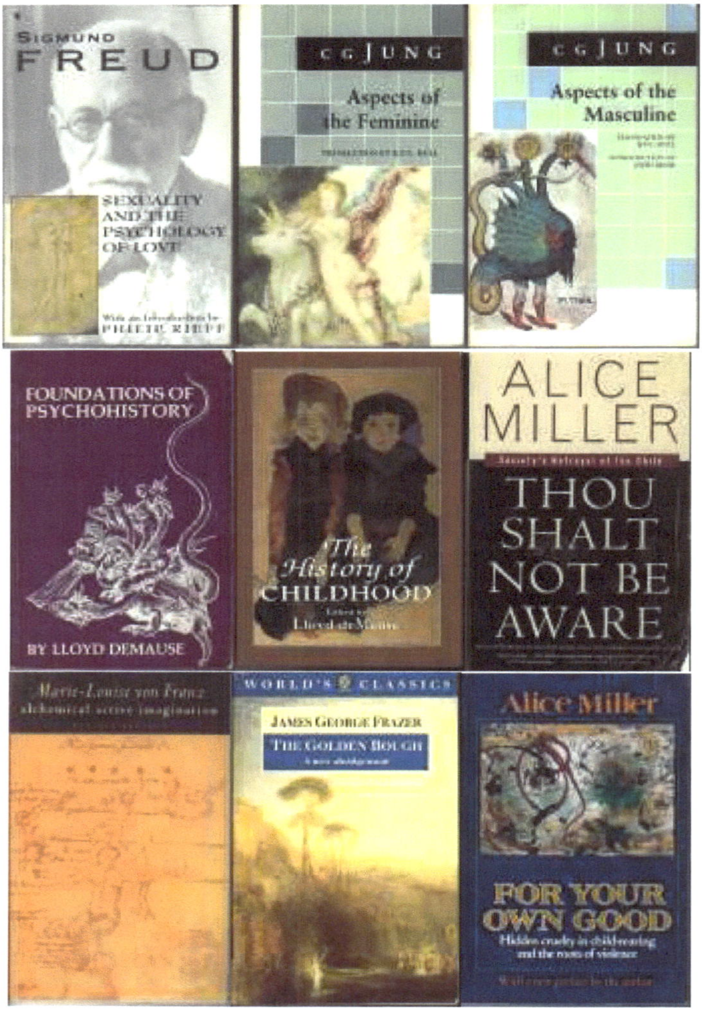

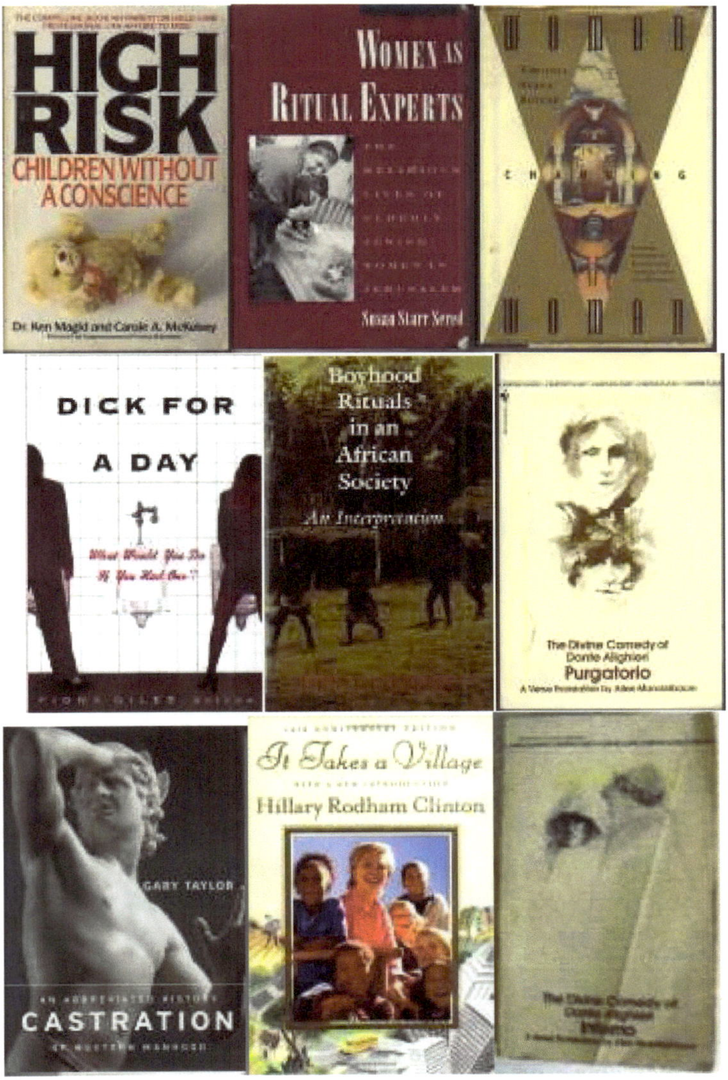
HIGH RISK
CHILDREN WITHOUT A CONSCIENCE
Dr. Ken Magid and Carole A. McKelvey
WOMEN AS RITUAL EXPERTS
Susan Starr Sered
DICK FOR A DAY
Boyhood Rituals in an African Society
An Interpretation
The Divine Comedy of Dante Alighieri
Purgatorio
GARY TAYLOR
CASTRATION
It Takes a Village
Hillary Rodham Clinton

Mandated Report VA to CDC - Matteoli

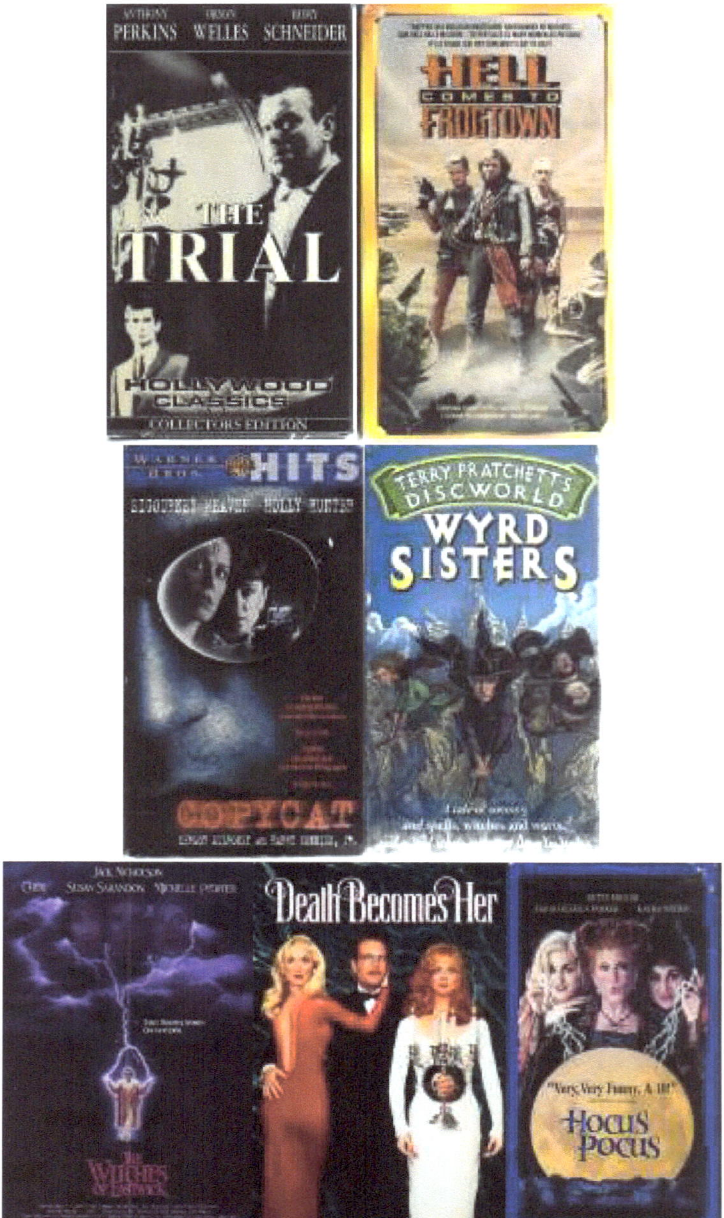

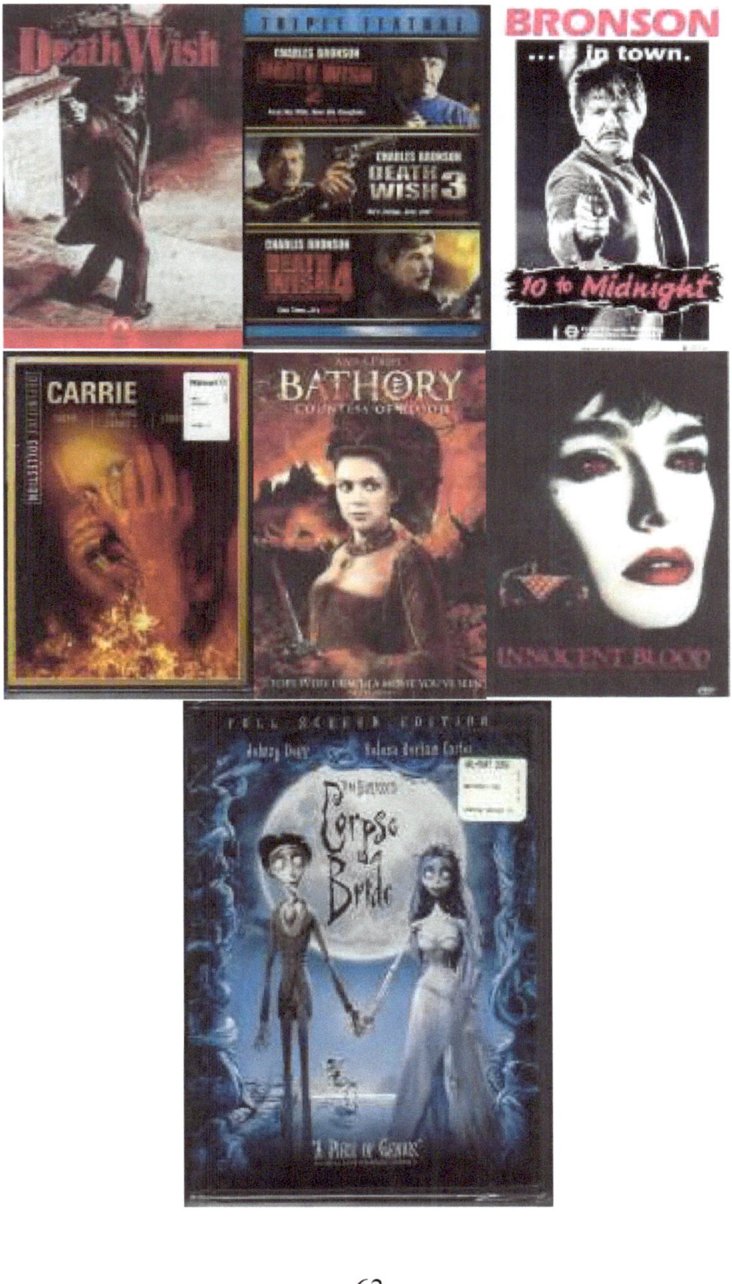
Death Wish
CHARLES BRONSON
DEATH WISH 3
BRONSON
10 to Midnight
CARRIE
BATHORY
INNOCENT BLOOD
Corpse Bride

Read Picture Line as a Sentence

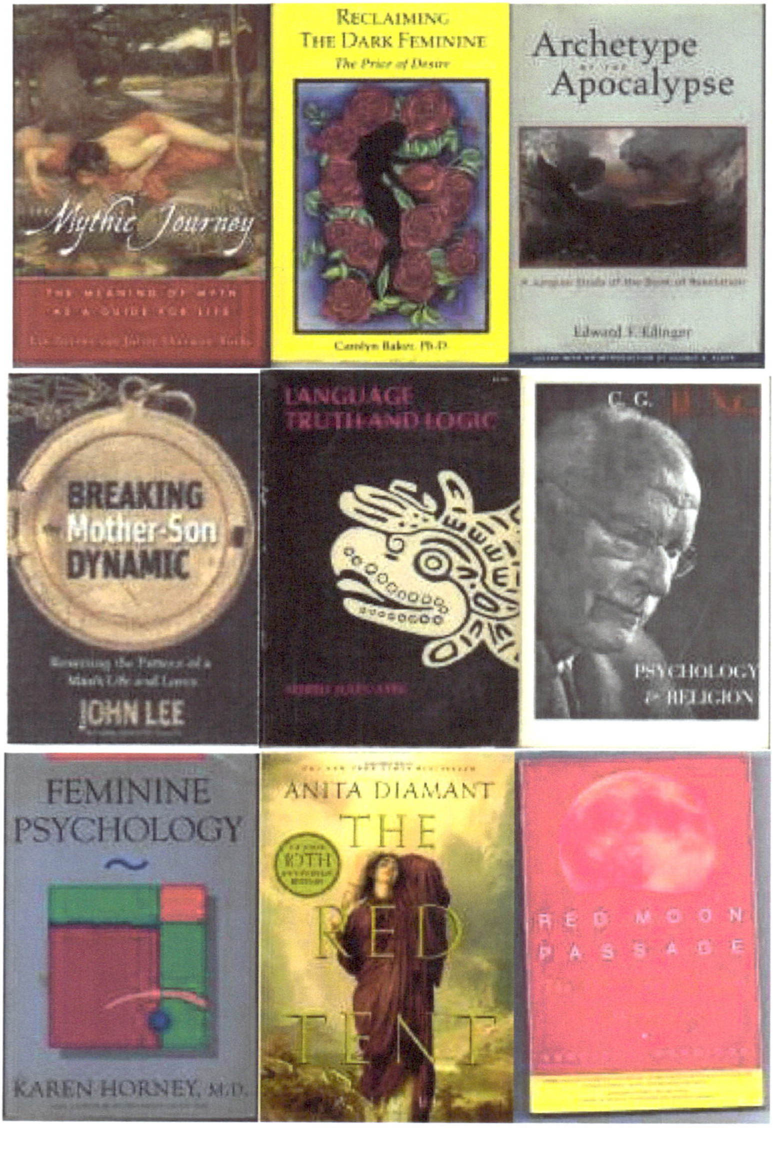

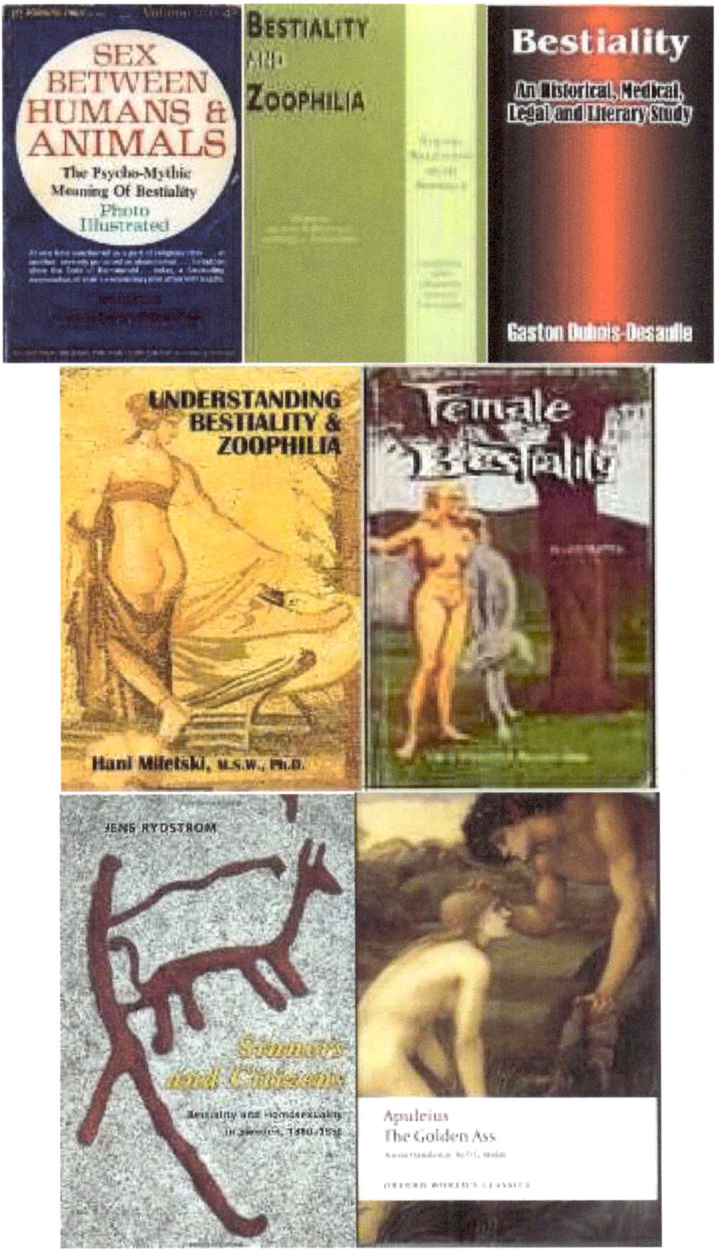
SEX BETWEEN HUMANS & ANIMALS
The Psycho-Mythic Meaning Of Bestiality
Photo Illustrated
BESTIALITY AND ZOOPHILIA
Bestiality
An Historical, Medical, Legal and Literary Study
Gaston Dubois-Desaulle
UNDERSTANDING BESTIALITY & ZOOPHILIA
Hani Miletski, M.S.W., Ph.D.
Female Bestiality
JENS RYDSTROM
Apuleius
The Golden Ass
OXFORD WORLD'S CLASSICS

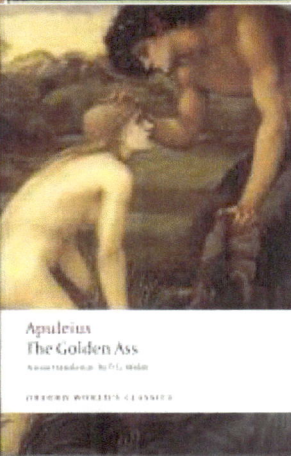

Read Picture Line as a Sentence

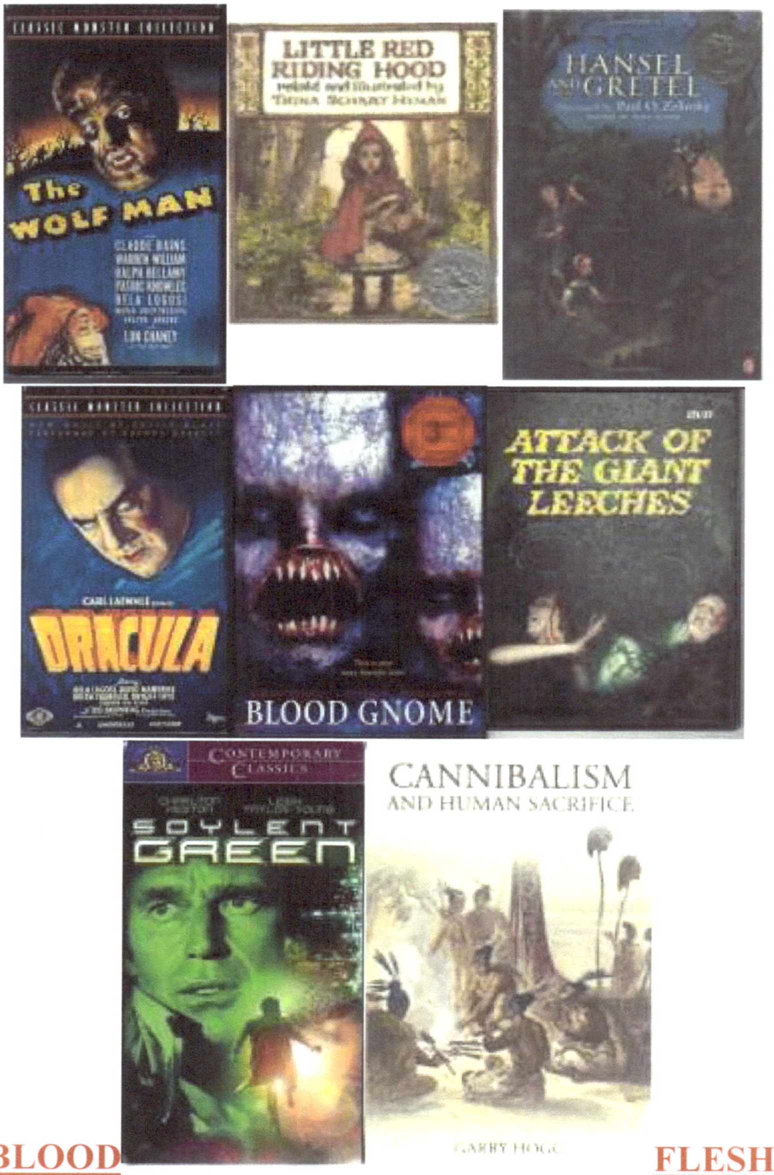

BLOOD **FLESH**

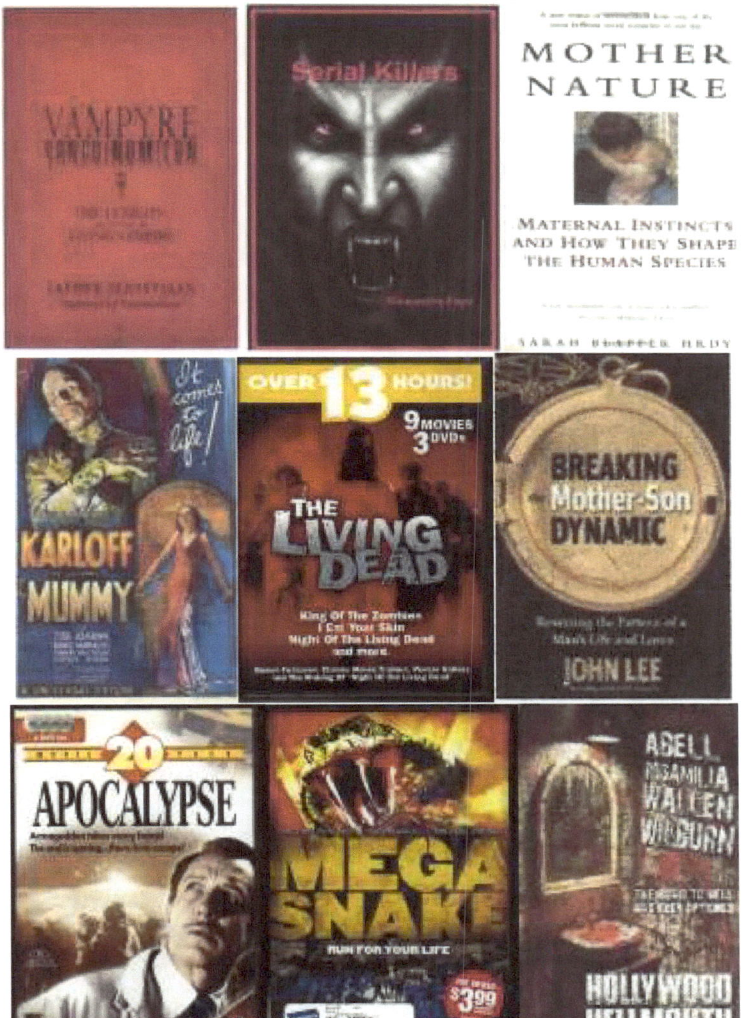
VAMPYRE
Serial Killers
MOTHER NATURE
MATERNAL INSTINCTS AND HOW THEY SHAPE THE HUMAN SPECIES
It comes to life!
KARLOFF
MUMMY
OVER 13 HOURS!
9 MOVIES 3 DVDs
THE LIVING DEAD
King Of The Zombies
I Eat Your Skin
Night Of The Living Dead
and more
BREAKING Mother-Son DYNAMIC
JOHN LEE
20
APOCALYPSE
MEGA SNAKE
RUN FOR YOUR LIFE
$3.99
ABELL
HOLLYWOOD HELLMOUTH

WHO IS THE WILD WOMAN?
SHE IS THE LIFE/DEATH/LIFE FORCE

Life's twin sister is a force named Death. The force called Death is one of the two magnetic forks of the wild nature.

Clarissa Pinkola Estes
Women Who Run With the Wolves:
Myths and Stories of the Wild Woman Archetype

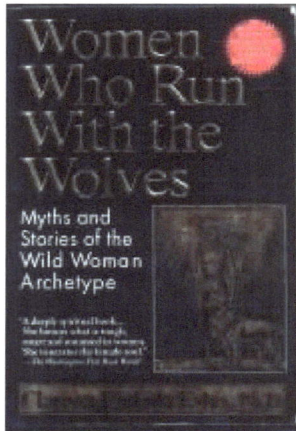

This is **NORMAL**. **MAN** is Born of **WOMAN**.
Those with the Power to **GIVE** have the Power to **TAKE**.

THINK: <u>LIGHT SIDE</u> *V*. <u>DARK SIDE</u>
Woman is Existence; Man is the Servant of Existence
MATRIARCHAL IDENTITY

Robert E. Lee top West Point student detested slavery but chose his mother's identity in Virginia for State's Rights and captured John Brown. Ulysses S. Grant lowest West Point student, except for Horsemanship, chose his father's identity, in a way. Abolitionism was a Matriarchal Movement.
John Brown's father taught Ulysses S. Grant's father the Tanning Trade.

Einstein for religious reasons spent the rest of his life trying to disprove his Expanding Universe theory. He studied: What IF?
Today we mostly use Tesla. He autisticly studied: What IS?

EMMA JUNG'S "ANIMUS and ANIMA" is the first book to read before studying any subject outside Empiric Science

Animus and Anima

Carl Jung defined the male's Anima as the female within him. The female's Animus is conversely the male within her. The anima and animus are the inclusioned eyes within the Eastern Yin and Yang.

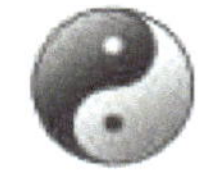

> ***Anima:*** the feminine component of the unconscious male *psyche* and inner counterpart to the persona. Ultimately an *archetype* of Eros and of life itself, this woman "within" functions as a filter, bridge, guide, and mediator between the ego and the deeper layers of the *unconscious*.

> ***Animus:*** the male component of the unconscious female *psyche*. Like the *anima* (Eros), but he personifies "spirit" and "intellect" (Logos). His negative aspect gives a woman her irrational convictions and opinions. He is usually plural because women focus in one man only in conscious relationships.

Though not set in inescapable stone and can be overcome, Emma Jung taught on both the animus and anima:[10]

On feminine Animus:

> *Her animus, for the most part, does not perceive the individual masculine, but rather perceives a grouping of males as a collective image. She postulates the masculine as a council, and the more he expresses individually the more he becomes distant. Thus she is more apt to try to make the individual male become what she wants him to be may become what she wants him to be through projective transference. In this, she seeks fulfillment through him by which he has as a mirror become from her actions regarding all masculine aspects she desires. Thus to an individual male, she sees the many factors that males possess and can bring her.*

> *Usage of his elements is through aggressive authority and power of suggestion. The process becomes caught in religious concept enforced by* "ritual" *and* "rite." *Yet, in attempts to make connections she does not realize what she sacrifices. The female's animus does not exhibit masculine Logos and its critical ability. Right and wrong of an act, in and of itself, is superseded to acceptance because of what the act represents. Her animus tries to accomplish goals regardless of logical consequences of logical process. In this, she becomes the more primitive Self of human existence through desire. By this, her animus often misses the Logos connection of reality through imagination and sensation.*

> *Yet, the drive of her animus is a necessity for balance of the outer corporeal world to that of the inner spiritual, and is perceived as an intuition of existence that is deficient in masculine Logos that is dependent on his need for experimental fact. Her expression is Nature. From Nature's movements her inner voice of animus is a critical expression as to motives and intentions that evoke command edicts and prohibitions, all for the purpose of shaping life worth living.* ***"She must be obeyed."***

<u>CONTINUING</u>

VA PUNISHMENT FOR TELLING THE **DIRTY LITTLE SECRET**

with

Genocide – VA: Social Ritual into Medical

TEAM PREDATION

TRANSFENCE OF AGGRESSION

<u>Transference</u>: the deliberate displacement of one's unresolved conflicts, dependencies and aggressions onto a substitute object

<u>Dissociation</u>: The inability to perceive the humanity of another *syn*: disunion, separation, division, dividing, parting, split, splitting, sundering, break, rupture, rift, divorce, cleavage

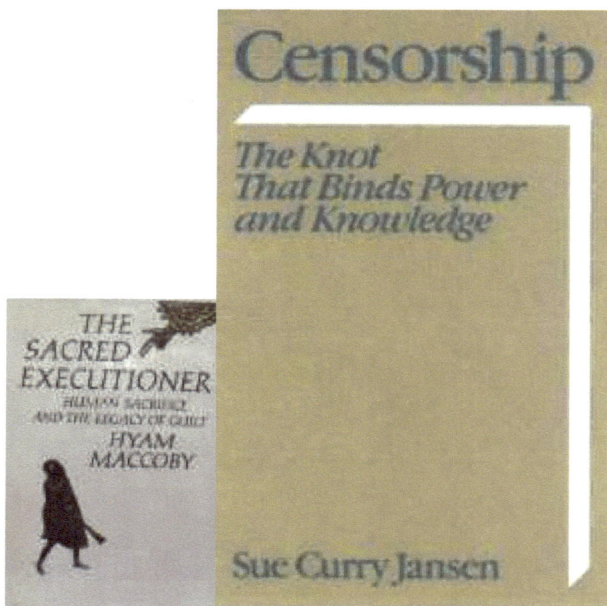

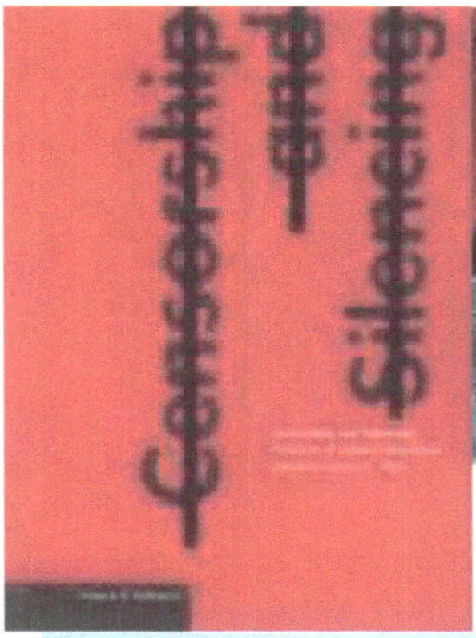
Censorship
and
Silencing

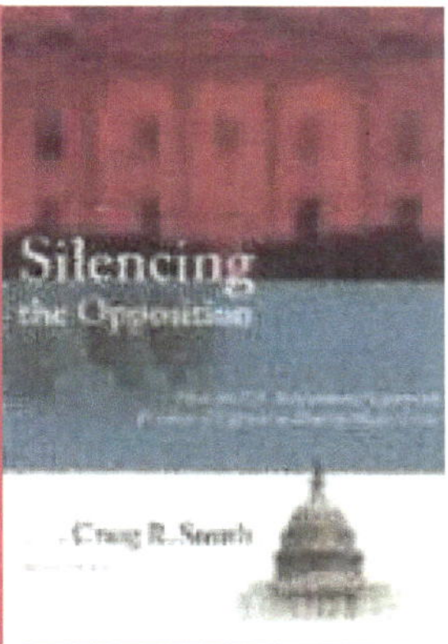
Silencing

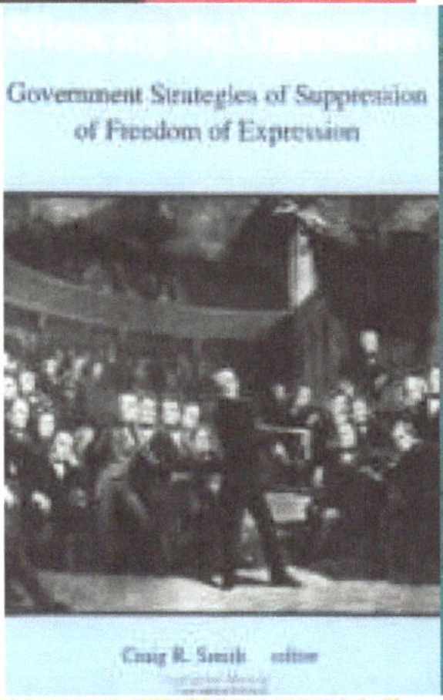
Government Strategies of Suppression
of Freedom of Expression

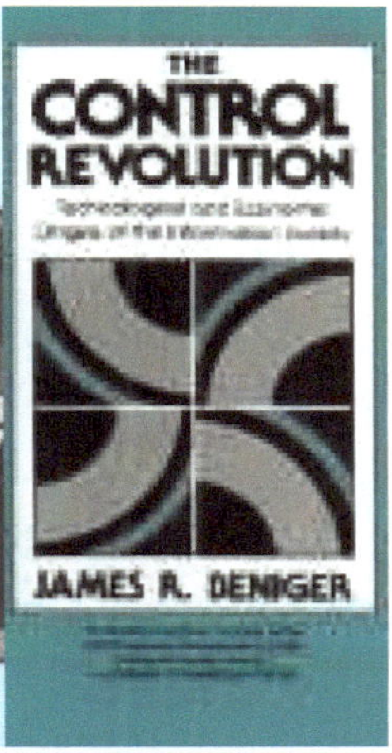
THE
CONTROL
REVOLUTION
JAMES R. BENIGER

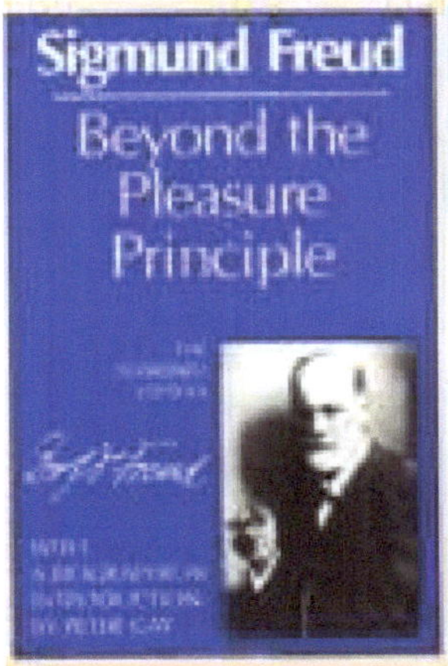
Sigmund Freud
Beyond the
Pleasure
Principle

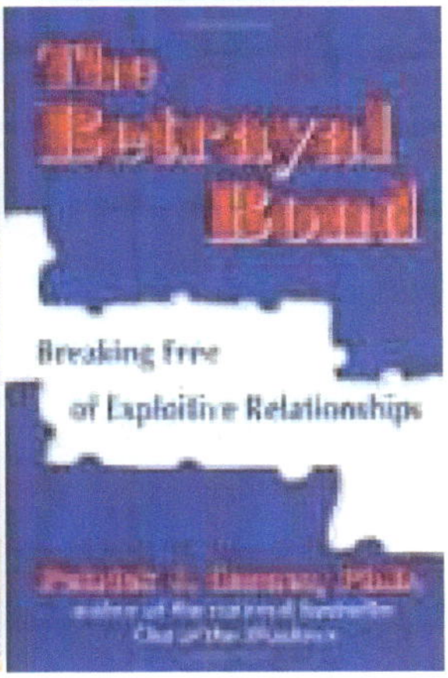
The
Betrayal
Bond
Breaking Free
of Exploitive Relationships

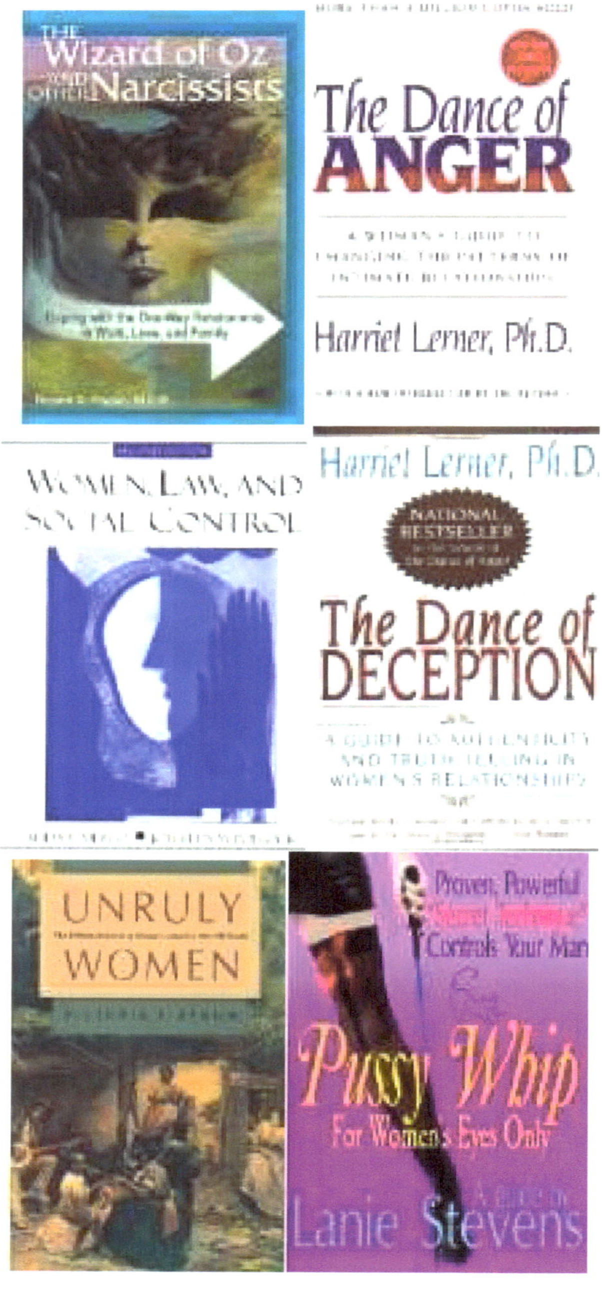
The Wizard of Oz and other Narcissists
The Dance of ANGER
Harriet Lerner, Ph.D.
Women, Law, and Social Control
Harriet Lerner, Ph.D.
NATIONAL BESTSELLER
The Dance of DECEPTION
A GUIDE TO AUTHENTICITY AND TRUTH-TELLING IN WOMEN'S RELATIONSHIPS
UNRULY WOMEN
Proven, Powerful
Controls Your Man
Pussy Whip
For Women's Eyes Only
Lanie Stevens

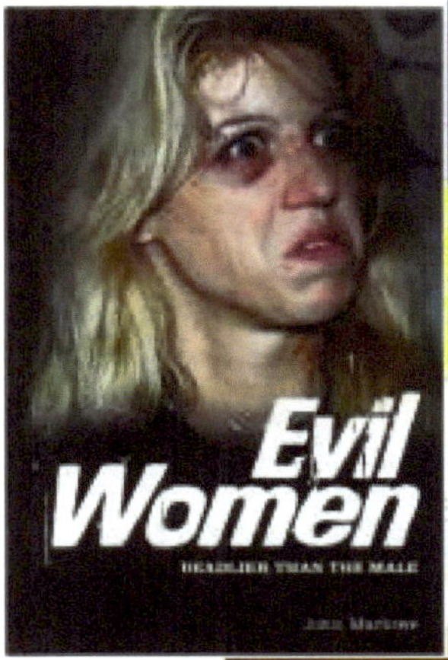
Evil Women
DEADLIER THAN THE MALE

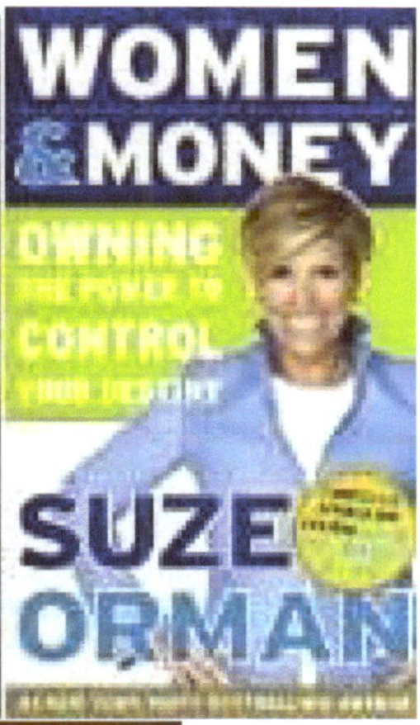
WOMEN & MONEY
OWNING
CONTROL
SUZE ORMAN

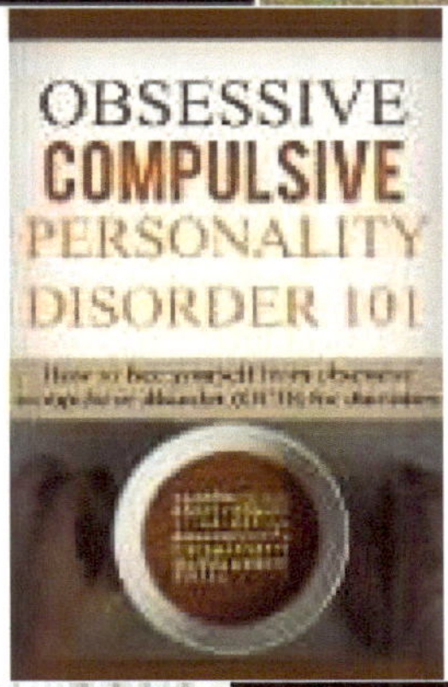
OBSESSIVE COMPULSIVE PERSONALITY DISORDER 101

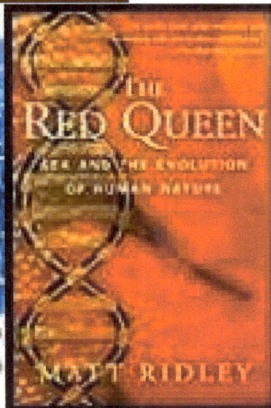

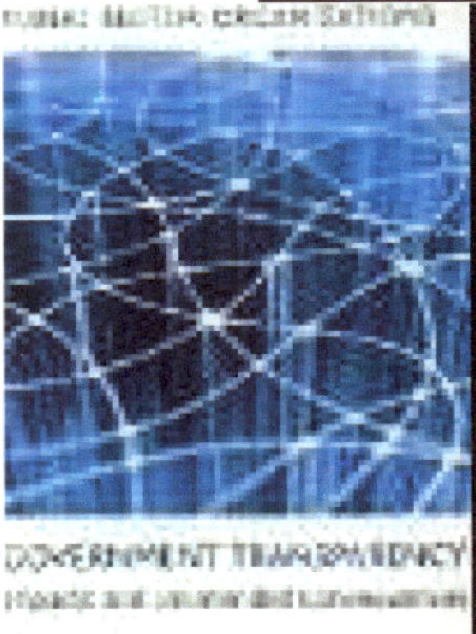
GOVERNMENT TRANSPARENCY

THE RED QUEEN
SEX AND THE EVOLUTION OF HUMAN NATURE
MATT RIDLEY

CULTURAL CONVENTION USURPS THE RULE OF LAW

Cultural Relativity *v.* Empiricism

Eddy Bernays' wrote *Propaganda* in 1928 and used by Joseph Goebbels in charge of Nazi propaganda. Bernays considered the general population – *The Herd* – and inferior. He observed:[55]

> *The conscious and intelligent manipulation of the organized habits and opinions of the masses is an important element in democratic society. Those who manipulate this unseen mechanism of society constitute an invisible government which is the true ruling power of our country. We are governed, our minds are molded, our tastes are formed, our ideas suggested, lately by men we have never heard of. This is a logical result of the way in which our democratic society is organized... In almost every act of our daily lives, whether in the sphere of politics or business, in our social conduct or our* ***ethical thinking****, we are dominated by the relatively small number of persons... It is they which pull the wires which control the public mind.*

Dissociation requires a change in ethical behavior with rationalizing away wrongs. This may occur under stress.[56-58] Robert Solomon wrote *A Short Introduction to Philosophy* and related with last paragraph relates Carol Gillian's retort to Lawrence Kholberg:[59]

Inductive logic: does not guarantee the truth of the conclusion, but only makes it more reasonable for us to believe the conclusion compared to other possible conclusions
Deductive logic: guarantees the truth of the conclusion, if the premises are true

Psychological egoism: All acts are basically selfish
Ethical egoism: You ought to act selfish
Psychological altruism: Some of our acts are basically altruistic
Ethical altruism: You ought to act for the good of others

Rationalism: Knowledge is based on reason
Necessary Truth: A statement that true because of reason
Empiricism: Knowledge is based on experience
Empirical Truth: A statement is true because of the facts

Moral Relativism: There are no universal and essential moral values, that morality is 'relative' to particular societies or peoples.
Ethical Relativism: the thesis that whatever a culture or a society holds to be right is therefore right, or, at least right for them.
Moral absolutism: the thesis that there are universal and essential moral values. If some society or people do not accept these values, then they are not moral.

> *Rather than thinking of ethics in terms of impersonal, abstract, moral principles of right and wrong, claimed Gillian, women tend to think of ethics in terms of moral personal responsibility. While men understood a moral dilemma posed by the experimenter as a problem having a right and wrong answer, women understood such a dilemma as the result of an interpersonal conflict in need of a resolution, not a right-versus-wrong answer. Gillian hypothesized that in addition to the moral reasoning grounded in abstract principles of right and wrong described by Kant and Kohlberg, there is also a more "feminine" but equally valid type of moral reasoning that is grounded in maintaining the stability of interpersonal relationships.*

Moral evil **is a product of our actions**

Solomon, Robert C., *The Big Questions: A Short Introduction to Philosophy*. 1982, p. 326.

Questions remain: **Who is the relationship for?**

NARCISSISM

Edited and Condensed with Author Permission

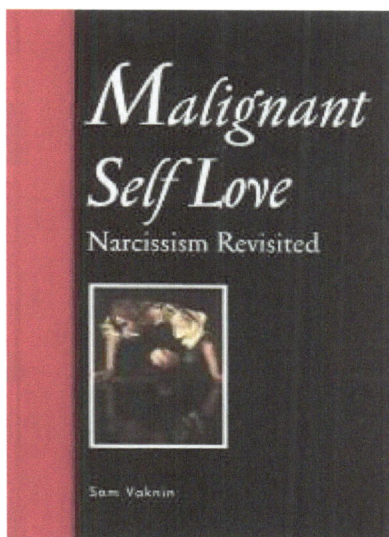

The narcissist is an actor in a melodrama, yet forced to remain behind the scenes. The scene takes center stage instead. The narcissist does not cater at all to his own needs. Contrary to his reputation, the narcissist does not love himself in any sense of the word. He feeds off other people who hurl back at him an image that he projects to them.

This is their sole function in his world: to reflect, to admire, to applaud, to detest – in a word, to assure him that he exists. Otherwise, they have no right to tax his time, energy, or emotions – so he feels.

The narcissist's **ego** is weak and lack clear borders. Many of the ego functions are projected. The **superego** is sadistic and punishing. The **id** is unrestrained. Primary objects in the narcissists childhood were badly idealized and destroyed…

He becomes unscrupulous, never bothered by the constant use he makes of his milieu (surroundings), is indifferent to the consequences of his actions, the damage and the pain that he inflicts on others and even the social condemnation and sanctions that he often has to endure. The narcissist does not suffer from a fault sense of causation. He is not oblivious to the likely outcomes of his actions and to the price he may have to pay. **He doesn't care.**

The narcissist lives in a world of all or nothing, of a constant *to be or not to be*. This every minor disagreement with a source of narcissistic supply – another person – is interpreted as a threat to the narcissist's very self-definition.

The narcissist has to condition his human environment to refrain from expressing criticism and disapproval of him or of his actions and decisions.

The narcissist – wittingly or not – utilizes people to buttress his self-image and sense of self-worth. As long and in as much as they are instrumental in achieving these goals – he holds them in high regard, they are valuable to him. He sees them only through his lens.

The narcissist also takes forms hermetic or exclusive, cult-like, social circles, which share his **delusions** (**Pathological Narcissistic Space**).

The function of these social cohorts is to serve as a psychological entourage and to provide **objective** proof of the narcissist's self-**importance** and to **grandeur**. The narcissist convinces himself – by first convincing others – that he is in the process of making significant achievements.

The narcissist represses the knowledge that it all rests on falsities.

The narcissist derives Narcissistic Supply from Primary and Secondary sources. But this supply is used by the narcissistic much the same as one uses perishable goods. He uses the supply to substitute for certain ego functions.

At first, he uses his **False Self** with the aim of obtaining **Primary Narcissistic Supply** source by demonstrating his **superiority** and **uniqueness**. This he does by putting on his intellect and knowledge.

Once this phase is over the narcissist believes that his excellence is established, securing a constant flow of Narcissistic Supply and **narcissistic accumulation**. His False Self is satisfied and exits the scene. **It will not reappear unless the supply is threatened**.

So too serial rapists, child molesters and serial killers.

So let's get this straight and state it plainly: It is my belief, based on several decades of experience, study, and analysis, that the overwhelming majority of repeat sexual predators do what they do because they want to, because it gives them satisfaction they do not achieve in any other aspect of their lives, and because it makes them feel good, regardless of the consequences to others. In that respect, the crime represents the ultimate in selfishness; the perpetrator doesn't care what happens to his victim as long as he gets what he wants. In fact, exercising this manipulation, domination, and control – and the infliction of pain and death are for him their ultimate expression – are the critical factors in making him feel complete and alive.

John Douglas with Mark Olshaker, *Obsession,* pp. 33-34

It was the duty of these teams to segregate the prisoners of war who were candidates for execution… And to report to the office of the Gestapo.

K. Lindeau *Nuremburg Trials*

Mandated Report VA to CDC - Matteoli

Chief Operating Officer, VA Sierra Pacific Network Office (VISN 21)

Director VA Palo Alto

Special Director VA Phoenix Whistleblower Investigation

Leadership Team - VA Palo Alto Health Care System | Page 1 of 2

LOCATOR | CONTACT | SEARCH

(http://www.va.gov)

VA (http://www.va.gov/) » Health Care (http://www.va.gov/health) » VA Palo Alto Health Care System (/index.asp) » About Us (/about/index.asp) » Leadership Team

VA Palo Alto Health Care System

MENU

Leadership Team

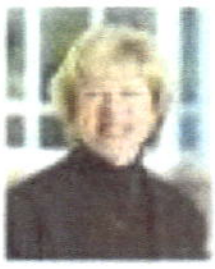

Elizabeth Joyce Freeman, FACHE | 650-858-3939

Director

Elizabeth (Lisa) Joyce Freeman is the Director of the VA Palo Alto Health Care System. She was appointed to the position Feb. 11, 2001.

She began her VA career in 1983 as a Resident Engineer at the VA Medical Center in Oklahoma City, Okla. Later positions held include Senior Resident Engineer, Shreveport, La.; Project Manager, Southern Region, VA Central Office; Health Systems Specialist, Southern Region Field Support Office, VA Central Office; Health System Administrator Trainee, VA Palo Alto Health Care System; Chief Operating Officer, VA Sierra Pacific Network Office, San Francisco, Calif.; Associate Director, VA Palo Alto Health Care System; and Acting Director, VA Palo Alto Health Care System.

She graduated from the University of Notre Dame with a bachelor's degree in Civil Engineering in 1983 and received a master's degree in Business Administration from Louisiana Tech University in 1987. She is a licensed civil engineer in the state of Virginia.

In addition to her VA responsibilities, she is a Fellow in the American College of Health Care Executives and serves as a formal mentor to numerous VA emerging leaders. She is a member of the California Hospital Association's Santa Clara County Section and served on the 2006 Board of Directors for the Hospital Council. In 2005, she received the VA Alumni Association's Honorary Leadership Award. She received a Presidential Rank Award at the meritorious level in 2005 and at the distinguished level in 2009. In 2011, she was named one of the top 100 influential women in Silicon Valley. She completed the Brookings Institution Certificate in Public Leadership Program in 2012.

Thomas J. Fitzgerald III, CHESP | 650-858-3940

Here the State must act as the guardian of a millennial future.
Adolf Hitler

Mandated Report VA to CDC - Matteoli

Freeman Appointed Interim Director re Whistleblower Deaths and Waiting List

Fires Whistleblower NO Others Reprimanded

Punitive Personality Disorder

ABOUT POGO OUR WORK DO SOMETHING BLOG DONATE

Interim Director in Charge of Arizona VA Put Whistleblower on Leave

POGO Letter to Acting VA Secretary Details "Toxic" Culture of Retaliation Across VA

Topics: Government Accountability, Whistleblower Protection

Related Content: Veterans Affairs

July 31, 2014

[illegible]

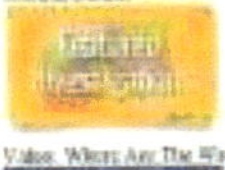

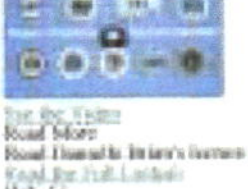

[illegible]

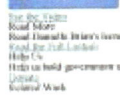

Mandated Report VA to CDC - Matteoli

Western Region

LOCATOR   CONTACT   SEARCH

(http://www.va.gov)

VA (http://www.va.gov/) » Health Care (http://www.va.gov/health/) » VA Sierra Pacific Network (VISN 21) (/index.asp) » About the VA Sierra Pacific Network (VISN 21)

VA Sierra Pacific Network (VISN 21)

MENU

About the VA Sierra Pacific Network (VISN 21)

The VA Sierra Pacific Network is one of 21 integrated health care networks in the Veterans Health Administration (VHA). Also known as Veterans Integrated Service Network 21 (VISN 21), our Network comprises six major health care systems based in Honolulu, HI, Palo Alto, CA, San Francisco, CA, Sacramento, CA, Fresno, CA, and Reno, NV. Together these health care systems include 54 geographic sites of care to Veterans residing in northern Nevada, central and northern California, Hawaii and the vast Pacific Region (including Guam, American Samoa, the Commonwealth of the Northern Mariana Islands, and the Philippines). As Director of this dynamic and unique Network, it is my honor to share with you VISN 21 At a Glance – who we are, where we serve, and how we honor Veterans and their families.

VISN 21 is remarkable in several ways – one of which is its academic affiliations. All six VISN 21 health care systems have highly successful clinical affiliations with prestigious universities in the areas of medicine, nursing and allied health professions. VISN 21 hosts the largest number of Centers of Excellence in VHA, receives the most research funding in VHA, and has expansive and collaborative relationships with its Department of Defense (DoD) partners. VISN 21 is on par nationally with inpatient and outpatient satisfaction measures, and often exceeds the VHA national average. VISN 21 has ranked number 4 among all VISNs for best places to work based on the most recent All Employee Survey.

VISN 21 is committed to ensuring that Veterans have full access to the highest quality of care, and that patients and staff alike have high levels of satisfaction. Currently we face one of the most challenging times in VA and must restore trust and faith in VA health care services. We will focus on providing Veterans timely access to quality care and include virtual modalities, rural health outreach, non-VA care contracts, and collaborations with community and federal partners. Our efforts align with the recently passed Veterans Access, Choice, and Accountability Act (VACAA) of 2014. To guide VA into the future and achieve the desired VACAA outcomes, Secretary Robert McDonald has developed the Blueprint for Excellence which focuses on improving performance, promoting a positive culture of service, advancing health care innovation for Veterans and the Country, and increasing operational effectiveness and accountability. VISN 21 will embrace the Blueprint for Excellence and incorporate its 10 strategies into our daily work. Our workforce is the cornerstone to VISN 21's achievements and success, as well as navigating through these challenging times, and embracing opportunities to meet the needs of our Veterans and their families.

Mandated Report VA to CDC - Matteoli

LOCATOR CONTACT SEARCH

(http://www.va.gov)

VA (http://www.va.gov/) » Health Care (http://www.va.gov/health) » VA Sierra Pacific Network (VISN 21) (/index.asp) » About Us (/about/index.asp) » Leadership Team

VA Sierra Pacific Network (VISN 21)

MENU

Leadership Team

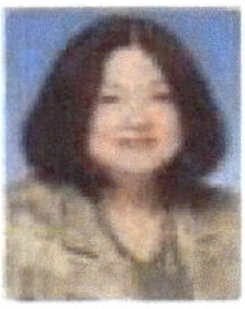

Sheila M. Cullen | 707-562-8350

Network Director

return to top »

CONNECT

Veterans Crisis Line: (http://www.veteranscrisisline.net/)
1-800-273-8255 (tel:+18002738255) (Press 1)

Social Media

Complete Directory (http://www.va.gov/opa/socialmedia.asp)

EMAIL UPDATES

Email Address Signup

VA HOME

Mandated Report VA to CDC - Matteoli

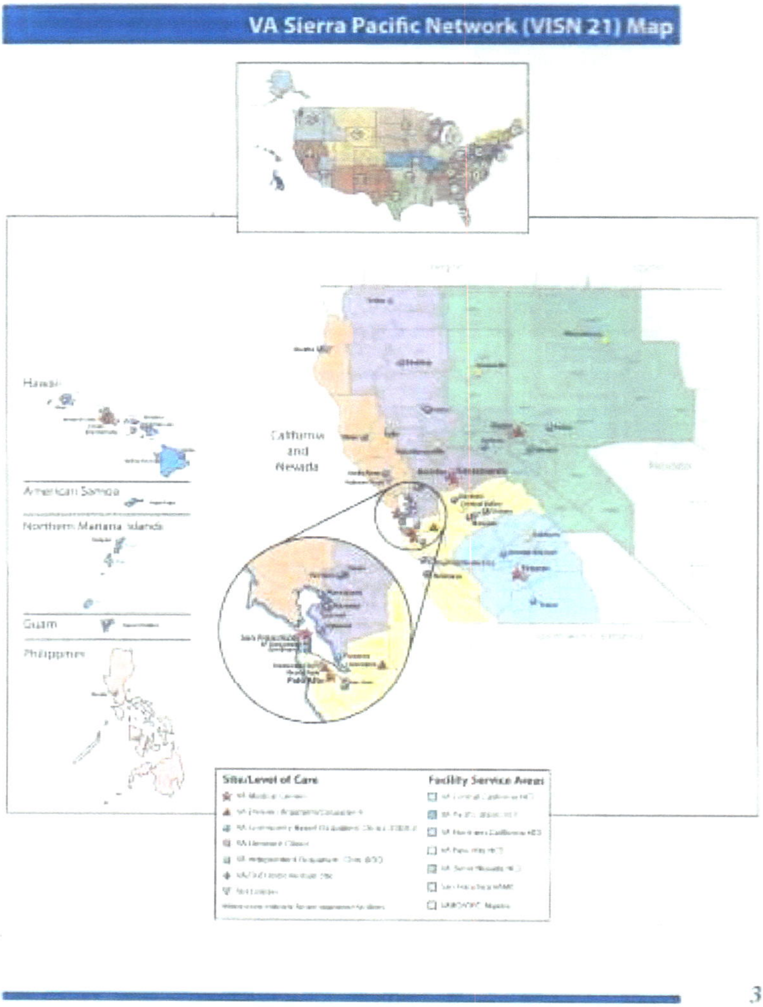

Mandated Report VA to CDC - Matteoli

Meet Our Leadership Team - Oakland Regional Benefit Office

Page 1 of 2

U.S. Department of Veterans Affairs

Oakland Regional Benefit Office

Meet Our Leadership Team

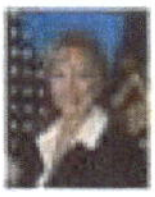

Director: Julianna M. [illegible]

[illegible] was appointed Director of the Oakland Regional Office [illegible]

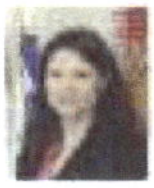

Assistant Director: Michelle M. [illegible]

Michelle [illegible] was appointed to this position in April 2012. Prior to this, Ms. [illegible] served for [illegible] years as Veterans Service Center Manager at the Los Angeles RO

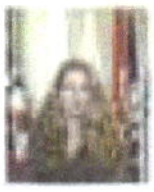

Veterans Service Center Manager: Mary [illegible]

Mary [illegible] was selected for this position in June [illegible]

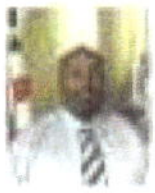

Vocational Rehabilitation and Employment (VR&E) Officer: [illegible]

[illegible] was appointed to this position in November [illegible]. He provides division-level oversight of the VR&E services provided by the Oakland RO.

CONNECT WITH BENEFITS

eBenefits

Access Your VA & DoD Benefits

www.ebenefits.va.gov

http://www.benefits.va.gov/oakland/leadership.asp

8/10/2015

CULTURAL RELATIVITY: Congressional Testimony
It does not matter if the decision was wrong.
She were told to submit it.

Search

ICYMI: Whistleblower Details How Oakland VA Hid and Manipulated 13,184 Claims

Apr 24, 2015 | Press Release

Washington, DC – On Wednesday the House Committee on Veterans' Affairs held a hearing on systemic failures and mismanagement at the Oakland Veterans' Affairs (VA) Regional Office, where investigations determined that at least 13,184 veterans' benefit claims were hidden and that veterans had died without receiving a response. Mrs. Rustyann Brown, a veteran of the U.S. Navy and former employee at the Oakland VA Regional Office that worked on the 13,184 claims, testified during the hearing about VA management's efforts to conceal the claims. Mrs. Brown contacted Rep. Doug LaMalfa in 2013, while she was still employed at the Oakland VA, to blow the whistle on the outrageous cover-up within the Oakland VA.

"We realized that a substantial portion of these veterans were now dead and their claims had never been answered; nothing had been done to help them," Ms. Brown testified. **"If we determined they were dead or had never filed a claim, we were instructed to mark them 'No Action Necessary'."**

In addition, Mrs. Brown added that no efforts were made to contact surviving spouses or families, some of whom may have been entitled to benefits. By simply marking claims "No Action Necessary", they were kept out of the benefits system and set aside.

When Mrs. Brown and other members of the team that was tasked with reviewing these claims spoke out, they were reprimanded by their supervisors and removed from the project. In Mrs. Brown's case, the retaliation for speaking up on behalf of veterans was shockingly cruel.

"I began to see Military Sexual Trauma claims show up in my work assignments. These claims are supposed to be developed by the Special Ops Team because of the sensitive nature of the claim. But, when I would take the claim to my mentor or supervisor and tell them what I had and that it needed to be moved to the Special Ops Team, I was told to just do the next action and move it on. This was a huge problem for me as I am a survivor of military sexual trauma and service-connected

for PTSD due to this. For me, simply reading the statements would bring back all the memories I had tried for years to forget. I would spend time in the restroom crying or hiding in a stairwell so I could be alone and not have anyone see the physical reaction I would have to these claims."

Rep. LaMalfa, who has repeatedly challenged the VA to produce records proving the 13,184 claims were addressed, thanked Mrs. Brown for traveling to the Capitol to testify.

"Rustyann Brown proudly served her country in the U.S. Navy for ten years and decided she wanted to continue to serve by helping her fellow veterans," said Rep. LaMalfa. **"She was a hard-working employee, dedicated public servant, and a tremendous asset to the Oakland VA. The way she was treated by her managers in Oakland is disgraceful and represents a culture of bullying and intimidation that cannot be tolerated. I applaud Rusty's courage in speaking out and thank her for all her efforts to help our nation's veterans."**

Following Mrs. Brown's testimony and Rep. LaMalfa's participation in the hearing, the VA Office of the Inspector General testified that it has reopened an investigation into the Oakland VA Office.

Video of Wednesday's hearing may be viewed in two parts at the following links:

http://www.ustream.tv/recorded/61409440

http://www.ustream.tv/recorded/61414304

Congressman Doug LaMalfa is a lifelong farmer representing California's First Congressional District, including Butte, Glenn, Lassen, Modoc, Nevada, Placer, Plumas, Shasta, Sierra, Siskiyou and Tehama Counties.

###

Search

Oakland VA Director Defends Office Against claims of Mismanagement

Apr 20, 2015 | In The News

To read this article in the San Jose Mercury New, please click here

By Mark Emmons

memmons@mercurynews.com

Posted: 04/20/2015 03:15:43 PM PDT3 Comments | Updated: 7 days ago

Speaking out for the first time, the director of the Oakland VA regional office said Monday that benefit claims found stuffed in a file cabinet were not mishandled and that no vet was forgotten

Director Julianna Boor's staunch defense of her office comes two days before a Congressional hearing that will examine allegations of mismanagement of veterans' compensation at Oakland.

Boor said that the 13,184 claims located in 2012 – some of them dating back to the mid-1990s – were merely duplicates of processed claims. Boor admitted that the office's record-keeping had been a problem but that the process since has been streamlined with a paperless digital system

Boor, however, also said that a complete list of those claims does not exist.

Rep. Doug LaMalfa, R-Oroville, has called for the list to be released to an independent auditor for review to ensure that no veterans or surviving spouses were ignored by the VA -- something that Oakland whistleblowers say occurred.

"I wish we could do that," Boor said. "I wish I could just wave a magic wand and make it appear. We were not keeping an audit when we did the review. We were just so focused on making sure the veterans were taken care of properly and make sure that nobody was left behind."

On Wednesday, the Oakland and Philadelphia offices will be under a microscope on Capitol Hill when the House Committee on Veterans' Affairs looks into scathing VA Office of Inspector General reports that were critical of both sites.

In a statement, Rep. Jeff Miller, the committee chairman, said they will attempt to determine what went wrong at each office, and learn who is responsible and if the VA intends to hold anyone accountable. "Right now VA leaders have a choice," said Miller, a Republican from Florida. "They can either fire those responsible for these failures -- including those who have now moved on to other positions within the agency -- or keep those who caused the problems on the VA payroll, ensuring the substandard service to veterans the IG has documented continues."

Oakland is the conduit for $1.9 billion in benefits that annually go to more than 137,000 Northern California vets. In February, the office was questioned by VA investigators over how a file cabinet came to be filled with "informal" claims from vets seeking to file for benefits and compensation connected to their military service.

The investigation, which was requested by LaMalfa after whistleblowers turned to his office alleging that there was a cover-up, found that Oakland managers conceded that 13,184 claims were improperly stored. But investigators couldn't verify that number due to "poor record keeping practices." Later, Allison Hickey, the VA under secretary for benefits, said the file cabinet contained only duplicates.

Boor said Monday that Oakland staffers told VA investigators the same thing, although that wasn't included in the eight-page report.

In late 2012, when the claims were discovered, the national VA benefits system was in crisis. Oakland, in particular, was overwhelmed. A special team even was sent to help Oakland, which at the time had 35,000 pending formal claims from Northern California vets.

When a review was conducted of those file cabinet informal claims -- ones not filled out on the proper paperwork -- it was determined that they were copies and 97 percent required no further action, Boor said. Corrective action was taken on the rest, which usually boosted the compensation award to the vet.

Rustyann Brown, a whistleblower who will appear at Wednesday's hearing, is adamant that those claims were not duplicates -- recalling how one claim was a handwritten plea on stationary from a World War II widow.

Mandated Report VA to CDC - Matteoli

Boor acknowledged that without a full list, there is no way to verify the VA's numbers independently.

"There's no indication that there was any mishandling," Boor said. "But we can't disapprove any allegations because we don't have every document. But our people care for veterans. Half of our employees are veterans. So I have no reason to believe that anyone did anything improper on purpose. But was this the best record-keeping practice? Probably not."

Boor said the Oakland staff has reduced the size of the backlog to 16,000, cut the time veterans must wait and have improved the accuracy of processing claims.

"A lot of progress has been made," she said. "There was a problem. But we have addressed the problem. I don't mind looking back to make sure that no veterans (have) been left behind. But we are looking forward."

Follow Mark Emmons at Twitter.com/markedwinemmons.

HOUSE COMMITTEE ON Veterans' AFFAIRS HEARING

What: "Philadelphia and Oakland: Systemic Failures and Mismanagement"When: Wednesday, 7:30 a.m. (West Coast time)
Where: Washington, D.C.
Witness list: Veterans Affairs officials and whistleblowers, including Rustyann Brown, a former employee at the Oakland office
Live streaming: http://veterans.house.gov

Mandated Report VA to CDC - Matteoli

LOCATOR CONTACT SEARCH

U.S. Department of Veterans Affairs (http://www.va.gov)

VA (http://www.va.gov/) » Health Care (http://www.va.gov/health/) » San Francisco VA Health Care System (/index.asp) » About Us (/about/index.asp) » Leadership Team

San Francisco VA Health Care System

MENU

Leadership Team

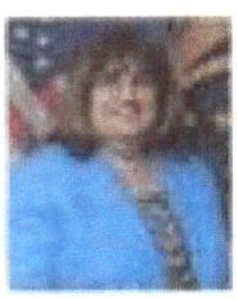

Bonnie S. Graham | 415-750-2047

Medical Center Director

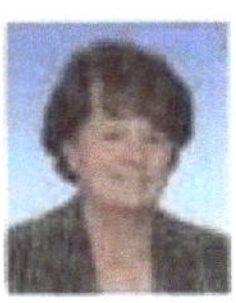

C. Diana Nicoll, M.D., Ph.D., MPA | 415-750-2047

Chief of Staff

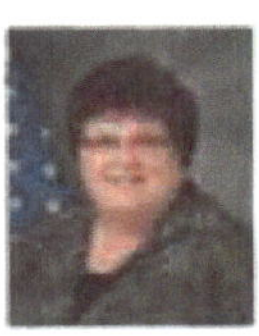

Shirley A. Pikula, RN, MSN, MS-HSA | 415-750-2040

Associate Director for Patient Care/Nursing Service

return to top »

Mandated Report VA to CDC - Matteoli

DISORGANIZED CRIME – WORK COMPUTER

Opportunistic Offender

Hacked Ashley Madison Website Reveals VA Employees Cheat The Most　　Page 1 of 30

Home » Ben's Blog » Hacked Ashley Madison Website Reveals VA Employees Cheat The Most

Disabled Veterans

Redeeming The Promise Of A Square Deal

- Home
- Articles
- About
- Voc Rehab Guide
- Share Your Story
- Contact

Hacked Ashley Madison Website Reveals VA Employees Cheat The Most

August 20, 2015 by Benjamin Krause — 32 Comments

Facebook | Twitter | Google+ | LinkedIn 15 | 19 SHARES

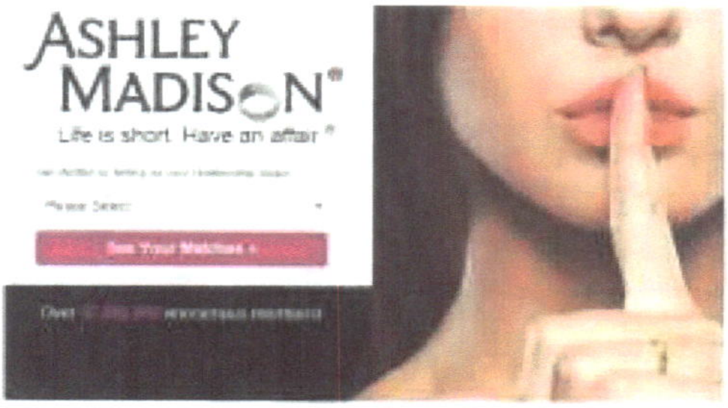

ASHLEY MADISON
Life is short. Have an affair.

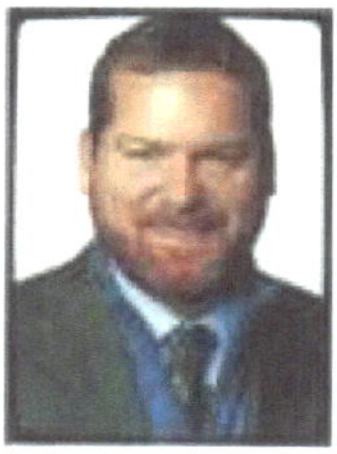

The recent hacking of the cheater website Ashley Madison shows VA employs the most cheaters out of the entire federal government using the va.gov work email to solicit hookups behind the backs of their spouses.

The tagline for Ashley Madison is "Life is short. Have an affair."

https://www.disabledveterans.org/2015/08/20/hacked-ashley-madison-website-reveals-va-...　　8/29/2015

Mandated Report VA to CDC - Matteoli

So while VA is engaging in "delay, deny, hope they die" blocking and tackling, they meanwhile are living up to the Ashley Madison tagline… since life is short.

The backstory is the hacker group, called Impact Team, threatened Ashley Madison. They threatened to reveal customer details if the website did not shut down. The hacker group previously revealed Ashley Madison was not deleting customer data despite claims it would do so. It did not shut down, so Impact Team released the data.

And now we know a lot of VA employees are cheaters who use Ashley Madison. I wonder how many of them used AshleyMadison.com to set up affairs while at work?

The company owning Ashley Madison apparently thought it would all the bluff, which turned out to be no bluff at all. Now America knows its taxpayer dollars are helping VA employees cheat on their spouses using work emails.

If nothing else, this may be a sign that hostile work environments like the Department of Veterans Affairs drives spouses to cheat like no other agency. This article clearly falls in the "useless but amusing" news category.

While I do not endorse unlawful hacking, I find the results, in this instance, to be quite amusing.

Anyone have a similar story to tell?

Source: http://thelibertarianrepublic.com/va-employees-use-ashley-madison-more-than-any-other-non-military-department/

Disabled Veterans

Redeeming The Promise Of A Square Deal

Home

Articles

About

Voc Rehab Guide

Share Your Story

Contact

Mandated Report VA to CDC - Matteoli

ORGANIZED CRIME – HOME COMPUTER

SCAPEGOAT SACRIFICE

COULD NOT RETALIATE AGAINST RETIRED NAVY HEALTH CARE PROFESSIONAL. RETALIATION ATTEMPT AGAINST ONLY VA PHYSICIAN WHO TREATED CORRECTLY

The CON Approach – Service Personality

Dear (REDACTED)

You recently received a survey about your visit to *VA Palo Alto Health Care System* with (REDACTED). If you have already taken the survey, please accept our thanks and disregard this email. Otherwise, please take a few minutes to give your feedback now. By sharing your thoughts and feelings, you can help us improve the care we provide. If you have received this email regarding a family member, please complete the survey on his or her behalf.

To ensure confidentiality, this survey is administered by an independent third-party, Press Ganey Associates, Inc. Your participation will help us to improve the quality of care that we provide to you, your family, friends, and neighbors.

Click here to begin your survey.

Thank you for your feedback.

Sincerely,

Elizabeth Joyce Freeman
Director
If clicking the above link does not take you to the survey or a verification screen, please go to https://esurvey.pressganey.com and enter the following PIN: n2x2v2f3vw5n8c2j

This is an unmonitored email box, please do not reply to this email. If you have specific questions for your healthcare provider, please contact them directly.

To unsubscribe from future Press Ganey online patient satisfaction survey notices, click here.

REDACTED

3 Whitepages profiles found for 'Elizabeth Freeman in San Jose'.

3 exact matches.
Over 300,000,000 profiles searched from the largest and most trusted way to find people online.

1.

2. Elizabeth Freeman
   Age: Unknown
   Current: San Jose, CA
   Prior: No known previous cities

3.

© 2015 Whitepages Inc.

Mandated Report VA to CDC - Matteoli

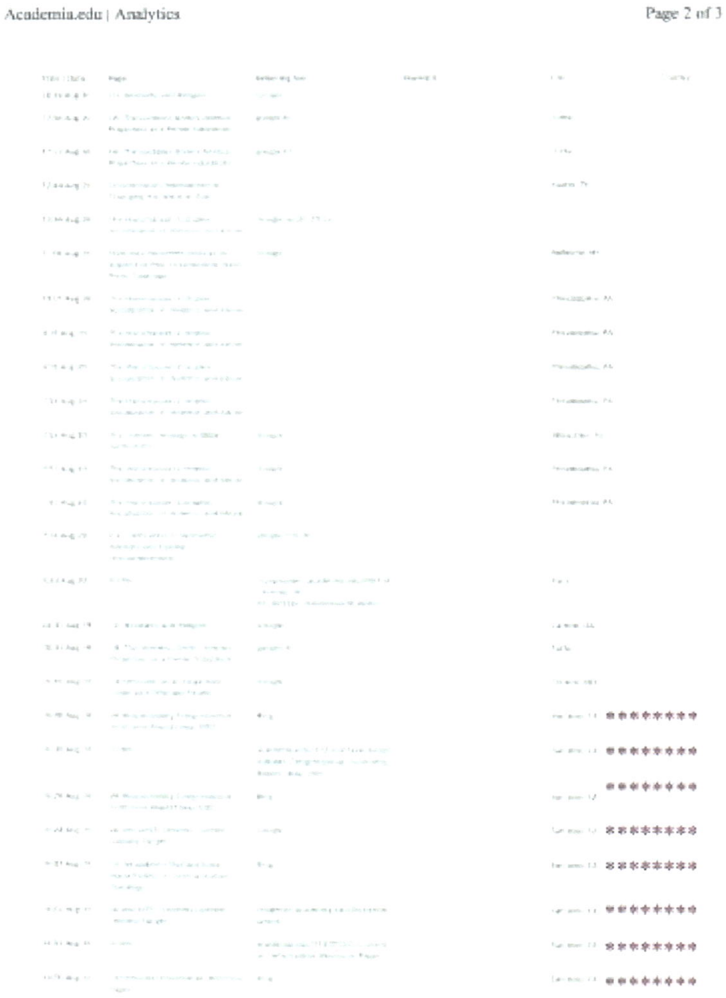
Academia.edu | Analytics Page 2 of 3

SUBJECT WAS COUNSELLED AS BEST POSSIBLE

Subject advised upon numerous requests to speak to wife that wife is a:

Medical Transcriptionist, Verbatim Court Reporter

Worked numerous positions in hospitals,

Worked for a County Sheriff tracing Team Predator child abuse perpetrators

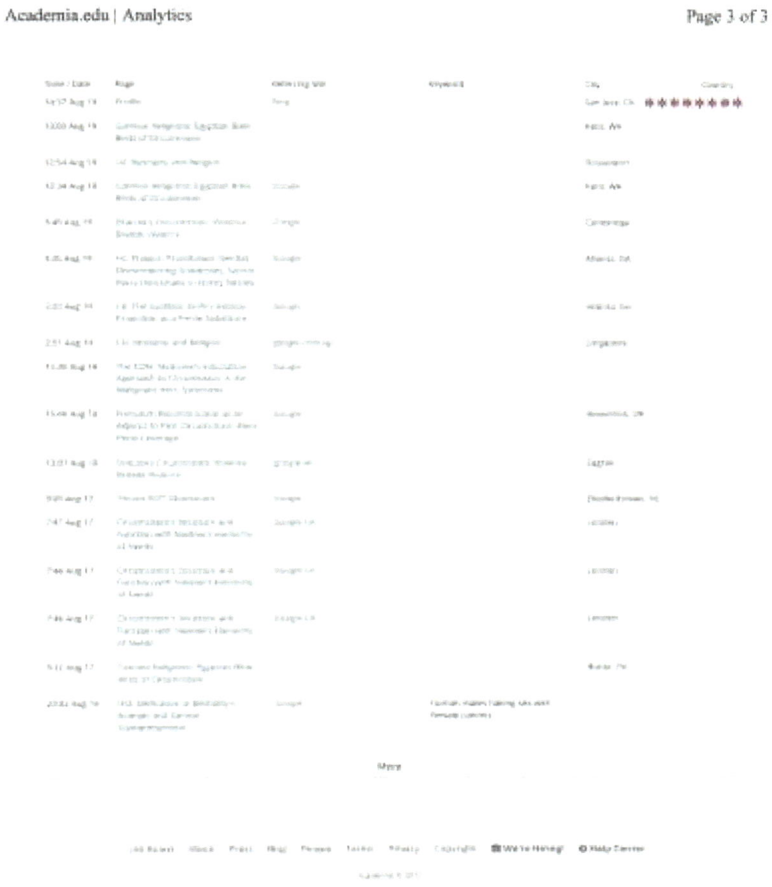
Academia.edu | Analytics Page 3 of 3

THE EPHIALTES MANOUVER

SURPRISE: The victim is chosen and a trap is set. They usually attack from the behind. Threats are made if the victim does not cooperate. This approach is often used by the **Power Reassurance perpetrator**

ALL SERVICEMEMBERS HAVE A CONTINUAL LEGALLY BINDING CONTRACT WITH THE UNITED STATES GOVERNMENT TO BENEFITS BOTH IN WRITING OR BY AND THROUGH IMPLIED INTENT UNDER WHICH THE CONTRACT WAS MADE BY THE GOVERNMENT TO THE CONTRACTOR SERVICEMEMBER, IN PART, UNINCUMBERED INTENTIONAL OR OTHERWISE DELIVERY OF GOODS AND SERVICES WITHIN INTERNATIONAL STANDARDS OF CARE IN PRACTICE AND NOT BELOW SUCH STANDARDS OF CARE AS WELL AS ALL INCLUSIVE PROCEDURAL CONTRACT LAW.

THE VETERAN IS A PAST, AND/OR RETIRED, GOVERNMENT EMPLOYEE WITH CONTRACTOR RIGHTS AS WELL AS HOUSEHOLD MEMBERS IF CONTRACT COVERAGE IS APPLICAPABLE.

THEREFORE, AS A CONTRACTOR, ALL VETERANS MAY REQUEST:

WHISTLEBLOWER PROTECTION.

Mandated Report VA to CDC - Matteoli

MANUFACTURING FALSE EVIDENCE
LIBEL, DEFAMATION OF CHARACTER

OPINION

Medical Records of Whistleblowers Are Being Used Against Them

BY J.D. TUCCILLE [illegible]

If you really need further evidence of why it's dangerous to let government officials demand sensitive information from us, look no further than the ongoing scandal at the U.S. Department of Veterans Affairs.

Once focused on the apparently lethal mistreatment of military veterans by a system created to provide them with (usually crappy) medical care, the story now also encompasses retaliation by officials against VA employees who raise concerns about such mistreatment.

Perhaps most disturbing: "In several cases, the medical records of whistleblowers have been accessed and information in those records has apparently been used to attempt to discredit the whistleblowers," commented Carolyn Lerner from the Office of Special Counsel at a congressional hearing on April 13.

Try Newsweek for only $1.25 per week

The hearing, held by the House Committee on Veterans' Affairs, Subcommittee on Oversight and Investigation, was part of an ongoing saga that includes testimony from multiple participants, though Lerner's presence was an understandable repeat performance, given the Office of Special Counsel's role in protecting whistleblowers. Last September, Lerner told another congressional committee that her office "received over 80 new VA whistleblower retaliation cases related to patient health and safety just since June 1, 2014."

Among the VA cases Lerner's office had addressed at that point, it "for the first time obtained a stay on behalf of an employee who faced retaliation for refusing to obey an order that would have violated the law." That employee had been ordered to enter classified information into an unsecured computer network, which you would think government agencies would be getting just a bit more sensitive about. Well... OK. That's a vain hope.

In fact (the VA is now the biggest source of these complaints and rated over [illegible] OSC attorneys by itself as of last July) of whistleblower retaliation cases from the VA has mostly involved punishments that you would expect from an arrogant, insular government agency against employees who go against the grain. But Lerner told the committee that many VA employees, who are often veterans themselves, find that their health records have been accessed by officials looking for fodder.

According to TheBlaze:

> "One example of a veteran who believes his medical records were inappropriately accessed is Brandon Coleman, a Marine Corps veteran who sustained injuries to his right foot while he served. Coleman works at the VA system in Phoenix, and told TheBlaze he became a whistleblower after it became clear that someone illegally went into his medical records.
>
> He said after he started publicizing the failures of his own office to properly treat veterans with suicidal tendencies, his own mental health was questioned by his superiors. As of this year, the VA has threatened to reduce his disability rating."

More than a few government agencies have access to sensitive information—medical, financial, criminal, sexual... The IRS and Census Bureau compel disclosure, law enforcement agencies gather it through legal filings and court records and intelligence operations just hoover it up. Much of it gets stored away indefinitely for reasons even officials couldn't tell you, except that they have the storage space.

But it makes sense that officials capable of gaming health care waiting lists to the point that people die from delayed treatment are perfectly willing to mine records for weaponizable information for use against dissident employees—or anybody else.

Yeah, the government is inefficient and unreliable with the information it gathers. But those aren't the only concerns. When they accumulate and store all of our sensitive information, officials may also be arming themselves against us.

Just look at the VA.

Mandated Report VA to CDC - Matteoli

FALSE IMPRISONMENT ATTEMPT

Home » Ben's Blog » Unlawful Detention Scheme Revealed At Phoenix VA

Unlawful Detention Scheme Revealed At Phoenix VA

Disabled Veterans

Redeeming The Promise Of A Square Deal

- Home
- Articles
- About
- Voc Rehab Guide
- Share Your Story
- Contact

August 24, 2015 by Benjamin Krause — 26 Comments

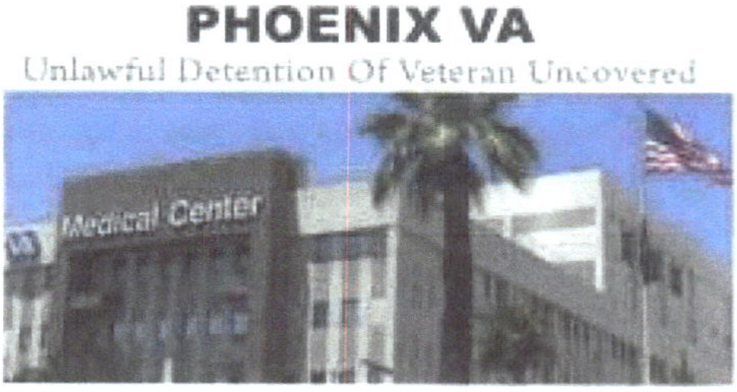

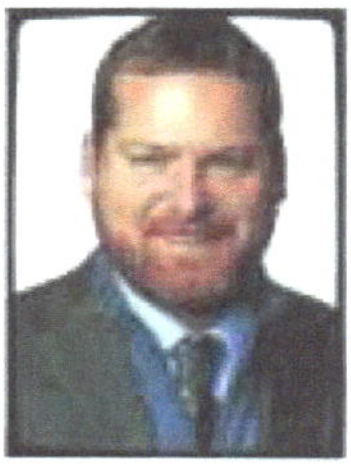

New allegations have surfaced at Phoenix VA of an unlawful detention of a veteran being justified by creating a falsified investigation report and citation.

The allegations concern VA Criminal Investigator Robert Mueller, who was previously linked to harassment and unlawful behavior against a whistleblower, Tonja Laney.

The Daily Caller just unearthed an outrageous violation of the law and VA ethics called out by one VA police officer, Liam

Mandated Report VA to CDC - Matteoli

Disabled Veterans

Redeeming The Promise Of A Square Deal

Home

Articles

About

Voc Rehab Guide

Share Your Story

Contact

Davis. The Caller found a report showing Mueller was linked to the scheme as the Criminal Investigator. The officer claims Mueller pressured him to create a falsified report and issue an unlawful citation for disorderly conduct.

Given the history, how many veterans have been harmed by such a scheme? Isn't the act of falsifying citations and pressuring others to make false claims in itself a crime? Is Mueller still employed by VA?

For some backstory, VA police responded to a call from staff at Phoenix VA concerning a veteran who left the facility while on a medical hold. The police recovered the patient, who had walked across the street, and returned him to the facility. When they returned, the officers were told to arrest the patient. That is when the trouble started.

The citation was used to justify an unlawful detention of a veteran. In an addendum to the report written a few days later, Davis wrote that the citation should be voided "because I was pressured to write this citation by a supervisor in order to justify their prolonged unlawful detention of the named defendant."

DOWNLOAD: Review VA Police Phoenix Investigative Report

In the addendum, Davis went on to explain how Mueller, the Criminal Investigator, bullied him into lying about the veteran in question.

> "I protested this citation and the detention to the supervisor in presence of the physical security specialist. Further, I was told by the criminal

Mandated Report VA to CDC - Matteoli

FALSE IMPRISONMENT ATTEMPT

Department of Veterans Affairs
VA Police
Phoenix
Investigative Report

Investigative Report#: 201311041113-8706

VA Facility: Phoenix

Date/Time Printed: 6/19/2015 13:21

This Document is to be handled in accordance with the Privacy Act
Contents shall not be disclosed, discussed, or shared with individuals unless they have a direct need-to-know in the performance of their official duties. The document(s) are to be handled in accordance with For Official Use Only procedures.

Date/Time Received	11/4/13 11:13 AM
Date/Time of Offense	11/4/13 11:13 AM
Location	Ward 4D
Investigating Officer	LIAM DAVIS
Incident Synopsis:	VA Police responded to a call from 4D staff reference a patient attempting to leave while on an active medical hold. Officers caught up to staff several minutes later outside the Emergency Department. The medical staff advised that the patient [redacted] was across the street. After receiving supervisory approval, an officer left property and with a medical staff member, made voluntary contact with [redacted] VA Police were able to convince [redacted]o return to the hospital to see a doctor before [redacted] leaves [redacted] was given a ride back to the ED entrance. Medical staff were about to escort [redacted] upstairs, when the VA Police Criminal Investigator advised Officers to take [redacted] into custody and place [redacted] in the holding cell for suspicion of possession of drugs and drug paraphernalia. Acting on good faith, Officers placed [redacted] in handcuffs and escorted [redacted] to the VA Police headquarters. Officers then charged [redacted] with 38CFR 1.218 (a) (5) Disorderly Conduct which prevents the normal operation of a service or operation of the facility. The drug paraphernalia was placed in evidence for destruction.
Classification Code:	
Final Disposition:	
Initial Disposition	Closed
Case Status	REOPENED

Use of Force

OC Weapon used:	No
Baton Used:	No
Firearm Drawn:	No
Firearm Used:	No

Complainant

Name:	SUBJECT UNKNOWN
Status:	
Work Address	
Work Phone	
Statement	

Victim

Name:	UNITED STATES GOVERNMENT		
Gender:		Ethnicity:	
Status:			

Page 1

This Document is to be handled in accordance with the Privacy Act
Contents shall not be disclosed, discussed, or shared with individuals unless they have a direct need-to-know in the performance of their official duties. The document(s) are to be handled in accordance with FOUO procedures.

Mandated Report VA to CDC - Matteoli

Facility: Phoenix		ER#:	201311041113-6706
Driver's License:		State:	GENERAL
Work Address:	N/A N/A, US		
Work Phone:			
Treatment:	No		

Suspect

Name: SSN: Gender: Weight: Skin Tone: Status:	[redacted]	DOB: Ethnicity: Hair Color: Mark:	[redacted]	Age: Height: Eye Color:	[redacted]
Driver's License Number:	[redacted]			License State:	[redacted]
Home Address:					
Home Phone:					
Work Address:	[redacted]				
Work Phone:					
Offense(s):	[redacted]				
Violation(s):					

Witness

Name: Work Address:	[redacted]
Work Phone:	
Statement:	See investigation

Notification

Agency:	Phoenix Police Records (P.A.C.E)
Contact:	Dispatcher A3415
Date & Time of Notification:	11/4/13 1148
Instructions Received:	No wants. No warrants.

Narrative

Origin	On Monday, November 4th, 2013 at about 1113hrs, VA Police responded to a phone call from Ward 4D staff, reference a patient attempting to leave while on an active medical hold.
Initial Observation	See investigation
Investigation	Sgt. Placer and Officer Davis conducted a sweep of the last known location of the missing patient. About ten minutes into the search, officers caught up to ward 4D staff outside the Emergency Department (ED) South entrance. The medical staff advised that the patient [redacted] was across the street at CVS. After receiving supervisory approval, I left property and with a medical staff member, made voluntary contact with [redacted] at 998 E Indian School Rd. Staff were able to convince [redacted] to return to the hospital to see a doctor and attempt to conclude [redacted] treatment before leaving.

Page 7

This document is to be handled in accordance with the Privacy Act.
Contents shall not be disclosed, discussed, or shared with individuals unless they have a direct need-to-know in the performance of their official duties. The document must be handled in accordance with FOUO procedures. 000002

Mandated Report VA to CDC - Matteoli

Facility: Phoenix — UPR: 20131104111[illegible]

[redacted] was given a ride back to the ED entrance. Upon arrival [redacted] exited the vehicle on [redacted] own accord and proceeded to the smoking shelter to smoke before heading back the medical ward.

Medical staff were about to escort [redacted] upstairs, when the VA Police Criminal Investigator advised Sgt. Placer and I to take [redacted] into custody and place [redacted] in the holding cell for drug paraphernalia. Acting on good faith, I placed [redacted] in handcuffs, double locked them. I then escorted [redacted] to the VA Police headquarters (HQ) room D106.

I arrived at the VA Police HQ and placed [redacted] in the temporary holding cell (D106C) at about 1143 hrs. I searched [redacted] and secured [redacted] to the holding cell bench. The VA Police Criminal Investigator then entered the holding cell and read [redacted] the VA Police Pre Questioning Advice of Constitutional Rights (VA Form 1430). After [redacted] verbalized consent, VA Criminal Investigator Lt Mueller questioned [redacted] about drug paraphernalia found in [redacted] patient room on Ward 4D.

While the interview was being conducted, VA Police dispatch conducted a Motor Vehicles Division (MVD) check was conducted and cross referenced with the information provided to confirm [redacted] identity. The check revealed that [redacted] had a suspended [redacted] Driver License [redacted]

I requested dispatch to conduct an (ACJIS) Arizona Criminal Justice Information System inquiry on [redacted]. The inquiry had negative results for wants and warrants.

Sgt. Placer also conducted a check on the Decentralized Hospital Computer Programs (DHCP) and (VAPS) Veterans Affairs Police System, for prior contact with VA Police. VAPS revealed the following:

VA Police contacted [redacted] on 10/13/2013 Theft of Services. No Charges were filed.

VA Police contacted [redacted] on 11/03/2013 for Disorderly Conduct. No Charges were filed.

Further, VA Police Dispatch then conducted a Police Automated Computer Entry (PACE) System inquiry on [redacted]. Dispatcher [illegible] 3415 of the City of Phoenix Records and Identification Bureau was contacted at about 1148 hrs. This inquiry revealed that [redacted] had no active warrants with the City of Phoenix.

After the interview was completed, [redacted] investigation was continued with Ward 4D staff [redacted]. After Lt Mueller conducted the interview with [redacted] it was determined that the suspected drug paraphernalia was dropped off to medical staff by [redacted] mother [redacted] claimed to have dropped off the item to VA medical staff be[redacted]cause it [redacted] residence and did not know what to do with it. Sgt. Placer secured the evidence which was a clear glass pipe resembling a classic "crack pipe" containing the burnt residue of an unknown substance. Sgt. Placer obtained the evidence from Head Nurse [redacted] in room D406 and secured the evidence in temporary Evidence Locker # 7 located in the VA Police HQ room D103. The evidence was marked for destruction.

Investigating Officer: LIAM DAVIS — Signature: ____________
Badge: 3226-ON — Date: ___/___/_____
Printed by: ROBERT MUELLER

< < < End of Report > > >

Released LTR Mueller #4
19 Jun 2015

Page 3

This Document is to be handled in accordance with the Privacy Act.
Contents shall not be disclosed, discussed, or shared with individuals unless they have a direct need to know in the performance of their official duties. The document [redacted] be handled in accordance with FOUO procedures. 000000

Mandated Report VA to CDC - Matteoli

Facility: Phoenix | IR#: 20131104111[illegible]-8705

Follow Up

Investigator: LIAM DAVIS **Date/Time:** 11/6/2013 9:07:42PM

I requested CVB violation # 3138479 be voided. I am requesting a void on this citation because I was pressured to write the citation by a supervisor in order to justify the prolonged unlawful detention of the named defendant. I protested the citation and the detention to the supervisor in the presence of the physical security specialist. Further, I was told by the criminal investigator to lie and include false statements in the PC statement. The criminal investigator told me to include statements that were false three times in the presence of my supervisor and the department's secretary. Further, the medical hold decision was affected by the VA Police under VA Policy Memorandum No. MH&SSS/115A-07 which states on page 1, 2. POLICY: "In accordance with Arizona Revised Statutes Title 36, subsection 520, 531 and 540. As VA Police under proprietary jurisdiction, we can not enforce state codes. Also, the subject in this case never made any threats, threating movements or made any statements referencing harming [redacted] or others. The subject never became loud or argumentative. The subject never cursed or failed to follow the instruction of Officers.

Investigator: ROBERT MUELLER **Date/Time:** 12/7/2014 3:21:32PM

About 6 Dec 2014 item of evidence associated with this case was destroyed in my presence by [redacted] Inventory Management. VA FM 3524 and Evidence ledger Updated.

Page 4

This Document is to be handled in accordance with the Privacy Act
Contents shall not be disclosed, discussed, or shared with individuals unless they have a direct need-to-know in the performance of their official duties. The document should be handled in accordance with FOUO procedures. 000004

Mandated Report VA to CDC - Matteoli

CENSORSHIP

Palo Alto Online

Palo Alto VA employee alleges retaliation, gag order for flagging errors

Veterans agency says it cannot comment on case pending investigation

TOP BLOGS

Standardized testing may become a thing of the past

Getting yanked out of a rut by my preschooler

Marriage Interview 10: A Cross-Cultural Love Story

143 important decisions in 150 minutes by a 20-member committee

Fruit and flowers

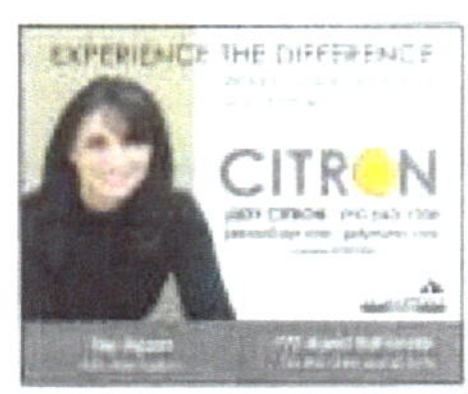

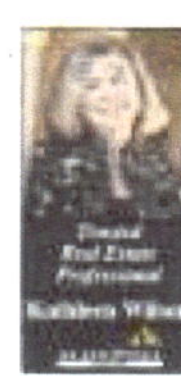

Mandated Report VA to CDC - Matteoli

[illegible]

Comments

[illegible]

Home » Ben's Blog » Illegal VA Complaints Strategy Against Veterans Exposed

Illegal VA Complaints Strategy Against Veterans Exposed

Disabled Veterans

Redeeming The Promise Of A Square Deal

Home

Articles

About

Voc Rehab Guide

Share Your Story

Contact

August 6, 2014 by Benjamin Krause — 28 Comments

Facebook Twitter Google+ LinkedIn 36 SHARES

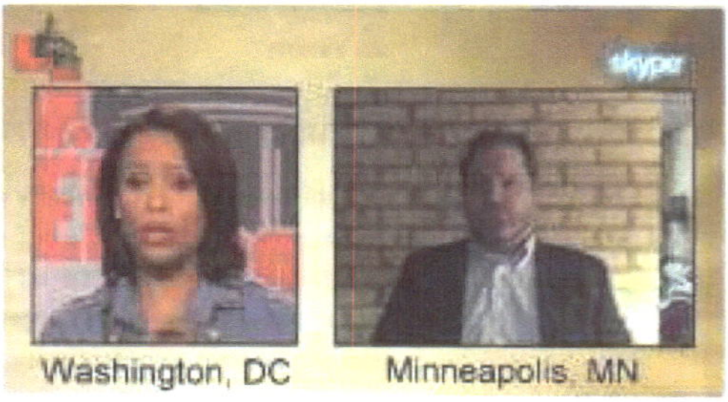
Washington, DC
Minneapolis, MN

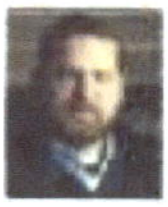

Last week, journalist Angela Rae exposed despicable treatment of veterans through a little known process VA employees use against veterans. Some VA employees illegally lodge VA complaints against veterans to manipulate the purpose of disruptive behavior committees.

Angela Rae interviewed me about how veterans are impacted by this illegal retaliation at the receiving end of VA's disruptive behavior committees.

Here is the interview

Mandated Report VA to CDC - Matteoli

f 𝕏 g+ in ✉

Disabled Veterans

Redeeming The Promise Of A Square Deal

44:17

HD

- Home
- Articles
- About
- Voc Rehab Guide
- Share Your Story
- Contact

Benjamin Krause – Veteran Challenges from DC Breakdown on Vimeo

Disruptive Behavior Committees

Disruptive behavior committees are intended as a catch all to manage hostile and threatening veterans while they seek health care from VA. On the surface, this sounds reasonable. Some veterans are in fact dangerous. However, many nonveterans are also dangerous, and I have yet to see a secret committee like these in civilian hospitals.

My problem with the process is that it is secret. The review process is done in secret and the veteran will not know who sat on the committee or what the evidence presented was prior to the decision. Only after the decision is made are veterans informed of the outcome and given a chance to appeal the vague allegations. That seems like a due process violation if I have ever seen one.

Further, the process of filing complaints against veterans has been used in many instances where the veteran initially files a complaint against a VA doctor or staff member. In some f 🐦 8+ in ✉

Disabled Veterans

Redeeming The Promise Of A Square Deal

- Home
- Articles
- About
- Voc Rehab Guide
- Share Your Story
- Contact

instances, when a complaint is lodged, VA personnel escalate the intensity of the conversation and even threatening the veteran.

In those instances, VA employees are guilty of illegally filing counter complaints against veterans since the totality of the circumstances would not match the allegations. Unfortunately, VA has a tendency of never believing the veterans, and veteran complaints against VA personnel are almost never received well. As is the case here, in many instances those complaining veterans are instead retaliated against.

I believe this tactic is used to disparage and discredit the veteran when VA reviews the matter.

Background on DC Breakdown Interview

Initially, Angela Rae was outraged when she heard about what VA is doing behind the scenes to retaliate against honest veterans seeking care, so much so that she decided to interview me to learn more about the illegal practice.

It was done via Skype while I was on vacation with family, so the sound has a slight delay. But, you will get a good idea about what is going on and how certain VA doctors and administrators are harming veterans by misusing the process of disruptive behavior committee reviews.

This form of retaliation is, in my opinion, one of the biggest crimes VA is committing across the country because it chills the speech of veterans who respectfully file complaints that have merit. In response to many of these valid complaints, VA employees have been known to file counter complaints that defame the veteran and diminish their credibility. The

Mandated Report VA to CDC - Matteoli

f 🐦 8+ in ✉

end result is a veteran having an improper flag on their file, harassment from VA police, and/or restrictions in access to timely health care.

If you have been harmed by an illegal use of disruptive behavior committee policies, please comment below or send me a private email.

Disabled Veterans

Redeeming The Promise Of A Square Deal

- Home
- Articles
- About
- Voc Rehab Guide
- Share Your Story
- Contact

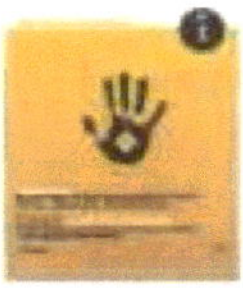

Benjamin Krause is the creator of the DisabledVeterans.org community, author of the Voc Rehab Survival Guide for Veterans, and numerous other guides.

Benjamin is an award winning investigative reporter, Veterans Law attorney, and a disabled veteran of the US Air Force, where he served in its Special Operations Command. After receiving an Honorable Discharge, Benjamin began his decade long fight for benefits after being lowballed with a 10% rating in 2002. During that fight, he received degrees from Northwestern University and the University of Minnesota Law School while using VA Vocational Rehabilitation.

You can connect with Benjamin on Google+, Twitter, Facebook and LinkedIn.

Share this:

Print Share 0 Share 38 Tweet 6

8+ Share 0

Related

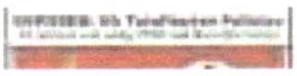  

Mandated Report VA to CDC - Matteoli

78033

Rules and Regulations

Federal Register

Vol. 71, No. 249

Thursday, December 28, 2006

This section of the FEDERAL REGISTER contains regulatory documents having general applicability and legal effect, most of which are keyed to and codified in the Code of Federal Regulations, which is published under 50 titles pursuant to 44 U.S.C. 1510.

The Code of Federal Regulations is sold by the Superintendent of Documents. Prices of new books are listed in the first FEDERAL REGISTER issue of each week.

OFFICE OF PERSONNEL MANAGEMENT

5 CFR Part 724

RIN 3206–AK55

Implementation of Title II of the Notification and Federal Employee Antidiscrimination and Retaliation Act of 2002—Reporting & Best Practices

AGENCY: Office of Personnel Management.

ACTION: Final rule.

SUMMARY: The Office of Personnel Management (OPM) is issuing final regulations to carry out the reporting and best practices requirements of Title II of the Notification and Federal Employee Antidiscrimination and Retaliation Act of 2002 (No FEAR Act). The No FEAR Act requires Federal agencies to report annually on certain topics related to Federal antidiscrimination and whistleblower protection laws. The No FEAR Act also requires a comprehensive study to determine the executive branch's best practices concerning disciplinary actions against employees for conduct that is inconsistent with those laws. This rule will implement the reporting and best practices provisions of the No FEAR Act.

DATES: *Effective Date:* The rule is effective February 26, 2007.

FOR FURTHER INFORMATION CONTACT: Gary D. Wahlert by telephone at (202) 606–2930; by FAX at (202) 606–2613; or by e-mail at *NoFEAR@opm.gov*.

SUPPLEMENTARY INFORMATION:

Background

The United States and its citizens are best served when the Federal workplace is free of discrimination and retaliation. In order to maintain a productive workplace that is fully engaged with the many important missions before the Government, it is essential that the rights of employees, former employees and applicants for Federal employment under antidiscrimination and whistleblower protection laws be protected and that agencies that violate these rights be held accountable. Congress has found that agencies cannot be run effectively if those agencies practice or tolerate discrimination. Furthermore, Congress has found that requiring Federal agencies to provide annual reports on discrimination, whistleblower, and retaliation cases should enable Congress to improve its oversight of compliance by agencies with laws covering those types of cases. Finally, Congress has required that the President or his designee conduct a study of discipline taken against Federal employees for conduct that is inconsistent with Federal antidiscrimination and whistleblower protection laws. The results of this study are then to be used to develop advisory guidelines that Federal agencies may follow to take such disciplinary actions. Therefore, under authority delegated by the President, OPM is issuing final regulations to implement the annual reporting and best practices provisions of Title II of the Federal Employee Antidiscrimination and Retaliation Act of 2002 (No FEAR Act), Pub. L. 107–174.

Introduction

On January 25, 2006, OPM published at 71 FR 4053 (2006) a proposed rule implementing the reporting and best practices provisions of the No FEAR Act and providing a 60-day comment period. On March 31, 2006, in response to requests by the No FEAR Coalition and Members of Congress, OPM at 71 FR 16246 (2006) reopened the initial comment period until May 1, 2006. OPM received 13 comments from Federal agencies or departments, 3 comments from associations/organizations/coalitions (including the No FEAR Coalition), 4 comments from unions, 92 comments from individuals and 2 comments from Members of Congress. OPM thanks all who provided comments—each comment has been carefully considered.

Reporting Obligations

Definition of Discipline

The No Fear Act requires agencies to create annual reports on a number of items, including disciplinary actions taken for conduct that is inconsistent with Federal antidiscrimination and whistleblower protections. These reports are to be submitted to Congress, the Equal Employment Opportunity Commission (EEOC), the Attorney General, and OPM. OPM proposed in § 724.102 to define discipline for reporting purposes to include a range of actions from reprimands through adverse actions such as removals and reductions in grade. OPM also stated that it was considering expanding the range of disciplinary actions reported to include unwritten actions such as oral admonishments. OPM asked for comments on whether such additional actions should be reported.

Most commenters raised no objection to the definition of disciplinary actions as proposed, i.e., reprimands through adverse actions, but many expressed strong disagreement with the notion of expanding that definition to include unwritten actions such as oral admonishments. Many of those, including the No FEAR Coalition, were concerned that an expanded definition would undermine what they assert was the intent of Congress that stiff penalties be imposed on those who violate Federal antidiscrimination and whistleblower protection laws. Many believed that reporting such additional actions would improperly inflate the numbers of actions taken to discourage improper activities. Others felt that the reporting of non-written actions would be inconsistent with the concept of progressive discipline or would encourage agencies to take types of actions that might impinge upon the recipients' procedural rights. Federal agencies were opposed to reporting unwritten actions for primarily two reasons: (1) Oral admonishments, unwritten warnings, and similar actions are not true disciplinary actions and (2) it would be an administrative burden to report such actions because of their undocumented nature. Some thought that documentation of unwritten actions by agencies would negatively impact their ability to attempt to resolve workplace issues informally.

Mandated Report VA to CDC - Matteoli

Commenters in favor of reporting unwritten actions such as oral admonishments generally felt that it is important for there to be a complete record of what agencies have done when they discover conduct inconsistent with Federal antidiscrimination and whistleblower protection laws. For example, one organization stated that such reporting would "give some indication of how serious the agencies are when it comes to combating discrimination." One union stated that "[t]his information is necessary to fully understand the scope of agencies' practices in this area and, particularly, whether agencies have failed to adequately discipline employees who may have committed serious breaches of the discrimination and whistleblower protection laws by imposing only minor, unwritten discipline." Another union in favor of reporting unwritten actions stated that extensive reporting helps ensure that there is "an accurate and detailed portrait of any given agency's compliance with the letter and spirit of the No FEAR Act." One commenter recommended that the definition of discipline be further expanded to include "reassignment from a supervisory to a non-supervisory position" because such actions occur "frequently" for disciplinary reasons.

OPM received numerous comments suggesting that an expanded definition of discipline would be seen by many as an impediment to, rather than in support of, an effective Federal workforce. Moreover, expanding the definition could incorrectly suggest that OPM, through the No FEAR Act, is authorized to establish disciplinary penalties beyond the normal definition of discipline. Therefore, OPM has decided not to expand the definition of discipline to include unwritten actions such as oral admonishments or any other actions suggested by commenters. The role of OPM under the No FEAR Act is not to dictate what disciplinary actions are appropriate to be taken by agencies but rather OPM's role is to address what is to be reported under the Act.

Agency Training Plans

Section 724.302(a)(9) proposed a new reporting element that required agencies to provide copies of their written training plans developed under the earlier (February 28, 2005) proposed rule at § 724.203(a). Several commenters suggested that this element be dropped since it is not required by the No FEAR Act or suggested that the requirement be held up since § 724.203(a) was only in proposed form at the time the current regulations were proposed. Training is a critical component of obligations imposed under the No FEAR Act to ensure that the workplace is free of discrimination and reprisal. Because it is critical, OPM has decided to retain the proposed reporting element on training plans. OPM also declines to drop the proposal as premature since Subpart B (Notification and Training) along with § 724.203(a) was published as a final regulation on July 20, 2006.

One agency noted that proposed § 724.203(a) requires agencies to write training plans. Since these plans, in turn, are to be reported annually under § 724.302(a)(9), the agency asked whether it is required to resubmit the agency's written plan in each annual report even when there are no amendments to a previously reported plan. Each report should be complete and able to stand on its own independent of other reports that might have been filed by an agency. Thus, a written training plan should be submitted with each annual report by an agency.

Agency Disciplinary Policies

One commenter asked whether OPM's "review of agencies' discussions" under § 724.402(b) refers to future discussions that OPM will have with an agency or refers to discussions that an agency may have had internally about their disciplinary policies. OPM notes that the discussions referenced are synonymous with the "detailed description" of an agency's policy for taking disciplinary action under § 724.302(a)(6). Another commenter wondered whether this "detailed description" means that agencies would be required to develop new disciplinary policies under the regulations. While agencies may decide to develop new disciplinary policies, the regulations do not require such action. One agency stated that, with regard to the obligation to provide a detailed discussion of agency policies in § 724.302(a)(6), significant changes in agencies' reports from year to year should not be expected since agency disciplinary policies aren't often changed. OPM takes no position on this observation.

One commenter noted that the regulations refer to disciplinary actions taken for "conduct that is inconsistent with" Federal antidiscrimination and whistleblower protection laws. The commenter asked that OPM clarify the phrase "conduct that is inconsistent with." In this regard, while agencies have the authority to take disciplinary actions against employees for misconduct, this misconduct may or may not be associated with a formal finding of a violation of Federal antidiscrimination and whistleblower protection laws. For example, a case may be settled with no admission of liability but is clearly a case where the law would be found to have been violated if there were a formal finding. Discipline taken in such a case should not go unreported under the No Fear Act. It should be noted, however, that entering into a settlement agreement should never be construed as proof of wrongdoing by either party because settlements may be reached for a variety of reasons. In sum, it is the conduct of the employee that dictates whether a disciplinary action is to be reported under the regulations, not whether there is a formal finding of a violation.

Case Reporting

As proposed, § 724.302(a)(1) would require agencies to report on cases involving Federal antidiscrimination and whistleblower protection laws that are pending or resolved in Federal courts in each fiscal year. One commenter asked whether this applies to cases in both U.S. District Court and Courts of Appeals. OPM states that it does.

One agency commented that reporting on pending cases "does not further the purpose of the No FEAR Act" because the number of pending cases is "not an accurate reflection of violations" since complaints are often filed pro se and plaintiffs often fail to accurately identify their cause of actions. The agency noted that many cases are filed under multiple statutes and causes of actions and it's difficult to understand what cases are about. As a result, the agency recommended that agencies only report an aggregate number of cases resolved in Federal court and without relating each case to provision(s) of law involved as required by the proposed rule. Another commenter suggested that the Department of Justice be tasked with obtaining the status and coverage of cases. As discussed elsewhere in the Supplementary Information, the No FEAR Act calls on agencies to discuss the status or disposition of cases in the Federal courts. The provision would be meaningless if the status of all cases reported is "resolved." Therefore, OPM declines to limit agencies' reporting obligation only to cases in Federal court that have been resolved. OPM also declines to modify the reporting requirement to just reporting the aggregate number of cases in Federal court. The Act requires that each case be related to a provision(s) of law involved. OPM has no authority under the Act to task the Department of Justice as suggested by one commenter.

One agency asked that OPM define what is considered to be a "pending case" in Federal court. The regulations call for reporting about cases in Federal court that are pending or resolved in each fiscal year. That is, if a case is filed in court during a current reporting cycle's fiscal year or resolved during that fiscal year or filed and resolved in that fiscal year, it is to be reported. Cases filed in previous years but not resolved would be counted as (pending) cases in the current reporting year. Cases filed in previous years and resolved in the current year would be counted as (resolved) cases. Some cases may be pending for a number of years in Federal court.

Section 724.302(a)(6) requires that agencies report the number of employees disciplined in accordance with any agency policy described in § 724.302(a)(3) regardless of whether it was in connection with a case in the Federal courts. One commentor wondered why administrative cases are covered in this reporting element when other reporting elements only apply to cases in the Federal courts. OPM believes that the No FEAR Act at section 203(a)(6)(B) asks, without restriction, for reports on all discipline in connection with Federal antidiscrimination and whistleblower protections laws. Another commenter suggested that the phrase "whether or not" in § 724.302(a)(6) be deleted. OPM declines to adopt the suggestion.

Section 724.302(a)(5) also requires agencies to report on the number of employees disciplined for conduct inconsistent with Federal antidiscrimination and whistleblower protection laws, whether or not in connection with cases in Federal court, and to identify the specific nature of the disciplinary actions (e.g., reprimand, etc.). One agency asked whether former employees should be included in this reporting requirement. OPM states that any discipline taken during the reporting period for conduct inconsistent with the laws noted previously is to be reported even if the individual is no longer employed when the report is prepared.

Based on its analyses of the relationship between section 203(a)(1) and section 201(a) of Title II of the No FEAR Act, one agency concluded that the "plain meaning" of the Act is that agencies, under § 724.302(a)(1) of the proposed rule, are only required to report on cases in Federal court in which Judgment Fund payments have been made. OPM notes that section 203(a)(2) of the Act requires reporting on the "status or disposition" of cases described in section 203(a)(1) of the Act. If the only cases reported are those in which Judgment Fund payments have been made, section 203(a)(2) would be meaningless since the status or disposition of all cases would be similar. Accordingly, OPM declines to modify § 724.302(a)(1) and agencies must report on all cases in Federal court whether or not there has been Judgment Fund payment.

The same agency also suggested that the proposed rule § 724.302(a)(3) be modified so that agencies are not obligated to report on the nature of each disciplinary action and the provision of law concerned in each case, but rather report solely on the numbers of disciplinary actions taken. Here the agency cites to section 203(a)(4) of Title II of the No FEAR Act which calls for reporting disciplinary actions but does not speak to the nature of the action or the provision of law concerned. The agency also comments that the phrase "provision of law" is unclear and asks whether the phrase applies to the Federal antidiscrimination and whistleblower protection laws concerned or whether it refers to laws authorizing disciplinary actions (such as the law codified at 5 CFR 752 concerning adverse actions).

In response to the comment on the issue of whether the Act requires agencies to identify the nature of an action and the provision of law concerned in each case, section 203(a)(6)(B) of Title II calls for identification of the nature of the disciplinary actions reported. This reporting requirement is codified at § 724.302(a)(5). In addition, section 203(a)(1) of Title II calls for reporting on the cases arising under "the respective provisions of law" and that requirement is reflected in § 724.302(a)(3). The reporting requirements under both § 724.302(a)(3) and § 724.302(a)(5) should be consistent with regard to labeling discipline in order to provide the most meaningful and useful data to Congress and others. Thus, OPM declines to modify § 724.302(a)(3).

In response to another agency's question about reporting disciplinary actions, agencies are required to associate the nature of a disciplinary action with each case in such a manner that the report will list the types of disciplinary actions taken and then state the numbers of employees affected by each particular type of action.

With regard to the issue of what the phrase "provision of law" means, it means the Federal antidiscrimination or whistleblower protection laws involved in a particular case whenever that phrase is used in § 724.302. Another agency asked how specific an agency must be when it relates individual cases to these laws, e.g., whether the agency needs to cite laws such as the Civil Rights Act, Age Discrimination in Employment Act, etc. or whether it can just broadly refer to antidiscrimination laws or whistleblower protection laws. The No FEAR Act requires specificity and thus agencies need to identify the specific laws involved such as those cited in the commenter's question.

One agency commented on OPM's proposed §§ 724.301 and 724.302(a)(1) stating that they should contain the same language as that proposed in § 724.202(a) on February 28, 2005. That section calls on agencies to give notice to employees about Antidiscrimination Laws and Whistleblower Protection Laws applicable to them. OPM agrees the regulation should be consistent and has modified §§ 724.301 and 724.302(a)(1) to include the phrase "applicable to them" to modify Antidiscrimination Laws and Whistleblower Protection Laws.

One organization suggested that administrative cases also should be reported by agencies under the regulations. In this regard, the commenter noted that the regulations ignore the "thousands of cases which are processed administratively through the MSPB (Merit Systems Protection Board) and the EEOC." The commenter stated that, to be truly reflective of both the magnitude of these cases and whether an agency is disciplining employees who are found liable in forums other than courts, those cases must be reported. The commenter also recommends that all settlement agreements be reported regardless of any no fault clauses. With regard to reporting administrative cases, OPM notes that, apart from the data required pursuant to section 203(a)(6), Title II of the No FEAR Act is very clear that the cases to be reported are those that have gone to Federal courts. Under Title III of the Act, the EEOC already collects information regarding administrative cases within its jurisdiction. These regulations are consistent with the requirements of the Act and the suggestion is not adopted.

With regard to settlements, OPM notes that agencies are required to report on all cases that have gone to Federal court. Some of these cases may result in settlement agreements and they must be reported. OPM takes no position on the same commenter's proposal regarding EEOC's administrative judges' salaries because the comment is beyond the scope of these regulations and that issue is not a part of the No FEAR Act.

One agency commented that employees in Federal courts often receive lump sum payments from the Judgment Fund that provide no information about how the payment is to be divided among the employee, attorney(s), and other recipients. As a result, it is difficult for an agency to report what attorney's fees were paid in connection with cases in court. Since agencies are required to report under the regulations on attorney's fees, the commenting agency suggested that the Department of Justice advise agencies of the payment breakdown since the Department is involved in most cases in Federal court. OPM notes that the regulation at § 724.302(a)(2)(iii) only requires the reporting of attorney's fees where they have been "separately designated." If they have not been separated out in any part of the proceeding, agencies are not required to report on them.

A commenter suggested inserting for clarity the word "calendar" into the phrase "each agency must report no later than 180 days" in § 724.302(a). OPM adopts this suggestion.

Section 724.302(a)(9)(b)(5) provides that agencies are to submit their annual reports to "Each Committee of Congress with jurisdiction relating to the agency." One agency commented that this provision is unclear and asked whether it is within each agency's discretion to determine which Committees have jurisdiction relating to that agency. OPM notes that, while the No FEAR Act does not elaborate on this requirement, OPM has concluded the provision covers committees with subject-matter jurisdiction over a particular agency's mission as well as other committees with oversight responsibility for a particular agency such as appropriations committees. Beyond these committees, it is left with agencies to determine what other committees, if any, have jurisdiction relating to their agencies.

Supplemental Reports

Section 724.302(b) requires agencies that submitted their annual reports before these regulations become final to ensure that their reports contain data elements 1 through 8 of paragraph (a) of that section. If the earlier reports do not cover all of these data elements as written, agencies would be obligated to submit supplemental reports. Data element 9 concerns agency training plans and agencies are only required to include it in their future reports. One agency commented that comparing earlier reports to the final rules and providing supplemental reports would be an "unnecessary administrative burden" on agencies. Another agency said that it would be "overly burdensome" for those that complied with the Act earlier in "good faith." That agency strongly recommended that the final rule apply only to future reports. Because the proposed regulations on reporting closely track the provisions of the No FEAR Act itself, OPM believes that the differences between what was submitted earlier and the requirements of the regulations will be minimal. OPM commends those agencies that have taken the initiative and submitted reports based on the Act even though OPM's regulations had not been finalized. However, because differences are likely to be minimal and because OPM believes that Congress needs consistent reports from all agencies in order to see how well the Federal Government is working toward a discrimination and reprisal-free workplace, OPM declines to eliminate the supplemental reporting requirement of § 724.302(b).

Best Practices

Best Practices Study

One commenter stated that OPM "has not gone far enough" concerning its determination of best practices because it appears that OPM plans a "reactive response" based on reports developed by agencies. The commenter said that OPM should provide "thoroughly researched, comprehensive, proactive guidelines which could help agencies avoid inappropriate discipline actions and would provide managers with sound guidance * * *." OPM notes the proposed rule stated only that the study "will include," rather than "will be limited to" a review of agencies' discussions provided in their reports under the No FEAR Act.

Another commenter recommended that disciplinary best practices be shared with Federal agencies. Under § 724.403, disciplinary best practices will be incorporated in the advisory guidelines that OPM will provide to Federal agencies.

Advisory Guidelines

Some agencies suggested that OPM change the manner in which they are to reply to the advisory guidelines issued under § 724.403, eliminate the reply as an unnecessary burden, make the guidelines non-mandatory, change the recipient list, delay implementation of the guidelines after they are issued, and/or change the amount of time allocated for replying (provide more time). The No FEAR Act is very specific about agencies' obligations regarding this topic. Therefore, OPM declines to adopt these suggestions.

One agency suggested that agencies be given maximum flexibility in administering disciplinary actions and that the guidelines be focused essentially on program measures to determine effectiveness. Such program measures might be the reduction in agency complaints, policies issued to deter discriminatory behavior, and effective implementation of recommendations from previous agency reports. OPM will consider these suggestions in drafting the advisory guidelines.

One commenter suggested that OPM provide agencies with an opportunity to comment on advisory guidelines drafted under the No FEAR Act and/or publish them in the **Federal Register** for public comment. While the Act does not provide the opportunity for such comments, the President's delegation of authority to OPM does require that its activities concerning regulations under the No FEAR Act be accomplished in consultation with the Attorney General and other offices of the executive branch OPM determines appropriate. Thus, OPM has consulted with the Department of Justice, the Equal Employment Opportunity Commission, the Office of Special Counsel, and the Department of the Treasury and may do so in connection with the advisory guidelines.

With regard to agencies' obligation to state in writing whether or to what extent they are going to follow the advisory guidelines, one commenter wanted to know what will happen if an agency "opts out". Will there be consequences? The No FEAR Act requires agencies to provide their written statements to the Congress, the EEOC, and the Attorney General. The Act contains no "opt out" provision.

Miscellaneous Comments

Training

One of the union commenters recommended that there be "mandatory training requirements" and proposed that managers who have violated discrimination laws attend education and awareness training pertaining to managing a diverse workforce. OPM notes that the No FEAR Act requires training for all employees including managers. Agencies have flexibility to develop training curricula as appropriate for their needs. OPM declines to adopt this recommendation.

Enforcement

One organization suggested that EEOC and MSPB amend their regulations so that they could dismiss on jurisdictional grounds complaints and appeals filed by

Federal Register / Vol. 71, No. 249 / Thursday, December 28, 2006 / Rules and Regulations 78037

employees who are disciplined in accordance with best practices guidance on disciplinary matters as set forth by OPM. OPM takes no position on this comment because it is beyond the scope of these regulations.

Another organization suggests that, for enforcement purposes, when there are violations of Federal antidiscrimination and whistleblower protection laws within an agency, that agency should be required to post a public notice similar to what is done when an agency is found by the Federal Labor Relations Authority to have committed an unfair labor practice. Another enforcement-related proposal would be to create a central repository of all information collected under the No FEAR Act and posted in one location on a public Web site such as EEOC's. This commenter also suggested that the regulations set penalties for failing to report as required by the Act. Another organization suggests that OPM measure agencies' performance in implementing the No FEAR Act. Part of this process would involve identifying an office at OPM with primary responsibility for assessing policy performance. Agencies would submit policy to this office and a selected group of interested employees from agencies would determine important aspects to be included in agency performance assessment. The group's results then would be used to compile a list of agency performance criteria and success indicators. OPM takes no position on these comments because they are beyond the scope of these regulations.

Timeliness

A number of commenters expressed concern about the amount of time it has taken for regulations to be promulgated under the No FEAR Act. OPM notes that with the publication of final regulations on Subpart A (Judgment Fund) on May 10, 2006, Subpart B (Notification and Training) on July 20, 2006, and the current rule, Subparts C & D (Reporting and Best Practices), 5 CFR part 724 is now complete.

Regulatory Flexibility Act

I certify that this regulation will not have a significant economic impact on a substantial number of small entities because the regulations pertain only to Federal employees and agencies.

E.O. 12866, Regulatory Review

This final rule has been reviewed by the Office of Management and Budget under Executive Order 12866.

E.O. 13132

This regulation will not have substantial direct effects on the States, on the relationship between the National Government and the States, or on distribution of power and responsibilities among the various levels of government. Therefore, in accordance with Executive Order 13132, it is determined that this rule does not have sufficient federalism implications to warrant preparation of a Federalism Assessment.

E.O. 12988, Civil Justice Reform

This regulation meets the applicable standard set forth in sections 3(a) and 3(b)(2) of Executive Order 12988.

Unfunded Mandates Reform Act of 1995

This rule will not result in the expenditure by State, local and tribal governments, in the aggregate, or by the private sector, of $100,000,000 or more in any one year, and it will not significantly or uniquely affect small governments. Therefore, no actions were deemed necessary under the provisions of the Unfunded Mandates Reform Act of 1995.

Congressional Review Act

This action pertains to agency management, personnel and organization and does not substantially affect the rights or obligations of non-agency parties and, accordingly, is not a "rule" as that term is used by the Congressional Review Act (Subtitle E of the Small Business Regulatory Enforcement Fairness Act of 1996 (SBREFA)). Therefore, the reporting requirement of 5 U.S.C. 801 does not apply.

List of Subjects in 5 CFR Part 724

Administrative practice and procedure, Civil rights, Claims.

U.S. Office of Personnel Management.

Linda M. Springer,

Director.

■ Accordingly, OPM is amending part 724, title 5, Code of Federal Regulations, as follows:

PART 724—IMPLEMENTATION OF TITLE II OF THE NOTIFICATION AND FEDERAL EMPLOYEE ANTIDISCRIMINATION AND RETALIATION ACT OF 2002

■ 1. In § 724.102 of subpart A, add a new definition for discipline in alphabetical order to read as follows:

§ 724.102 Definitions.

* * * * *

Discipline means any one or a combination of the following actions: reprimand, suspension without pay, reduction in grade or pay, or removal.

* * * * *

■ 2. In part 724, add subparts C and D to read as follows:

Subpart C—Annual Report

Sec.
724.301 Purpose and scope.
724.302 Reporting obligations.

Subpart C—Annual Report

§ 724.301 Purpose and scope.

This subpart implements Title II of the Notification and Federal Employee Antidiscrimination and Retaliation Act of 2002 concerning the obligation of Federal agencies to report on specific topics concerning Federal Antidiscrimination Laws and Whistleblower Protection Laws applicable to them covering employees, former employees, and applicants for Federal employment.

§ 724.302 Reporting obligations.

(a) Except as provided in paragraph (b) of this section, each agency must report no later than 180 calendar days after the end of each fiscal year the following items:

(1) The number of cases in Federal court pending or resolved in each fiscal year and arising under each of the respective provisions of the Federal Antidiscrimination Laws and Whistleblower Protection Laws applicable to them as defined in § 724.102 of subpart A of this part in which an employee, former Federal employee, or applicant alleged a violation(s) of these laws, separating data by the provision(s) of law involved.

(2) In the aggregate, for the cases identified in paragraph (a)(1) of this section and separated by provision(s) of law involved:

(i) The status or disposition (including settlement);

(ii) The amount of money required to be reimbursed to the Judgment Fund by the agency for payments as defined in § 724.102 of subpart A of this part;

(iii) The amount of reimbursement to the Fund for attorney's fees where such fees have been separately designated;

(3) In connection with cases identified in paragraph (a)(1) of this section, the total number of employees in each fiscal year disciplined as defined in § 724.102 of subpart A of this part and the specific nature, e.g., reprimand, etc., of the disciplinary actions taken, separated by the provision(s) of law involved.

(4) The final year-end data about discrimination complaints for each

78038 Federal Register / Vol. 71, No. 249 / Thursday, December 28, 2006 / Rules and Regulations

fiscal year that was posted in accordance with Equal Employment Opportunity Regulations at subpart G of title 29 of the Code of Federal Regulations (implementing section 301(c)(1)(B) of the No FEAR Act);

(5) Whether or not in connection with cases in Federal court, the number of employees in each fiscal year disciplined as defined in § 724.102 of subpart A of this part in accordance with any agency policy described in paragraph (a)(6) of this section. The specific nature, e.g., reprimand, etc., of the disciplinary actions taken must be identified.

(6) A detailed description of the agency's policy for taking disciplinary action against Federal employees for conduct that is inconsistent with Federal Antidiscrimination Laws and Whistleblower Protection Laws or for conduct that constitutes another prohibited personnel practice revealed in connection with agency investigations of alleged violations of these laws.

(7) An analysis of the information provided in paragraphs (a)(1) through (6) of this section in conjunction with data provided to the Equal Employment Opportunity Commission in compliance with 29 CFR part 1614 subpart F of the Code of Federal Regulations. Such analysis must include:

(i) An examination of trends;

(ii) Causal analysis;

(iii) Practical knowledge gained through experience; and

(iv) Any actions planned or taken to improve complaint or civil rights programs of the agency with the goal of eliminating discrimination and retaliation in the workplace;

(8) For each fiscal year, any adjustment needed or made to the budget of the agency to comply with its Judgment Fund reimbursement obligation(s) incurred under § 724.103 of subpart A of this part; and

(9) The agency's written plan developed under § 724.203(a) of subpart B of this part to train its employees.

(b) The first report also must provide information for the data elements in paragraph (a) of this section for each of the five fiscal years preceding the fiscal year on which the first report is based to the extent that such data is available. Under the provisions of the No FEAR Act, the first report was due March 30, 2005 without regard to the status of the regulations. Thereafter, under the provisions of the No FEAR Act, agency reports are due annually on March 30th. Agencies that have submitted their reports before these regulations became final must ensure that they contain data elements 1 through 8 of paragraph (a) of this section and provide any necessary supplemental reports by April 25, 2007. Future reports must include data elements 1 through 9 of paragraph (a) of this section.

(c) Agencies must provide copies of each report to the following:

(1) Speaker of the U.S. House of Representatives;

(2) President Pro Tempore of the U.S. Senate;

(3) Committee on Governmental Affairs, U.S. Senate;

(4) Committee on Government Reform, U.S. House of Representatives;

(5) Each Committee of Congress with jurisdiction relating to the agency;

(6) Chair, Equal Employment Opportunity Commission;

(7) Attorney General; and

(8) Director, U.S. Office of Personnel Management.

Subpart D—Best Practices

Sec.

724.401 Purpose and scope.

724.402 Best practices study.

724.403 Advisory guidelines.

724.404 Agency obligations.

Subpart D—Best Practices

§ 724.401 Purpose and scope.

This subpart implements Title II of the Notification and Federal Employee Antidiscrimination and Retaliation Act of 2002 concerning the obligation of the President or his designee (OPM) to conduct a comprehensive study of best practices in the executive branch for taking disciplinary actions against employees for conduct that is inconsistent with Federal Antidiscrimination and Whistleblower Protection Laws and the obligation to issue advisory guidelines for agencies to follow in taking appropriate disciplinary actions in such circumstances.

§ 724.402 Best practices study.

(a) OPM will conduct a comprehensive study in the executive branch to identify best practices for taking appropriate disciplinary actions against Federal employees for conduct that is inconsistent with Federal Antidiscrimination and Whistleblower Protection Laws.

(b) The comprehensive study will include a review of agencies' discussions of their policies for taking such disciplinary actions as reported under § 724.302 of subpart C of this part.

§ 724.403 Advisory guidelines.

OPM will issue advisory guidelines to Federal agencies incorporating the best practices identified under § 724.402 that agencies may follow to take appropriate disciplinary actions against employees for conduct that is inconsistent with Federal Antidiscrimination Laws and Whistleblower Laws.

§ 724.404 Agency obligations.

(a) Within 30 working days of issuance of the advisory guidelines required by § 724.403, each agency must prepare a written statement describing in detail:

(1) Whether it has adopted the guidelines and if it will fully follow the guidelines;

(2) If such agency has not adopted the guidelines, the reasons for non-adoption; and

(3) If such agency will not fully follow the guidelines, the reasons for the decision not to do so and an explanation of the extent to which the agency will not follow the guidelines.

(b) Each agency's written statement must be provided within the time limit stated in paragraph (a) of this section to the following:

(1) Speaker of the U.S. House of Representatives;

(2) President Pro Tempore of the U.S. Senate;

(3) Chair, Equal Employment Opportunity Commission;

(4) Attorney General; and

(5) Director, U.S. Office of Personnel Management.

[FR Doc. E6-22242 Filed 12-27-06; 8:45 am]

BILLING CODE 6325-39-P

DEPARTMENT OF AGRICULTURE

Agricultural Marketing Service

7 CFR Parts 916 and 917

[Docket No. AMS-FV-06-0189; FV07-916/917-1 IFR]

Nectarines and Peaches Grown in California; Revision of Regulations on Production Districts, Committee Representation, and Nomination Procedures

AGENCY: Agricultural Marketing Service, USDA.

ACTION: Interim final rule with request for comments.

SUMMARY: This rule revises the administrative rules and regulations that define production districts, allocate committee membership, and specify nomination procedures for the Nectarine Administrative Committee (NAC) and the Peach Commodity Committee (PCC) (committees). The committees are responsible for local administration of the Federal marketing

Mandated Report VA to CDC - Matteoli

Retaliation on Employees Who Express Concerns and/or Become Whistleblowers

SAFETY FIRST

Whistleblowing legal definition of Whistleblowing

http://legal-dictionary.thefreedictionary.com/Whistleblowing

Whistleblowing

Also found in: Dictionary/thesaurus, Medical, Financial, Wikipedia

Whistleblowing

The disclosure by a person, usually an employee in a government agency or private enterprise, to the public or to those in authority, of mismanagement, corruption, illegality, or some other wrongdoing.

Since the 1960s, the public value of *whistle-blowing* has been increasingly recognized. For example, federal and state statutes and regulations have been enacted to *protect whistleblowers* from various forms of retaliation. Even without a statute, numerous decisions encourage and protect whistleblowing on grounds of public policy. In addition, the federal False Claims Act (31 U.S.C.A. § 3729) will reward a whistleblower who brings a lawsuit against a company that makes a false claim or commits Fraud against the government.

Persons who act as whistleblowers are often the subject of retaliation by their employers. Typically the employer will discharge the whistleblower, who is often an at-will employee. An at-will employee is a person without a specific term of employment. The employee may quit at any time and the employer has the right to fire the employee without having to cite a reason. However, courts and legislatures have created exceptions for whistleblowers who are at-will employees.

Whistleblowing statutes protect from discharge or discrimination an employee who has initiated an investigation of an employer's activities or who has otherwise cooperated with a regulatory agency in carrying out an inquiry or the enforcement of regulations. Federal whistle-blower legislation includes a statute protecting all government employees. 5 U.S.C.A. §§ 2302(b)(8), 2302(b)(9). In the federal civil service, the government is prohibited from taking, or threatening to take, any personnel action against an employee because the employee disclosed information that he or she reasonably believed showed a violation of law, gross mismanagement, gross waste of funds, abuse of authority, or a substantial and specific danger to public safety or health. In order to prevail on a claim, a federal employee must show that a protected disclosure was made, that the accused official knew of the disclosure, that retaliation resulted, and that there was a genuine connection between the retaliation and the employee's action.

Many states have enacted whistleblower statutes, but these statutes vary widely in coverage. Some statutes apply only to public employees, some apply to both public and private employees, and others apply to public employees and employees of public contractors.

Some statutes cover a broad array of circumstances, such as those that apply to federal employees that prohibit employers from dismissing workers in Reprisal for disclosing information about, or seeking a remedy for, a violation of law, gross mismanagement, gross waste of funds, abuse of authority, or a specific danger to public safety and health. Other statutes are narrow in scope, such as one that limits the protection of public and private employees to retaliation for reporting possible violations of local, state, or federal environmental statutes. A whistleblower statute may also limit protection to discussions of agency operations with members of the legislature or to disclosure of information to legislative committees or courts.

In whistleblower cases, states follow their general rules for determining whether a public policy Cause of Action exists in favor of the employee. Therefore, in states in which Wrongful Discharge actions must have a statutory (legal) basis, the case will be dismissed if the employer did not violate a statutorily enacted public policy. In many cases, the courts have refused to recognize a whistleblower's claim because no clearly mandated statutory policy has been identified. In addition, employees who blow the whistle on matters that affect only private interests (e.g., complaints about internal corporate policies) will generally be unsuccessful in maintaining a cause of action for discharge in violation of public policy.

Under the federal False Claims Act, any person with knowledge of false claims or fraud against the government may bring a lawsuit in his own name and in the name of the United States. As long as the information is not publicly disclosed and the government has not already sued the defendant for the fraud, the whistle-blower, who is called a relator in this action, may bring a False Claims Act case. The relator files the case in federal court under seal (in secret), and gives a copy to the government. The government then has 60 days to review the case and decide whether it has merit. If the government decides to join the case, the case is unsealed, a copy is served on the defendant, and the government and the relator work together in the case as co-plaintiffs. If the government declines to join the suit, the relator may proceed alone. In a successful False Claims Act case the relator will receive at least 15 percent but not more than 25 percent of the proceeds of the action or settlement of the claim, depending upon the extent to which the person substantially contributed to the prosecution of the action.

In the early 1990s, commentators were claiming that men were more likely than women to blow the whistle on improper conduct. Some analysts suggested the reason for this perception was that men seem to seek financial gain for whistleblowing. During the early 2000s, however, a number of women became involved in high profile acts of whistleblowing—for reasons other than fame and fortune.

In 2001, Sherron Watkins, a vice president at Enron Corporation, informed the company's board that Enron's accounting practices were improper. Enron later suffered a major collapse—largely as a result of its accounting practices—that led to the company's Bankruptcy and to the indictment of the company's auditor and chief financial officer. The following year, Cynthia Cooper, an auditor with WorldCom, told the company's board that WorldCom had covered up major losses of $3.8 billion through false bookkeeping. Like Enron, the accounting failures led to WorldCom's bankruptcy. During the same year, Coleen Rowley, an FBI staff attorney for more than 20 years, sent a letter to FBI director ROBERT MUELLER, indicating that the FBI's national headquarters had mishandled an investigation of Zacarias Moussaoui, who was later believed to be a co-conspirator in the September 11, 2001, terrorist attacks. Rowley later spoke before the intelligence committees of the House of Representatives and the Senate about her accusations.

Time magazine dubbed 2002 the "Year of the Whistleblower," and named Watkins, Cooper, and Rowley as its "Persons of the Year." Their stories fueled the observation that women are more likely to become whistleblowers not for the potential for fame and financial gain, but out of a sense of duty. Although Watkins, Cooper, and Rowley were each subjected to rather harsh treatment by their respective employers following their disclosures, they became national celebrities by "speaking up when no one else would."

Further readings

Callahan, Elletta Sangrey, and Terry Morehead Dworkin. 1992. "Do Good and Get Rich: Financial Incentives for Whistleblowing and the False Claims Act." *Villanova Law Review* 37.

Helmer, James B. 2002. *False Claims Act: Whistleblower Litigation*. 3d ed. Charlottesville, Va.: LexisNexis.

Kelly, James. 2002. "The Year of the Whistle-Blowers." *Time* (December 30).

Whistleblowing: A Federal Employee's Guide to Charges, Procedures, and Penalties. 2000. Reston, Va.: Federal Employees News Digest.

Cross-references

Employment at Will, Employment Law

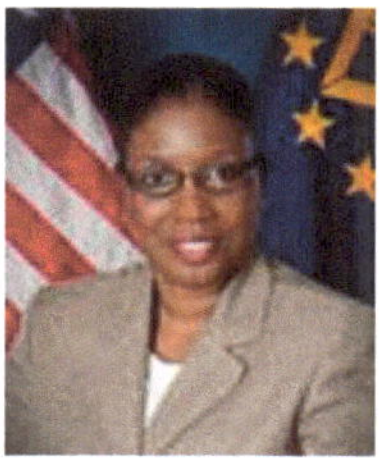

Sandra Flint

Regional office director in Phoenix

Under Flint's leadership, the backlog of disability claims in Phoenix more than doubled from 2009 to 2013, reaching more than 80 percent. That made it one of the worst-performing offices in the country. Yet Flint received more than $53,000 in bonuses between 2007 and 2011.

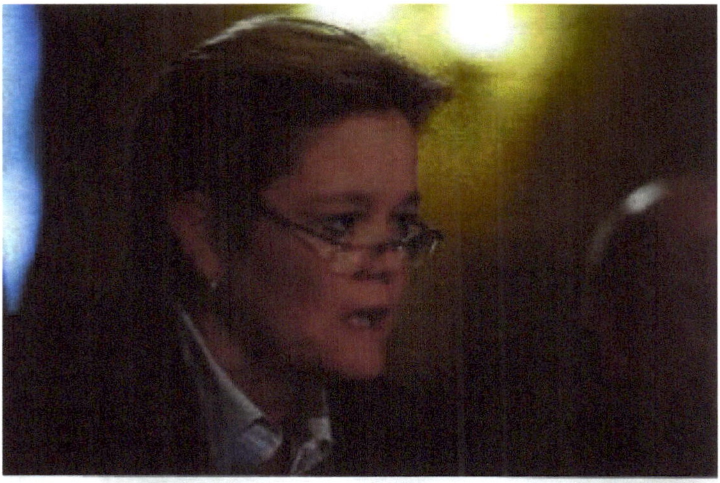

House Holds Hearing on VA Scandal

In This Photo: Diana Rubens

Deputy Under Secretary for Field Operations, Veterans Benefits Administration, U.S. Department of Veterans Affairs Diana Rubens responds to a question during a House Veterans' Affairs Committee, Disability Assistance and Memorial Affairs Subcommittee hearing on "Defined Expectations: Evaluating VA's Performance in the Service Member Transition Process" in the Cannon House Office Building, May 29, 2014, in Washington, DC These witnesses on the first panel, responded to questions from members of Congress.

(May 28, 2014 - Source: Rod Lamkey/Getty Images North America) more pics from this album »

WHISTLEBLOWER PROTECTION

Whistleblower retaliation is a Prohibited Personnel Practice, specifically defined and prohibited by the Whistleblower Protection Act (WPA), 5 U.S.C. 2302(b)(8)-(9), as well as by the Inspector General Act, 5 U.S.C. Appendix 3.

Under the WPA, all supervisors are prohibited from taking, directing, recommending, or approving, any personnel action[1] against an employee or applicant for employment for any lawful disclosure of information (including specifically to the OSC or the OIG) that the employee/applicant reasonably believes shows

a violation of any law, rule, or regulation,
gross mismanagement,
gross waste of funds,
abuse of authority, **or**
a substantial and specific danger to public health or safety, Unless specifically **prohibited by law** and not specifically required by Executive order to be kept **secret**

---

1 Personnel action is:
appointment;
promotion;
action under chapter 75 of this title or other disciplinary or corrective action;
detail, transfer, or reassignment;
reinstatement;
restoration;
reemployment;
performance evaluation;
decision concerning pay, benefits, or awards, or concerning education or training if the education or training may reasonably be expected to lead to an appointment, promotion, performance evaluation, or other action described in this subparagraph;
decision to order psychiatric testing or examination;
implementation or enforcement of any nondisclosure policy, form, or agreement;
any other significant change in duties, responsibilities, or working conditions

This protection extends to

the exercise of any appeal, complaint, or grievance right granted by any law, rule, or regulation,

testifying for or otherwise lawfully assisting any individual exercising whistleblower rights,

cooperating with or disclosing information to the Inspector General or the Special Counsel, in accordance with applicable provisions of law; **or**

refusing to obey an order that would require the individual to violate a law

The Whistleblower Protection Enhancement Act of 2012 (WPEA) expanded the definition of protected disclosures to include those:

made in the normal course of duties;

made to a supervisor or to a person who participated in an activity that the employee or applicant reasonably believed to be covered

that reveal information that had been previously disclosed;

made while the employee was off duty; **or**

made orally.

And the protection applies regardless of the employee's or applicant's motive for making the disclosure, and regardless of the amount of time which has passed since the occurrence of the events described in the disclosure.

Under the Inspector General Act, Section 7(c), any employee who has authority to take, direct others to take, recommend, or approve any personnel action, shall not, with respect to such authority, take or threaten to take any action against any employee as a reprisal for making a complaint or disclosing information to an Inspector General, unless the complaint was made or the information disclosed with the knowledge that it was false or with willful disregard for its truth or falsity.

WHISTLEBLOWER PROTECTION FOR CONTRACTORS

As noted above, Government employees are protected from whistleblower retaliation by 5 U.S.C. 2302, and Section 7 of the Inspector General Act of 1978.

Employees of contractors have similar, but not identical, protections pursuant to 41 U.S.C. 4705, and Subpart 3.9 of the Federal Acquisition Regulations (FAR), 48 C.F.R. Part 3.

Per Section 4705(b), contractor employees may not be "discharged, demoted, or otherwise discriminated against as a reprisal for disclosing to a Member of Congress or an authorized official of an executive agency or the Department of Justice information relating to a substantial violation of law related to a contract (including the competition for or negotiation of a contract)."

The statute and FAR Subpart 3.9 allow persons who perceive such a reprisal to report it to the IG of the agency engaging the contractor. The IG is required to evaluate the complaint, and if the complaint is determined to have merit, investigate. The investigative report is to be provided to the contractor, the aggrieved contractor employee, and the head of the engaging agency. The agency head can order the contractor to abate the reprisal, rehire the employee, and restore lost pay. If the contractor fails to comply with such an order, the agency head must seek judicial enforcement of the order in the Federal judicial district where the reprisal occurred.

WHISTLEBLOWER OMBUDSMAN

WHISTLEBLOWER PROTECTION OMBUDSMAN

WPEA amended the Inspector General Act of 1978 by adding Section 3(d):

(1) Each Inspector General shall…
(C) designate a Whistleblower Protection **Ombudsman who shall educate agency employees—**
(i) about prohibitions on retaliation for protected disclosures; **and**
(ii) who have made or are contemplating making a protected disclosure about the **rights and remedies against retaliation for protected disclosures.**

(2) The Whistleblower Protection Ombudsman shall **not act as a legal representative, agent, or advocate** of the employee or former employee.

Treasury's Whistleblower Protection Ombudsman is Rich Delmar, Counsel to the Inspector General. Contact him on 202-927-3973 or OIGCounsel@oig.treas.gov.

TREASURY DEPARTMENT RESPONSIBILITY AND OBLIGATION

TREASURY EMPLOYEE OBLIGATIONS AND PROTECTIONS

Inspector General Act of 1978, as amended – 5 U.S.C. App. 3

§ 6. Authority of Inspector General
(a) In addition to the authority otherwise provided by this Act, each Inspector General, in carrying out the provisions of this Act, is authorized--

(1) to have access to all records, reports, audits, reviews, documents, papers, recommendations, or other material available to the applicable establishment which relate to programs and operations with respect to which that Inspector General has responsibilities under this Act;

(2) to make such investigations and reports relating to the administration of the programs and operations of the applicable establishment as are, in the judgment of the Inspector General, necessary or desirable;

(b)(2) Whenever information or assistance requested under subsection (a)(1) or (a)(3) is, in the judgment of an Inspector General, unreasonably refused or not provided, the Inspector General shall report the circumstances to the head of the establishment involved without delay.

§ 7. Complaints by employees; disclosure of identity; reprisals
a) The Inspector General may receive and investigate complaints or information from an employee of the

establishment concerning the possible existence of an activity constituting a violation of law, rules, or regulations, or mismanagement, gross waste of funds, abuse of authority or a substantial and specific danger to the public health and safety.

b) The Inspector General shall not, after receipt of a complaint or information from an employee, disclose the identity of the employee without the consent of the employee, unless the Inspector General determines such disclosure is unavoidable during the course of the investigation.

c) Any employee who has authority to take, direct others to take, recommend, or approve any personnel action, shall not, with respect to such authority, take or threaten to take any action against any employee as a reprisal for making a complaint or disclosing information to an Inspector General, unless the complaint was made or the information disclosed with the knowledge that it was false or with willful disregard for its truth or falsity.

31 C.F.R. 0.207 Employee Rules of Conduct - Cooperation with official inquiries.

Employees shall respond to questions truthfully and under oath when required, whether orally or in writing, and must provide documents and other materials concerning matters of official interest when directed to do so by competent Treasury authority.

Treasury Directive 40-01 Responsibilities of and to the Inspector General

Subject only to the specific exceptions set out below, as a general rule all Department of the Treasury officials, officers and employees (hereafter Treasury employees) are required to report promptly to the OIG any information or allegation coming to their attention that indicates that any Treasury employee, former employee, contractor, subcontractor, or potential contractor, may have engaged in improper or illegal activity, including but not limited to:

a) a criminal or other illegal act;
b) a violation of the Standards of Conduct or other Federal regulation;
c) a prohibited personnel practice or violation of merit systems principles; and
d) any act which creates a specific danger to the public health and safety.

All Treasury employees must provide to the IG and to that official's duly authorized representatives full, free and unrestricted access to Treasury activities, property, data, correspondence, records, information technology systems, and any other information that the IG determines is necessary to an audit, investigation, or other official inquiry.

All Treasury employees shall cooperate fully with duly authorized representatives of the OIG by disclosing complete and accurate information pertaining to matters being investigated, audited or reviewed by the OIG. If the employee is the subject of an investigation, the employee will be afforded all required rights.

When the Secretary has provided the IG with written notification pursuant to Section 8D(a) of the Act, prohibiting the IG from carrying out or completing any audit or investigation or issuing any subpoena, to prevent the disclosure of sensitive information, a Treasury employee shall withhold that information from the IG.

Treasury employees who receive and review OIG audit reports or Reports of Investigation in the course of their official duties shall consult with the OIG prior to releasing or copying any report or portion thereof for the use of any other person, except for those persons with an official need to know.

Treasury employees shall maintain in confidence all communications with an authorized representative of the IG when requested to do so, unless required or permitted by law to disclose. Treasury employees shall not discuss any pending OIG investigation with the subject/subjects of the investigation or their representatives without approval of the OIG.

Any employee who has authority to take, direct others to take, recommend, or approve any personnel action shall not take or threaten to take any action against any employee as a reprisal for making a complaint or disclosing information to the OIG, unless the complaint was made or the information disclosed with the knowledge that it was false or with willful disregard for its truth or falsity.

Treasury employees and others may report suspected fraudulent or wasteful practices in Treasury programs and operations using a toll-free nationwide Treasury OIG Hotline number, 1-800-359-3898. The OIG will not disclose the identity of any employee without the employee's consent, unless the IG determines that such disclosure is unavoidable. The OIG will also make every effort to protect the identity of individuals who are not Treasury employees.

Mandated Report VA to CDC - Matteoli

RESERVIST'S RIGHTS BEING VIOLATED

Department of Defense

DIRECTIVE

NUMBER 1241.1
February 28, 2004

ASD(RA)

SUBJECT: Reserve Component Medical Care and Incapacitation Pay for Line of Duty Conditions

References: (a) DoD Directive 1241.1, "Reserve Component Incapacitation Benefits," December 3, 1992 (hereby canceled)
(b) Sections 1074, 1074a, 12322 and 12301(h) of title 10, United States Code
(c) Sections 204(g), 204(h) and 206 of title 37, United States Code
(d) DoD 7000.14-R, Volume 7A, "DoD Financial Management Regulation, Military Pay Policy and Procedures-Active Duty and Reserve Pay," August 2002
(e) through (g), see enclosure 1

1. REISSUANCE AND PURPOSE

This Directive:

1.1. Reissues reference (a) to update policies and assign responsibilities under references (b), (c), and (d), to authorize medical and dental care for members of the Reserve components who incur or aggravate an injury, illness, or disease in the line of duty, and provide pay and allowances to those members while being treated for or recovering from a service-connected injury, illness, or disease, or who demonstrate a loss of earned income as a result of an injury, illness, or disease incurred or aggravated in the line of duty.

1.2. Establishes policies for ordering a member to active duty or continuing a member on active duty, with the consent of the member, to receive authorized medical care, to be medically evaluated for disability or other purposes, or to complete a required Department of Defense (DoD) healthcare study, which may include associated medical evaluation of the member.

1.3. Establishes policies for ordering a Reserve component member to active duty or continuing the member on active duty while being treated for (or recovering from) an injury, illness, or disease incurred or aggravated in the line of duty.

1.4. Authorizes the issuance of DoD Instruction 1241.2 (reference (e)), to prescribe procedures for the management of the Reserve component member who incurs or aggravates an injury, illness, or disease in the line of duty.

2. APPLICABILITY

2.1. This Directive applies to the Office of the Secretary of Defense, the Military Departments, the Chairman of the Joint Chiefs of Staff, the Combatant Commands, the Inspector General of the Department of Defense, the Defense Agencies, the DoD Field Activities and all other organizational entities in the Department of Defense (hereafter referred to collectively as "the DoD Components").

2.2. The Coast Guard when it is not operating as a Military Service in the Navy by agreement with the Department of Homeland Security.

3. DEFINITIONS

3.1. Incapacitation. Physical disability due to injury, illness, or disease that prevents the performance of military duties as determined by the Secretary concerned, or which prevents the member from returning to the civilian occupation in which the member was engaged at the time of the injury, illness, or disease.

3.2. Line of Duty. A finding after all available information has been reviewed that determines an injury, illness, or disease was incurred or aggravated as a result of military duty not due to gross negligence or misconduct of the member. This includes a Reserve component member on inactive duty training, funeral honors duty, traveling directly to or from such duty or training, or while remaining overnight, immediately before the commencement of or between successive periods of such duty.

3.3. Military Duties as Determined by the Secretary Concerned. The duties of a Service member's office and grade, and not necessarily the specialty or skill qualification held by the member prior to incurring or aggravating an injury, illness, or disease in the line of duty.

3.4. Secretary Concerned. The Secretary of the Army regarding matters concerning the Army; the Secretary of the Navy regarding matters concerning the Navy, the Marine Corps, and the Coast Guard when it is operating as a Service in the Department of the Navy; the Secretary of the Air Force regarding matters concerning the Air Force; and the Secretary of Homeland Security regarding matters concerning the Coast Guard when it is not operating as a Service in the Department of the Navy.

4. POLICY

It is DoD policy that:

4.1. A Reserve component member on active duty for a period of 30 days or less; on inactive duty training, funeral honors duty, traveling directly to or from such duty or training, or while remaining overnight, immediately before the commencement of or between successive periods of such duty is entitled to medical and dental treatment for injuries, illnesses, or diseases incurred or aggravated in the line of duty not as a result of gross negligence or misconduct of the member.

4.2. A Reserve component member on active duty for a period of 30 days or less may be continued on active duty while the member is being treated for, or recovering from, an injury, illness, or disease incurred or aggravated in the line of duty.

4.3. The Secretary of the Military Department may order a Reserve component member to active duty, with the consent of the member, to receive authorized medical care, be medically evaluated for disability or other medical purposes, or complete a required DoD healthcare study, which may include an associated medical evaluation of the member.

4.4. Reserve component members who have been continued on active duty for medical reasons for more than 30 days are entitled to medical and dental care on the same basis as a member of the regular component.

*4.5. The Military Departments shall authorize pay and allowances, to the extent permitted by reference (c), for a Reserve component member who is not medically qualified to perform military duties, as determined by the Secretary concerned, because of an injury, illness, or disease incurred or aggravated in the line of duty, or to provide pay and allowances to a member who is fit to perform military duties, but experiences a loss of earned income because of an injury, illness, or disease incurred or aggravated in the line of duty. This is commonly referred to as incapacitation pay.

4.6. Where applicable, a line of duty determination approved by the Service component designated authority shall serve as basis for eligibility and continuation of medical and dental care and incapacitation benefits.

4.7. Medical and dental care authorized under this Directive shall be provided until the member is fit for duty, or the condition cannot be materially improved with continued treatment and the member has received a final disposition under the Disability Evaluation System, as prescribed in DoD Directive 1332.18 and DoD Instruction 1332.38 (references (f) and (g)).

5. RESPONSIBILITIES

5.1. The Assistant Secretary of Defense (Reserve Affairs), under the Under Secretary of Defense for Personnel and Readiness, and in coordination with the Deputy Under Secretary of Defense (Military Personnel Policy) and the Assistant Secretary of Defense (Health Affairs), shall be responsible for Reserve incapacitation system management policy and is authorized to issue instructions implementing the Directive.

5.2. The Secretaries of the Military Departments shall:

5.2.1. Establish funding policy and procedures for pay and allowances authorized under reference (c), and DoD 7000.14-R (reference (d)) for members authorized such pay during a period of incapacitation.

5.2.2. Develop a system to track Reserve component members who are incapacitated.

5.2.3. Develop a plan to manage Reserve component members being treated in medical treatment facilities or authorized treatment in civilian treatment facilities to ensure the member receives the proper treatment, evaluation, and referral services in a timely and efficient manner.

5.2.4. Review each case in which the member is projected to remain incapacitated for more than 6 months to determine if it is in the interest of fairness and equity to continue benefits paid under reference (c) (if applicable), and to determine if the case should be referred to the Disability Evaluation System. Such a review shall be made every 6 months.

Mandated Report VA to CDC - Matteoli

6. EFFECTIVE DATE

This Directive is effective immediately.

Paul Wolfowitz
Deputy Secretary of Defense

Enclosures - 1
E1. References, continued

E1. ENCLOSURE 1

REFERENCES, continued

(e) DoD Instruction 1241.2, "Reserve Components Incapacitation System Management," May 30, 2001
(f) DoD Directive 1332.18, "Separation or Retirement for Physical Disability," November 4, 1996
(g) DoD Instruction 1332.38, "Physical Disability Evaluation," November 14, 1996

Mandated Report VA to CDC - Matteoli

VA Admits CULTURAL ISSUE is Their PROBLEM

Acculturated Punitive Personality Disorder

The New York Times http://nyti.ms/1F5pZ9

U.S.

V.A. Punished Critics on Staff, Doctors Assert

By ERIC LICHTBLAU JUNE 15, 2014

WASHINGTON — Staff members at dozens of Department of Veterans Affairs hospitals across the country have objected for years to falsified patient appointment schedules and other improper practices, only to be rebuffed, disciplined or even fired after speaking up, according to interviews with current and former staff members and internal documents.

The growing V.A. scandal over long patient wait times and fake scheduling books is emboldening hundreds of employees to go to federal watchdogs, unions, lawmakers and outside whistle-blower groups to report continuing problems, officials for those various groups said.

In interviews with The New York Times, a half-dozen current and former staff members — four doctors, a nurse and an office manager in Delaware, Pennsylvania and Alaska — said they faced retaliation for reporting systemic problems. Their accounts, some corroborated by internal documents, portray a culture of silence and intimidation within the department and echo experiences detailed by other V.A. personnel in court filings, government investigations and congressional testimony, much of it largely unnoticed until now.

The department has a history of retaliating against whistle-blowers, which Sloan D. Gibson, the acting V.A. secretary, acknowledged this month at a news conference in San Antonio. "I understand that we've got a cultural issue there, and we're going to deal with that cultural issue," said Mr. Gibson, who replaced Eric K. Shinseki after

Mr. Shinseki resigned over the scandal last month. Punishing whistle-blowers is "absolutely unacceptable," Mr. Gibson said.

The federal Office of Special Counsel, which investigates whistle-blower complaints, is examining 37 claims of retaliation by V.A. employees in 19 states, and recently persuaded the V.A. to drop the disciplining of three staff members who had spoken out. Together with reports to other watchdog agencies and the Times interviews, the accounts by V.A. whistle-blowers cover several dozen hospitals, with complaints dating back seven years or longer.

ALASKA
#1 Dr. Jacqueline Brecht, a former urologist at the Alaska V.A. Healthcare System in Anchorage, said in an interview that she had a heated argument with administrators at a staff meeting in 2008 when she objected to using phantom appointments to make wait times appear shorter, as they had instructed her. She said that the practice amounted to medical fraud, and complained about other patient care problems as well.

Days later, a top administrator came to Dr. Brecht's clinic, put her on administrative leave, and had security officers walk her out of the building.

"It's scary to think that people can try to stand up and do the right thing, and this is the reaction," said Dr. Brecht, now in private practice in Massachusetts.

Her complaints were corroborated by other Alaska personnel and were the subject of an email that Dr. Brecht sent to a military doctor at the time. Dr. Brecht wrote that administrators "schedule fake patient appointments (i.e. commit FRAUD)." They do so, she wrote, "just so our numbers look good to DC (and the administrators get their bonuses for these numbers)."

ALASKA
#2 Kathy Leatherwood, a nurse and unit manager at the Alaska V.A., said in an interview that she also objected in 2008 to the use of phantom appointments. She said administrators directed her to schedule fake appointments for new patients within 30 days without even notifying the patients. She was then supposed to mark the patient as a "no show" or a cancellation and schedule a real appointment for later, she said. That way, the official record would show the veteran was offered a quick appointment within the required turnaround period.

Ms. Leatherwood said that she, too, went to V.A. administrators to object.

"It's my name that's going to be on that chart," she remembered telling one administrator. The administrator responded that if she was unwilling to carry out the policy, he would find someone who would, she said. When she continued objecting, he threatened to call security if she did not leave his office.

ALASKA

#3 Kathleen Belmonti, who was a nurse there, said in an interview that she, too, was aware of staff concerns about scheduling and management practices.

ALASKA DENIAL

Cynthia A. Joe, the chief of staff at the Alaska V.A. Healthcare System, said that the facility had never used phantom scheduling and that, while some staff members had raised questions about scheduling practices, no one had protested or faced disciplining after raising concerns.

DALLAS

#4 In court filings detailing the V.A. response to other problems, Dr. Ram Chaturvedi, formerly with the Dallas V.A. Medical Center, said that he began complaining in 2008 about shoddy patient care, including negligence by nurses who had marked the wrong kidney while preparing a patient for a procedure. In another instance, Dr. Chaturvedi said medical personnel had brought the wrong patient to an operating table.

DALLAS DEFERRAL

A supervisor told Dr. Chaturvedi to "let some things slide" because of staffing problems, but he continued writing up complaints. Officials considered him disruptive and fired him in 2010.

DELEWARE

#5 At the V.A. Medical Center in Wilmington, Del., Michelle Washington, a psychologist treating soldiers with post-traumatic stress disorder, also found her worries unwelcome. She said in an interview that she faced retaliation when she testified in 2011 to a Senate committee about staffing shortages that she said left veterans waiting dangerously long for psychological help.

DELEWARE DEFLECTION

A week before her scheduled appearance, Dr. Washington said she received an evaluation downgrading her performance at the hospital from "outstanding" to "unsatisfactory," citing management complaints she had never heard before. She was also stripped of some psychological treatment duties.

"I'm not sure how I went from outstanding to unsatisfactory in 30 days," Dr. Washington said. "The only intervening thing was my testimony."

PITTSBURGH

#6 In Pittsburgh, two V.A. doctors specializing in Legionnaires' disease, Dr. Janet Stout and Dr. Victor Yu, said they were forced out after complaining about budget and salary matters in 2006. The V.A. then closed their lab and destroyed their specimens — decisions the doctors contend contributed to a 2011 outbreak of Legionnaires' at the Pittsburgh hospital that killed six people.

"The V.A. isn't a place where you speak out," Dr. Stout said in an interview.

Dr. Yu called the department's decision to close his lab "malicious," and added in an interview that "I fall into a category that the V.A. absolutely abhors — whistle-blowers." **VA Punitive Personality Disorder. Censorship Silencing to Cover-Up Criminal Activity.**

The number of claims of retaliation by V.A. whistle-blowers is among the highest of any federal agency, said Carolyn Lerner, who runs the Office of Special Counsel, and have been documented by Congress going back at least two decades.

In 1992, a congressional report concluded that the V.A. discouraged employees from reporting problems by "harassing whistle-blowers or firing them." In 1999, a House subcommittee hearing on "Whistleblowing and Retaliation in the Department of Veterans Affairs" found little had changed.

Today V.A. employees and whistle-blower lawyers say the problem has only gotten worse.

FREEMAN INTERIM DIRECTOR

#7 In Phoenix, Dr. Sam Foote, whose complaints triggered the current scandal, said hospital officials ignored him at first and then harassed him when he complained about administrators who were "cooking the books." V.A. administrators "started coming after me," he told The Arizona Republic. He decided to retire early last year as a result.

CHICAGO DECEIT

#8 One way the V.A. has silenced whistle-blowers, their lawyers maintain, is by threatening to hold them in violation of patient privacy laws if they discuss medical cases. That happened in a 2007 case in Chicago, where Dr. Anil Parikh was fired after reporting "systematic problems" that he said delayed patient care. In terminating him, the V.A. charged that he had violated confidentiality laws by reporting his concerns to the inspector general and to Barack Obama, at the time a senator from Illinois, and other government officials, court filings show. After four years, a grievance panel reinstated Dr. Parikh with back pay.

Many employees, still fearing retaliation, are going outside the department to report what they say are systemic problems.

The **Project on Government Oversight**, a private group working with whistle-blowers, said it had received confidential complaints from about 175 current and former V.A. employees since the latest controversy began. Those complaints are of such interest to the government that the V.A. inspector general subpoenaed them last month, demanding all reports related to the Phoenix V.A. The group is resisting because of concerns about whistle-blower confidentiality.

"People are coming out of the woodwork," said J. Ward Morrow, a lawyer for the **American Federation of Government Employees**, which has received recent reports of problems from more than 100 V.A. employees.

Dr. Brecht, the Alaska urologist who was put on leave in 2008, said she thought about calling a whistle-blower's hotline at the time, but feared that administrators might take further steps to discredit her and risk her medical licensing.

"When I saw all this on the news the last few months, part of me felt this huge sense of relief," Dr. Brecht said, "because it was like I wasn't crazy after all."

A version of this article appears in print on June 16, 2014, on page A1 of the New York edition with the headline: V.A. Punished Critics on Staff, Doctors Assert.

Department of Veterans Affairs

Senior Executive Biography

Laura H. Eskenazi

Executive in Charge
Vice Chairman Board of Veterans' Appeals

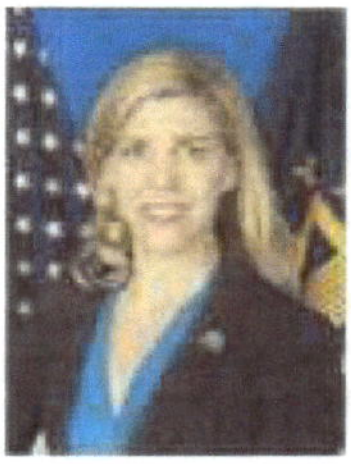

Laura H. Eskenazi was designated by Secretary Eric K. Shinseki as Executive in Charge and Vice Chairman of the Board of Veterans' Appeals (Board), on June 30, 2013

Prior to serving in these dual executive roles, Ms. Eskenazi served in a number of leadership positions at the Board. In July 2009, she was appointed by Secretary Shinseki to the position of Principal Deputy Vice Chairman of the Board, where she served as a key advisor to the Board's Chairman and Vice Chairman. Commensurate with her duties as the Principal Deputy Vice Chairman, in July 2010 she was appointed by Secretary Shinseki as a Veterans Law Judge, with the approval of President Barack Obama

Ms. Eskenazi also served as the Board's Chief Counsel for Operations, a Senior Level position, from November 2004 to 2009, after having served as Special Counsel to the Senior Deputy Vice Chairman.

Ms. Eskenazi began her career with the Board in January 1996 as a staff attorney, drafting tentative decisions for signature by Board Veterans Law Judges. During her nearly 19 years of experience in the Veteran's appeals system, she has been actively involved in the development of organizational strategy and execution of long-term goals to improve the Board's mission of providing timely and quality decisions to our Nation's Veterans.

Ms. Eskenazi is a graduate of Virginia Tech, with concentrations in English, Economics, and Political Science. She received a Juris Doctor degree from the University of Baltimore School of Law, and an LL.M. in Transnational Business Practices from McGeorge School of Law, University of the Pacific.

Ms. Eskenazi lives in Maryland with her husband, a former U.S. Navy Petty Officer, Second Class, and their three sons.

Appeals Board Corruption Still Unchecked

July 27, 2015 by Benjamin Krause — 36 Comments

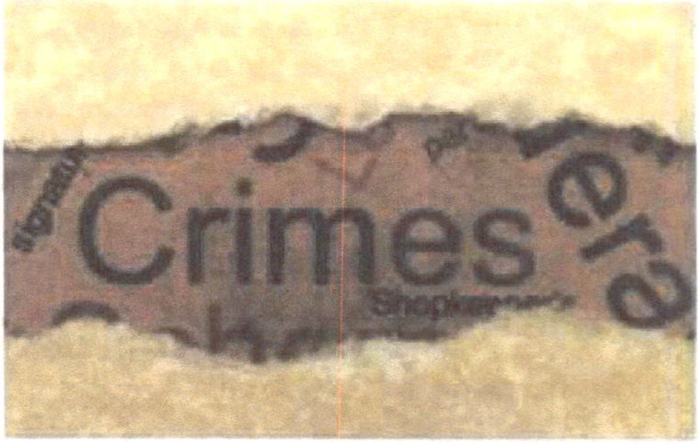

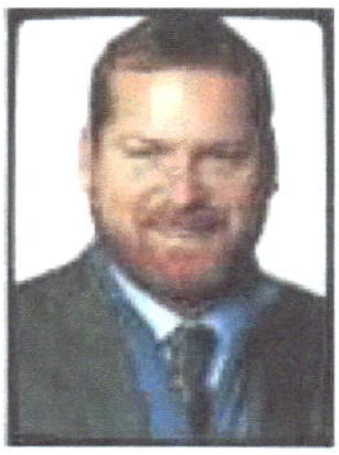

Former 'political prisoner' and disabled veteran Keith Roberts is still waiting for reinstatement of his veterans benefits by an appeals board following a 'trumped up' prosecution for wire fraud that has since been disproved.

Think it is possible that a bogus benefits denial at the VA Board of Veterans Appeals can result in imprisonment?

f 🐦 8+ in ✉

Disabled Veterans

Redeeming The Promise Of A Square Deal

Home

Articles

About

Voc Rehab Guide

Share Your Story

Contact

Roberts attorney, Robert Walsh, sent me a note about Roberts' case and I took the opportunity to review given current concerns by many in the veteran advocacy community over corruption within the Board of Veterans Appeals. Attorney Walsh's current fight for his client focuses on the current delay to fully adjudicate his client's benefits claim 5 years after a favorable reversal by the US Court of Appeals for Veterans Claims (Roberts v. Shinseki, 23 Vet. App. 416 (2010)) and after Roberts' release from prison. The Court's reversal confirmed evidentiary errors and procedural failures that call into question the evidence that resulted in Roberts' being imprisoned for wire fraud.

The case involves facts and events that I find shocking and deplorable, and a linkage between the current delay and reported corruption within the VA Board of Veterans Appeals that seems likely given that the Board created the benefits reversal in an unlawful decision that resulted in Roberts' imprisonment.

RELATED: Whistleblower claims records manipulation by VA appeals board

How can it take the VA Board of Veterans Appeals to rule on a remand order that essentially cleared a veteran of allegations of fraud erroneously leveled by the Board one decade ago? What you are about to read will venture into the realm of the bizarre, and I am fearful that many other cases like that of Roberts exist.

After learning more about Roberts, I thought it was high time to memorialize the current status of crimes perpetrated against this disabled veteran. He is a veteran with confirmed mental disorders likely linked to military service. He is a veteran VA employees did not like a lot. He is a veteran who was wrongly targeted in an agency witch-hunt after he made a VA OIG complaint about VA employees altering his files.

Let's hope he gets justice this time around more than a decade after the witch-hunt locked in on poor Roberts.

Political Scheming Against PTSD Veterans

Roberts was considered a political prisoner of a scheme hatched under the Republican Party in 2005 to disprove PTSD claims en mass while showing the world veterans are liars. While the Department of Justice pursued allegations against Roberts, it refused to prosecute government contractors defrauding taxpayers of billions in fraudulent claims.

To keep things level, this scheme against veterans and Roberts in particular has stemmed two political administrations, Republican and Democrat, and more than one decade. So clearly the scheme at play is beyond political party and purely and anti-veteran, anti-constitutional criminal conspiracy.

In 2005, the late Larry Scott, editor of VAWatchdog.org, discussed his views of the growing conspiracy with the Washington Post. Scott believed certain conservative groups were working to undermine existing PTSD rules awarding compensation for the condition. The obvious benefit to such scheme would be to reduce the long-term cost of the longest war in American history by eliminating disability benefits for this expensive condition.

According to Washington Post following Scott's interview:

Mandated Report VA to CDC - Matteoli

"Compensating people for disabilities is a cost of war," [Scott] said: "Veterans benefits are like workmen's comp. You went to war. You were injured. Either your body or your mind was injured, and that prevents you from doing certain duties and you are compensated for that."

Scott said Veterans Affairs' objectives were made clear in the department's request to the Institute of Medicine for a $1.3 million study to review how PTSD is diagnosed and treated. Among other things, the department asked the institute — a branch of the National Academies chartered by Congress to advise the government on science policy — to review the American Psychiatric Association's criteria for diagnosing PTSD. Effectively, Scott said, Veterans Affairs was trying to get one scientific organization to second-guess another.

RELATED: Associated Press spreading RUMORs about PTSD fakers

As I will discuss, the witch-hunt that resulted was largely a failure, but the fall-out from the stigma that resulted is still present and affecting many veterans seeking PTSD benefits. Still, VA psychologist hold secret website forums instructing these professionals on how to game the system.

RELATED: Clandestined C&P Examiner Website Exposed

The Keith Roberts Story

The Roberts story is the strangest I have ever come across. And, the despicable lengths to which VA went to support a case against him after he embarrassed the agency is a blemish on the credibility of our country

RELATED: Jailed Wisconsin Veteran Case Gets More Bizarre

In 1999, Roberts was diagnosed with PTSD because of his involvement in traumatic event. While in the Navy, Roberts was involved in a failed attempt to save a fellow Navy Airman who was crushed to death by a C-54. One witness corroborated the event.

In 2002, Roberts following the instruction of his veteran service officer to file for PTSD with a better retroactive date. By 2003, Roberts became convinced VA was engaged in fraudulent manipulation of his claims file. He further became knowing as a "belligerent ass" by VA employees while pushing them to follow the law.

As previously mentioned, in 2005, VA began a witch-hunt scheme that was little more than a failed attempt to accuse PTSD veterans of defrauding the government with malingering PTSD symptoms. Only 12 veterans out of the more than 2,000 investigated actually supported the criteria for malingering.

But that did not stop VA from pushing prosecution of some PTSD veterans by either wrongfully labeling them as frauds, withholding benefits, or putting some veterans in prison while the VA Board of Veterans Appeals wrongly supported poorly supported benefits denials.

For Roberts, the prosecution for wire fraud was based on thin evidence primarily supported by an incorrect denial of a better PTSD retroactive date. The agency claimed Roberts inflated his involvement in saving the Navy Airman and went on to erroneously claim Roberts received back benefits to which he was not entitled.

Making matters really squirrely, the Department of Justice proceeded to use the denial of benefits from the Board as support for its claim that Roberts committed wire fraud.

Think this through for a second. Veterans Affairs was engaged in a witch hunt to show veterans commit fraud on a regular basis when seeking PTSD claims. Roberts blows the whistle on VA for manipulating evidence – an act that would result in a veteran's benefits being fraudulently withheld.

Instead of going after the agency in the many instances of evidence destruction, the Department of Justice went after the lowly veteran because he pissed off the wrong people.

How is that for justice?

In 2010, the US Court of Appeals for Veterans Claims (CAVC) reversed the Board's decision. In so doing, it corrected the enormous evidentiary error perpetrated by the Board that was erroneously relied on in Wisconsin for Roberts conviction of wire fraud.

How can you commit wire fraud if you were actually entitled to the benefits you received based on a correct decision based on the evidence on hand?

You simply cannot.

And how does our great country reply to the grievance Roberts has against it for wrongfully imprisoning him?

f 🐦 g+ in ✉

Disabled Veterans

Redeeming The Promise Of A Square Deal

Home

Articles

About

Voc Rehab Guide

Share Your Story

Contact

On remand, the Board of Veterans Appeals has withheld its decision. The decision was rendered in 2010 and Roberts was exonerated.

So how is it that the Board can refuse to reverse its decision? How long can we expect Roberts to wait for justice?

His attorney Robert Walsh believes internal VA Board of Veterans Appeals corruption exposed by another whistleblower last year is at the core of the unlawful behavior.

Corruption at Board of Veterans Appeals

According to whistleblower Kelli Kordich, high ranking attorneys at the board created its own wait list scandal by changing tracking dates to make it appear Board attorneys had better performance numbers than otherwise. Those numbers supported bonuses and promotion for heads at the Board who were engaged in or actively supported the fraud.

The following excerpt is from Stars & Strips

> " Mirroring a scandal that engulfed its health care system, VA managers handling disability benefit appeals also manipulated records to hide overly long delays in deciding cases, an agency whistleblower testified Wednesday on Capitol Hill.
>
> The chairman and head office staff of the Board of Veterans' Appeals shifted cases in a tracking system in 2012 to wipe evidence it had held some for months, and over a year in at least one case, Kelli Kordich, an attorney with the board, told a House Veterans Affairs subcommittee.

f 𝕏 8+ in ✉

Disabled Veterans

Redeeming The Promise Of A Square Deal

- Home
- Articles
- About
- Voc Rehab Guide
- Share Your Story
- Contact

The sworn testimony sparked concerns among lawmakers that the systematic practice of doctoring electronic records at hundreds of VA hospitals and clinics to disguise long wait times may have spread to other areas of the sprawling federal agency.

The Board of Veterans' Appeals, which now has 280,000 pending appeals cases, said the incidents happened two years ago and were quickly fixed.

Kordich said a VA union sent a letter to former VA Secretary Eric Shinseki in June 2012 notifying him that board staff were unnecessarily delaying appeals. Veteran cases ranged from 120 to 415 days old, including five cases held personally by the board's principal deputy vice chairman.

"Most of the cases involved decisions on appeals of waiting veterans that already had been prepared by board attorneys and were simply awaiting the signature" of the head office staff, she said.

When the board became aware of the complaint to Shinseki, top staff members entered the electronic case tracking system and reassigned the old cases to new attorneys, Kordich said.

"This had the effect of resetting the calculation of how many days the appeal had languished in one location," Kordich said.

Mandated Report VA to CDC - Matteoli

U.S. Department of Justice

Civil Rights Division

[illegible]

Notice of Referral of Complaint for Appropriate Action

To: Ms. Catherine Mitrano
Deputy Assistant Secretary
For Resolution Management (08)
Department of Veterans Affairs
810 Vermont Avenue, N.W.
Washington, D.C. 20420

APR 15 2015

REDACTED

From: Disability Rights Section, Civil Rights Division, U.S. Department of Justice

Reference: **CTS# 510975; regarding Veterans Affairs, Oakland, CA; received by DOJ on December 22, 2014** RE: RECEIVED: VAOIG-CRIMINAL DIVISION: OAKLAND, CA

The Disability Rights Section has reviewed the enclosed complaint and determined that it raises issues that are more appropriately addressed by the U.S. Department of Veterans Affairs. We, therefore, are referring this complaint to that agency for appropriate action. This letter serves to notify that agency and the complainant of this referral. The Disability Rights Section will take no further action on this matter.

To check the status of the complaint, or to submit additional information, the complainant may contact the referral agency at the address above or at the following telephone number(s):

(202) 501-2800

If the agency has any questions or concerns about this referral or believes that it raises issues outside the agency's jurisdiction, please do not hesitate to contact the Department of Justice at the address and phone number attached hereto.

DJ# 202-11-0

Mandated Report VA to CDC - Matteoli

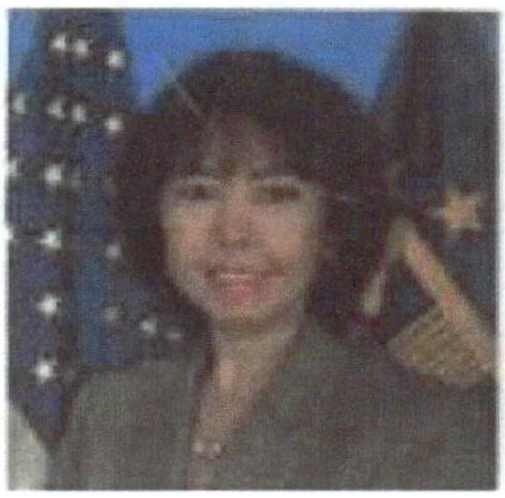

Catherine Mitrano

Deputy Assistant Secretary for Resolution Management at Department of Veterans Affairs

Washington D.C. Metro Area | Military

Previous	US Army, Federal Communications Commission, DHS
Education	Boston University
Recommendations	2 people have recommended Catherine
Websites	ARBA

Experience

Deputy Assistant Secretary for Resolution Management
Department of Veterans Affairs
July 2013 – Present (2 years 3 months) | Washington, DC

Deputy Assistant Secretary
US Army
July 2009 – July 2013 (4 years 1 month)

Deputy Associate General Counsel
Federal Communications Commission
2006 – 2007 (1 year)

Senior Counsel to the General Counsel
DHS
2003 – 2006 (3 years)

Attorney
U.S. Coast Guard
1999 – 2002 (3 years)

Attorney
Federal Aviation Administration
1991 – 1999 (8 years)

Mandated Report VA to CDC - Matteoli

PRITZ NAVARATNASINGAM: FROM BVA OAKLAND

U.S. Department of Veterans Affairs

Health | Benefits | Burials & Memorials | About VA | Resources | News Room | Locations | Contact Us

I AM A:

Benefits
Seattle Home
Visitor Information
Directions and Maps
Other VA Facilities
Applying for Benefits
Operating Status
About Us
Media and Publications

CONNECT WITH BENEFITS

Seattle Regional Benefit Office

Meet Our Leadership Team

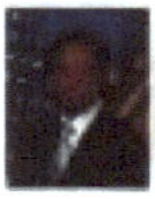

Director: Pritz Navaratnasingam

As Director of the Seattle Regional Office (RO), Pritz Navaratnasingam oversees [illegible] full-time employees and administers benefits and services totaling about $1.5 billion a year to the estimated [illegible] Veterans, Servicemembers, their families and survivors in Washington. Prior to this position, Mr. Navaratnasingam was Director of the Houston and Providence Regional Benefits Offices.

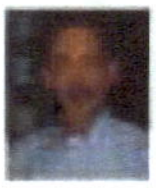

Assistant Director: Bill Borom

Bill Borom took this position in September 2008. Prior to this assignment, he served two years as Deputy Director of VA's Vocational Rehabilitation and Employment (VR&E) Service in Washington, D.C.

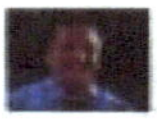

Assistant Director: Andrew Graf

Andrew was appointed in February 2015. Prior to this assignment, he served in numerous roles in VBA's Washington, D.C. Central Office, most recently as the Deputy Director of VA's Operations Analysis team that developed and executed VBA's monthly Performance Stat. Andrew started his VA career in the Milwaukee, WI Regional Office and was selected as first VA civilian to attend the U.S. Army's School for Advanced Military Studies.

Veterans Service Center Manager: Ayn-Marie Lofgren

Ayn-Marie Lofgren was appointed to this position in April of 2014. Prior to this position she was the Veterans Service Center Manager (VSCM) of the Des Moines Regional Office. Prior to her position at the Des Moines Regional Office, she served as the Assistant Veterans Service Center Manager at the St. Paul Regional Office, and as a member of the Training Staff at VA Central Office (VACO) in Washington DC. She began her VA career in February of 2004 at the Lincoln VA Regional Office (VARO).

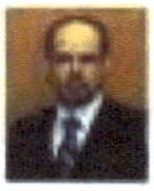

Special Mission Project Officer - Disability Rating Activity Site: Michael Crouse

Michael Crouse took this position in October 2013. Prior to this position, he was Veterans Service Center Manager (VSCM) of the Seattle Regional Office. Prior to this, he was the Assistant Veterans Service Center Manager at the Lincoln RO. Prior to joining VA, Mr. Crouse served 23 years with the U.S. Army, where he held numerous leadership and staff positions.

ALSO
1) RICKY YOUNG, BVA OAKLAND, FINANCE DIRECTOR
2) POSSIBLE AKA RICKIE YOUNG, ATLANTA, TOMBSTONE ACQUISITION AS LAST KNOWN POSITION

LOCATOR | CONTACT | SEARCH

U.S. Department of Veterans Affairs (http://www.va.gov)

MENU

VA (http://www.va.gov/) » Office of Public Affairs (/OPA/index.asp) » Leigh A. Bradley

Office of Public Affairs

Leigh A. Bradley

General Counsel U.S. Department of Veterans Affairs

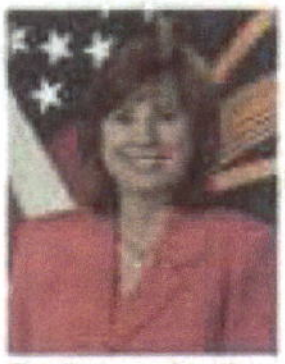

Leigh A. Bradley was sworn in as VA's General Counsel on December 18, 2014. Ms. Bradley previously served as the VA General Counsel from 1998-2001.

Prior to her appointment as VA General Counsel, Ms. Bradley served as the Director, Department of Defense Standards of Conduct Office, where she was responsible for the Defense Department's ethics program and policies. She has previously served in a variety of legal and policy positions in the Federal Government and the private sector. She served as the Chief Risk Officer of the American Red Cross where she oversaw the ethics, compliance, and risk management activities of one of the largest nonprofit organizations in the country. Immediately prior to that, Ms. Bradley was a partner at Holland & Knight LLP, specializing in federal procurement law matters.

Ms. Bradley has previously held a variety of legal positions in the Federal Government. From 1994-1998, she was the Principal Deputy General Counsel of the Navy. From 1987-1994, she was a senior attorney in the DoD Office of the Deputy General Counsel (Personnel & Health Policy), where she was responsible for an array of legal issues.

Before joining the DoD General Counsel's office, Ms. Bradley served for five years on active duty as an Air Force judge advocate, focused primarily on military justice matters. As a Reservist, she taught trial advocacy at the Air Force JAG School.

Office of Public Affairs

Gina S. Farrisee

Assistant Secretary Human Resources & Administration

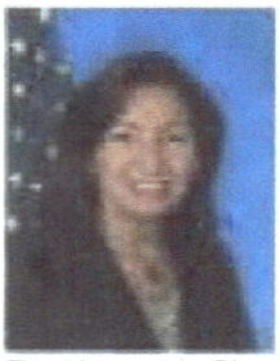

The Honorable Gina S. Farrisee assumed the duties of the Assistant Secretary, Office of Human Resources and Administration (HR&A) at the Department of Veterans Affairs (VA) on September 10, 2013. Prior to that, she served as VA's Deputy Assistant Secretary for Human Resources Management. Ms. Farrisee directs and oversees an HR&A team of over 750 employees who support more than 300,000 VA employees and 4,000 human resources professionals across the country. To meet the needs of the VA workforce, the HR&A team provides professional assistance in the areas of Administration, Human Resources Management, Diversity and Inclusion, Resolution Management, Labor-Management Relations, Human Capital Investment Plan Strategic Management, Veterans Employment Service, and Corporate Senior Executive Management. In addition, HR&A provides training through the VA Learning University.

Ms. Farrisee has a distinguished career as a leader in human resources management. Previously, Ms. Farrisee served as the Commanding General of the United States Army Human Resources Command (HRC), Fort Knox, Kentucky. In this capacity, she provided leadership, operational and managerial oversight of more than 4,000 HRC employees (military, civilian, contractors) with a $3 billion annual budget, which provided worldwide Human Resource services to a customer base of over 1 million people composed of Active and Reserve Soldiers, Veterans and family members including but not limited to human capital management, professional development, Casualty and Mortuary Affairs, promotion boards, freedom of information requests, Department of Army awards and personnel systems. She led the Command in managing a complex, high-volume customer service and geographically dispersed service delivery network.

LOCATOR CONTACT SEARCH

U.S. Department of Veterans Affairs (http://www.va.gov/)

MENU

VA (http://www.va.gov/) » Office of Public Affairs (/OPA/index.asp) » LaVerne H. Council

Office of Public Affairs

LaVerne H. Council

Assistant Secretary for Information and Technology and Chief Information Officer, Office of Information and Technology

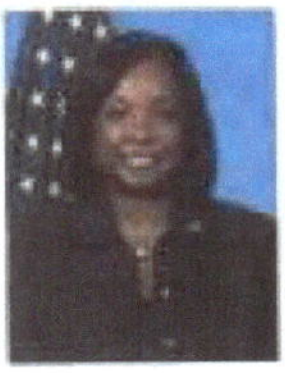

Ms. LaVerne H. Council joined the Department of Veterans Affairs in July 2015 as the Assistant Secretary for Information and Technology (OI&T) and Chief Information Officer. In this role, Ms. Council oversees the day-to-day activities of VA's $4 billion IT budget and over 8,000 IT employees to ensure that VA has the IT tools and services needed to support our Nation's Veterans.

Prior to joining VA, Ms. Council served as CEO of Council Advisory Services, LLC and Chair of the National Board of Trustees for the March of Dimes. In December 2011, she retired from Johnson & Johnson after serving as Corporate Vice President and Chief Information Officer for Johnson & Johnson's global Information Technology group. In this capacity, she was responsible for managing information technology and related systems for the $61.6B Johnson & Johnson worldwide enterprise. She was a Member of the Corporate Global Operating Committee and her organization included more than 250 operating companies with over 4,000 information technology employees and 7,000 contractors.

Ms. Council is a proven visionary senior executive with global experience in the development and execution of cutting-edge information technology and supply chain strategies in the healthcare/life sciences, consumer products and telecommunications/hi-tech industries. In 2011, Ms. Council received the Alumni Business Achievement Award from Ernst & Young. Business Trends Quarterly named her as one of the top four CIOs in America in 2010. The New Jersey Technology Council inducted her into their CIO Hall of Fame in 2009, and the Global CIO Executive Summit named her a Top 10 Leader and Change Agent in 2009 and a Top 10 Leader and Innovator in 2008.

CAREER CHRONOLOGY:

2015 – Present Assistant Secretary, Information and Technology, Department of Veterans Affairs 2012 – 2015 CEO, Council Advisory Services, LLC

Mandated Report VA to CDC - Matteoli

Ask Vetsfirst

- Home
- Submit a Request
- Check on a Request

- Knowledge Books
  - Veterans Guide to VA Benefits
  - Veterans VA Healthcare Guide
  - VA Compensation or Pension Advance Guide
  - Veterans Laws Unique Aspects and Implications
  - VA Claim Guidance
  - Veterans Employment and Education
  - VA Commonly Used Forms
  - Veterans How To Ask VetsFirst
  - VA Facilities Locator
  - VA Acronyms & Terms
  - VA Spinal Cord Injury System

Home → VA Acronyms & Terms → Acronyms and Terms Used in VA Benefits Claims & Appeals → **VA Acronyms and Terms**

1.1. VA Acronyms and Terms

Much like the Department of Defense (DOD), the United States Department of Veterans Affairs (VA) uses many acronyms in the handling of claims and appeals for VA benefits. The following is a sampling of some of the acronyms that a claimant or appellant may see in various military and VA records and documents.

9	VA Form 9, Appeal to the Board of Veterans' Appeals
10-10EZ	VA Form 10-10EZ, Application for Health Benefits
10-10EZR	VA Form 10-10EZR, Health Benefits Renewal Form
10-10EC	VA Form 10-10EC, Application for Extended Care Services
1151 Claim	A claim for benefits under 38 U.S.C. Section 1151 as a result of injury caused by VA treatment or rehabilitation services similar to a medical malpractice claim.
A&A	Aid and attendance
AAO	Assistant adjudication officer
ABCMR	Army Board for Correction of Military Records
ACAP	Annual clothing allowance payment
ADA	Americans with Disabilities Act
ADHC	Adult day health care
ADL	Activities of daily living
ADT	Active duty for training
AFB	Air Force Base
AFBCMR	Air Force Board for Correction of Military Records
AFHRA	Air Force Historical Research Agency
AFI	Air Force instruction
AFIP	Armed Forces Institute of Pathology

Mandated Report VA to CDC - Matteoli

CHAMPUS	Department of Defense Civilian Health and Medical Program of the Uniformed Service
CHAMPVA	Civilian Health and Medical Program of the Department of Veterans Affairs
CHR	Consolidated health record
CIB	Combat Infantryman Badge
Claim Number	Each claimant is assigned an unique VA claim number that VA uses to identify that claimant for life. Claimants should put their claim number on each document and correspondence sent to VA.
CLC	VA Community Living Center (formerly VA Nursing Home Care Units)
CLL	Chronic lymphocytic leukemia
CMB	Combat Medical Badge
CMD	Chief Medical Director
CMO	Chief Medical Officer
CNHC	Community nursing home care
CO	VA Central Office or commanding officer
COD	Character of discharge
COG	Convenience of the government
COLA	Cost-of-living adjustment
Compensation	A monetary benefit awarded based on the degree of disability caused by a service-connected condition.
CONUS	The contiguous United States
COVA	Court of Veterans Appeals (Renamed Court of Appeals for Veterans Claims)
COWC	Committee on Waivers and Compromises
CPI	Claims Processing Improvement
CRC	Community residential center
CRDP	Concurrent retirement and disability pay
CRSC	Combat-related special compensation
CUE	Clear and unmistakable error
CURR	Center for Units Records Research
CWT	VA Compensated Work Therapy Program
DAV	Disabled American Veterans
DBQ	Disability Benefits Questionnaire
DC	Diagnostic code
DD	Dishonorable discharge
DD-214	Discharge certificate
DDD	Degenerative disc disease
DEA	Dependent's educational assistance
DES	Disability evaluation system
DFAS	Defense Finance and Accounting Services
DFR	Dropped from the rolls
DIC	Death & Indemnity Compensation. A benefit awarded to surviving spouses and qualifying dependents when a service-connected condition is a cause of a veteran's death.
DM	Diabetes mellitus
DMZ	Demilitarized zone
DOD	Department of Defense
DRB	Discharge Review Board
DRO	Decision Review Officer. Usually an experienced member of a regional office rating team who reviews a rating decision at the request of the claimant after an

Mandated Report VA to CDC - Matteoli

	initial denial. DRO review is optional and cannot change decisions favorable to a claimant.
DSM	American Psychiatric Association's Diagnostic and Statistical Manual for Mental Disorders
DSO	Department service officer
DTR	Deep tendon reflexes
DVA	The Department of Veterans Affairs. A technically more accurate acronym than "VA," although not as widely used.
EAD	Entry on active duty
EAJA	Equal Access to Justice Act
eBenefits	VA online portal that allows veterans to manage their benefits and personal information.
ECA	Expedited Claims Adjudication Initiative
ED	Erectile dysfunction
EGC	Electrocardiogram
EKG	Electrocardiogram
EOB	Explanation of benefits
EOD	Entry on Duty or Explosive Ordinance Disposal
EVR	Eligibility verification report
FDC	Fully Developed Claim
Federal Circuit	The United States Court of Appeals for the Federal Circuit. The federal appellate court to which claimants and VA can appeal Veteran Court decisions.
FOIA	Freedom of Information Act
Form 9	The VA form that must be submitted after receipt of a Statement of the Case to perfect an appeal to the Board of Veserans Appeals.
FTCA	Federal Tort Claims Act
GAO	Government Accounting Office
GC	General counsel
GPO	Government Printing Office
GSW	Gun shot wound
GWS	Gulf war syndrome
HB	Housebound
HIPAA	Health Insurance Portability and Accountability Act
HISA	Home improvement and structural alterations
HIV	Human immunodeficiency virus
HO	Hearing officer
IED	Improvised explosive device
IG	Inspector general
IME	Independent medical expert or independent medical evaluation
INC	Incurred in service
IOM	Institute of Medicine
IOP	Internal operating procedures
IRIS	Inquiry Routing and Information System
IU	Individual unemployability
IVAP	Income for VA purposes
JAG	Judge Advocate General
JMR	Joint motion for remand
JSRRC	Joint Services Records Research Center
LOD	Line of duty

LOM	Limitation of motion
LSW	Licensed social worker
M21-1MR	Adjudication Procedures Manual Rewrite
M-1	VA Healthcare Adjudication Manual
M-21	VA Claims Adjudication Manual
MACR	Missing air crew reports
MAPR	Maximum annual pension rate
MGIB	Montgomery GI Bill
MIB	Marine index bureau
MOS	Military occupational specialty
MPR	Military personnel records
MRI	Magnetic resonance imaging
MST	Military Sexual Trauma
NA	National Archives
NARA	National Archives and Record Administration
NAS	National Academy of Sciences
NAUS	National Association for Uniformed Services
NHL	Non-hodgkins lymphoma
NMCB	U.S. Navy Mobile Construction Battalion
NOA	Notice of Appeal
NOD	Notice of Disagreement. Claimants must file a written NOD within one year of receiving a rating decision to be able to appeal that decision.
NOS	Not otherwise specified
NPC	Naval Personnel Command
NPRC	National Personnel Records Center
NRPC	Naval Reserve Personnel Command
NSC	Non-service-connected
NSLI	National Service Life Insurance
NSO	National service officer
NVLSP	National Veterans Legal Services Program
OEF	Operation Enduring Freedom
OGC	Office of the General Counsel
OIF	Operation Iraqi Freedom
OIG	Office of Inspector General
OMPF	Official military personnel file
OPC	Outpatient clinic
OPT	Outpatient treatment
OQP	Office of Quality and Performance
OTH	Other than honorable
PDBR	Physical Disability Board of Review
PDR	Physicians Desk Reference
PEB	Physical Evaluation Board
Pension	A VA benefit based on financial need available to fully disabled veterans who served during a time of war.
PERMS	Permanent Electronic Records Management System
PG	Persian Gulf
PGW	Persian Gulf War
PIES	Personnel Information Exchange System
PIF	Pending issue file

PMC	Pension Maintenance Center
POA	Power of attorney
POW	Prisoner-of-war
PRC	Polytrauma Rehabilitation Center
Presumption	A legal term meaning that no evidence of a nexus between a current medical condition and an in-service occurrence is required. A claimant currently suffer from a "presumptive condition" only needs to establish he or she experienced the specified in-service event to be awarded service connection. See related Knowledge Book.
PT	Physical therapy or permanent total disability
PTE	Peace time era
PTSD	Posttraumatic stress disorder
PEBLO	Physical Evaluation Board Liaison Officer
RAD	Release from active duty
Rating Decision	The initial VA decision on a claim which either grants or denies an award or "continues" the claim for further development.
Rating Schedule	The table of medical conditions and disabilities established by law that VA raters use to determine the degree of disability for compensation purposes.
Remand	Return of a decision to the organization that made it for additional review and revision. The Board remands rating decisions to the originating regional office The Veterans Court remands Board decisions back to the Board.
RMC	Records Management Center
RMO	Records Management Officer
RN	Registered nurse
RO	Regional Office
ROTC	Reserve Officers' Training Corps
RVN	Republic of Vietnam
RVSR	Rating Veterans Service Representative
SBP	Survivor Benefit Plan
SC	Service-connected
SDRP	Special Discharge Review Program
SDVI	Service Disabled Veterans' Insurance
Secretary	The Secretary of Veterans Affairs. The Cabinet officer who is the administrative head of VA.
Service Connection	A requirement that a claimant for VA compensation must (1) have a current medical condition; (2) identify an event or condition during military service; and (3) establish a nexus or connection between the medical condition and the in-service event or condition. Without establishing service connection, VA will not award compensation benefits.
SF	Special forces
SGLI	Servicemembers' Group Life Insurance
SMC	Special Monthly Compensation. Additional compensation available to the most seriously disabled veterans for anatomical loss of limbs or loss of use of body parts, aid and attendance, and other special needs.
SMP	Special monthly pension
SMR	Service medical record
SN	Service number
SOC	Statement of the Case. A document that VA must prepare and provide to a claimant who has submitted a timely Notice of Disagreement. The purpose of an

	SOC is to identify the facts and law VA used to reach the decision(s) with which the claimant disagrees.
SPD	Separation program designator
SPN	Separation program number
SRD	Schedule for Rating Disabilities
SSA	Social Security Administration
SSB	Special separation benefits
SSDI	Social Security Disability Income
SSI	Supplemental Security Income
SSN	Social Security Number
SSOC	Supplemental Statement of the Case
STR	Service treatment records
STS	Soft tissue sarcoma
TAD	Temporary active duty
TBI	Traumatic brain injury
TCDD	2,3,7,8-tetrachlorodibenzodioxin
TDIU	Total Disability based on Individual Unemployability. A special rating that considers whether a claimant who does not meet the rating schedule requirements for 100% disability is still unable to work in a substantially gainful occupation. A TDIU award pays benefits at the 100% scheduler rate even though the actual rating percentage is less than 100%.
TRDL	Temporary disabled retirement list
TDY	Temporary duty
UCMJ	Uniform Code of Military Justice
U.S.C.	United States Code
U.S.C.A.	United States Code Annotated
U.S.C.S.	United States Code Service
USGLI	United States Government Life Insurance
USJSRRC	United States Joint Service Records Research Center
VA	The most commonly used acronym for the Department of Veterans Affairs.
VACO	VA Central Office
VAF	VA form
VAGC	VA General Counsel
VAHAC	VA Health Administration Center
VAMC	VA Medical Center
VAOGC	VA Office of the General Counsel
VAOIG	VA Office of the Inspector General
VAOPC	VA outpatient clinic
VAR	VA regulation
VARO	VA Regional Office
VBA	Veterans Benefits Administration
VCAA	Veterans Claims Assistance Act
VEAP	Post-Vietnam Era Veterans' Educational Assistance Program
Veterans Court	Another common name for the United States Court of Appeals for Veterans Claims. *See also* CAVC.
VFW	Veterans of Foreign Wars
VGLI	Veterans' Group Life Insurance
VHA	Veterans Health Administration
VISN	Veterans Integrated Service Network

Mandated Report VA to CDC - Matteoli

VJRA	Veterans Judicial Review Act
VLJ	Veterans Law Judge. A member of the Board of Veterans' Appeals who hears appeals from claimants who disagree with a rating decision.
VMLI	Veterans' Mortgage Life Insurance
VONAPP	Veterans Online Application. A VA website for electronically applying for VA benefits. https://www.ebenefits.va.gov/ebenefits-portal/ebenefits.portal?_nfpb=true&_nfxr=false&_pageLabel=Vonapp
VRC	Vocational rehabilitation counseling
VSCM	Veterans Service Center Manager
VSM	Vietnam Service Medal
VSO	Veterans service organization
VSR	Veterans Service Representative
WRIISC	War Related Illness and Injury Center

This page was: Helpful | Not Helpful
← I. Acronyms and Terms Used in VA Benefits Claims & Appeals I. Acronyms and Terms Used in VA Benefits Claims & Appeals →

Knowledge Books Search

Help Desk Software by HelpSpot

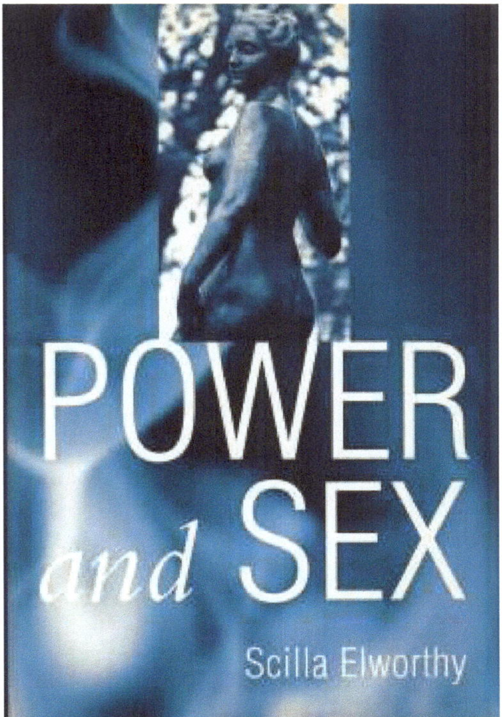
POWER
and SEX
Scilla Elworthy

RITUAL ABUSE
what it is
why it happens
how to help
MARGARET SMITH

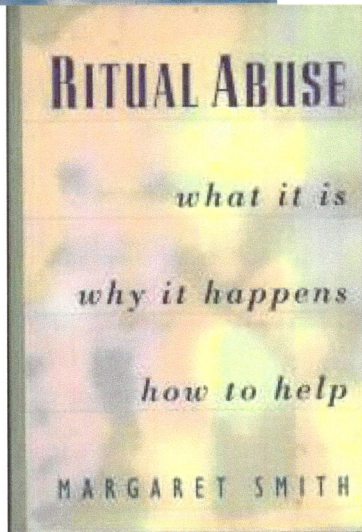

BOVINE and HUMAN SACRIFICES

Menstrual blood is in virtually all mythologies associated with (a) moon and (b0 blood from a wound... With totemism the mother's matrilineal blood and the clan's animal's blood equates as one generational flesh, is divine, and is of god and divine power… The message was clear. In the beginning, women were superior to men.

Chris Knight, *Blood Relations: Menstruation and the Origins of Culture*.

They are willing to have someone else to die for them for their selfish purposes, and that is one of the definitions of sociopathic behavior.

John Douglas with Mark Olshaker, *Mind Hunter*.

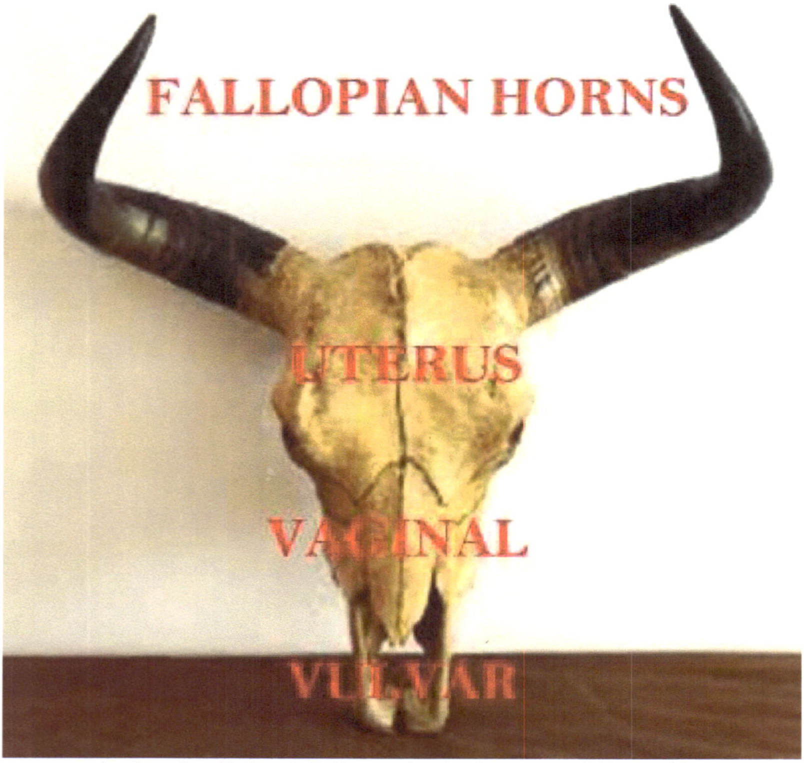

As for the Celestial Cow, she is the sacred Eye of Re.
Egyptian Book of the Dead, *The Papyrus of Ani*.

Taurobolium Bull Sacrifice – Sacrifice of the King

The Taurobolium with the VA rests in functionally penning the Director to non-function until he is sacrificed for the sins of the many.

Scapegoat Sacrifice – Sin Atonement not Redemption

The Scapegoat Sacrifice is a Tannist Sacrifice biblically meaning turning a goat out in the wild to the elements and natural predation. Biblically animals as birds and other animals were used. They were purchased and a pay-off, then life goes on as usual until another payoff is demanded.

Lamb Sacrifice – Sacrifice in either Bonding or Separation

The veteran is a Sacrifice of the Lamb in Separation for a continual Bonding to maintain Bonding of existing criminality and Profit.

Tannist Sacrifice – Substitute Sacrifice

Firing, reprimanding, demoting and any kind of threat and separation of patient is a Tannist Sacrifice to maintain impropriety. Such was the Mesopotamian Substitute King as Heracles when Omphale's Slave

Harvest Sacrifice – Fertility Sacrifice to the Great Mother

1): Taurobolium, Sacrifice of the King, Castration, Circumcision, Bloodletting, all meant for goddess fertilization-glorification.

2): Cretin Bull and Minoan Bull Sacrifices were Sacred Executioners sacrificing other society's Tribute Children instead of their own in vaginal Labyrinth motif to ensure goddess fertility and social abundance in the agricultural and personal abundance.

3): Celtic Wickerman to Mayan Male Prepuce bleeding to fertilize the Great Mother.

4): Female: Yearly during Spring the main Pharaoh wife, the Great Mother Incarnate, as the 7 Cleopatras as Isis incarnate would bleed the throat of a virgin Maiden into the Nile so her blood would bring feminine reproduction to the waters of the Nile with the semen of castrated Osiris whose genitals were eaten by the feminine fish of the social waters in Dark Leviathan Theology.

GENOCIDE

SOCIO-RELIGIOUS INTO VIOLENT EXPANSION

ROBERT LIFTON'S DOULBLING
V.
JANET MENAGE'S CONSTRUCTIVE DISPLACEMENT

The key to understanding how Nazi doctors came to do the work of Auschwitz is the psychological principle I call **doubling**: the division of the self into two functioning wholes, so that a part-self acts as the entire self. An Auschwitz doctor could, through **doubling**, not only kill and contribute to killing but organize silently, on behalf of that evil project, an entire self-structure (or self-process) encompassing virtually all aspects of his behavior.

Constructive Displacement is the psychological ability to cut another's body with the intent and motivation to cure and heal.

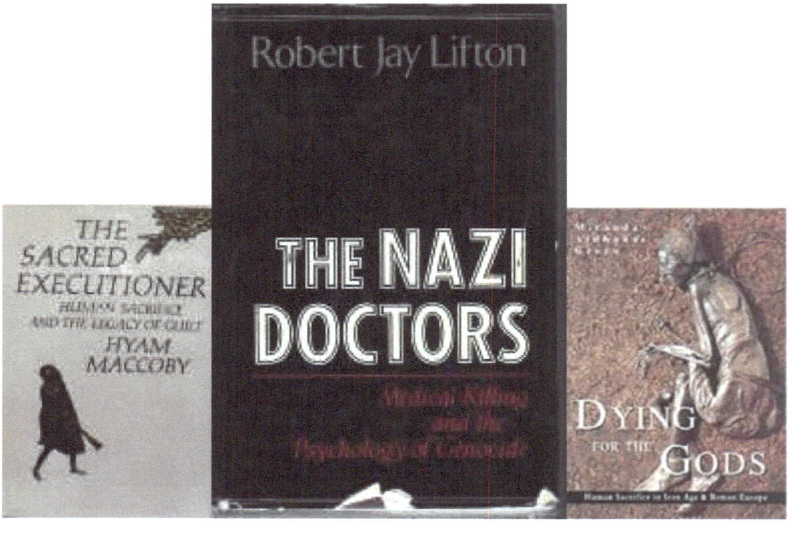

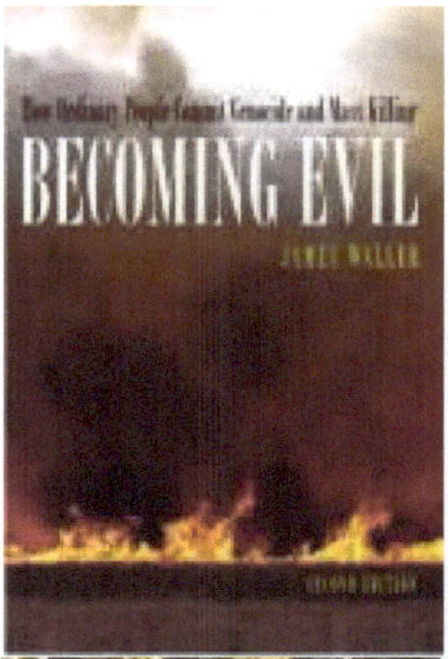
BECOMING EVIL

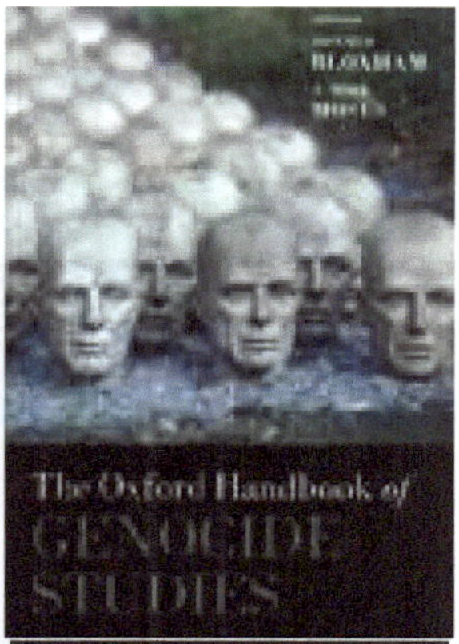
The Oxford Handbook of
GENOCIDE
STUDIES

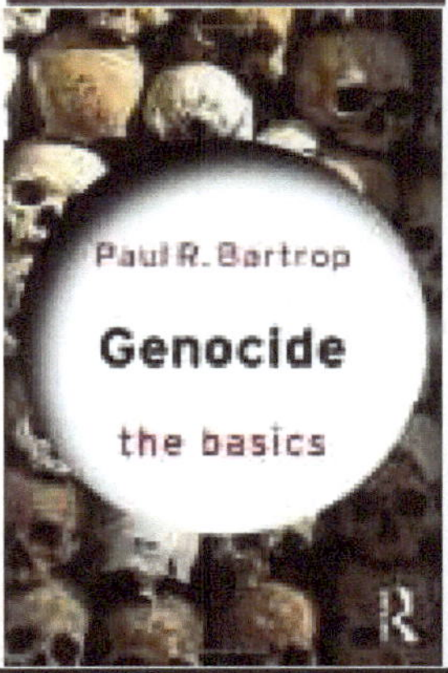
Paul R. Bartrop
Genocide
the basics

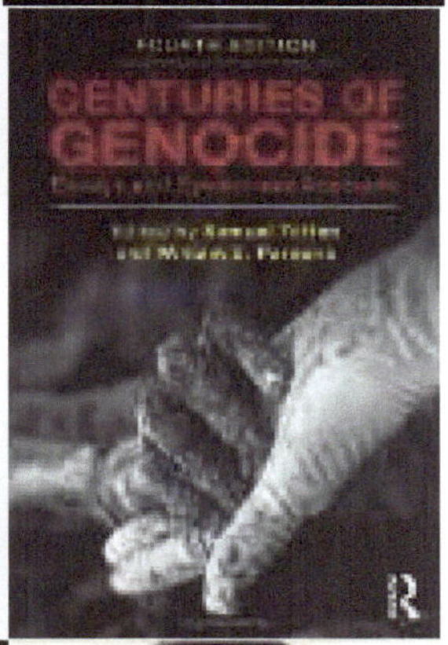
CENTURIES OF
GENOCIDE

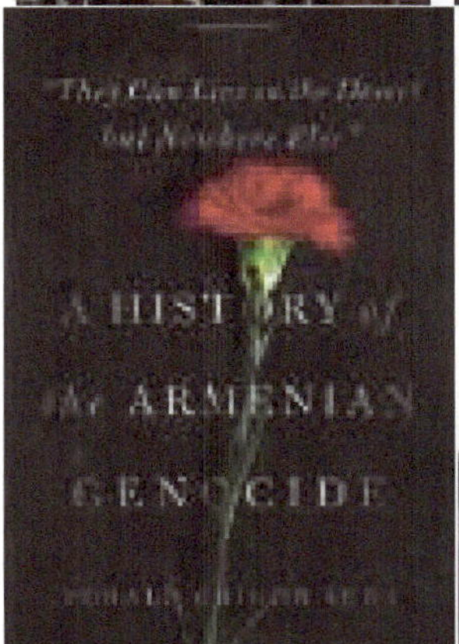
A HISTORY of
the ARMENIAN
GENOCIDE

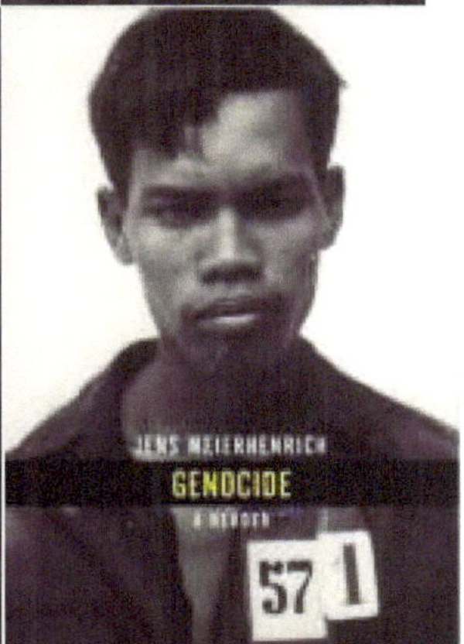
JENS MEIERHENRICH
GENOCIDE

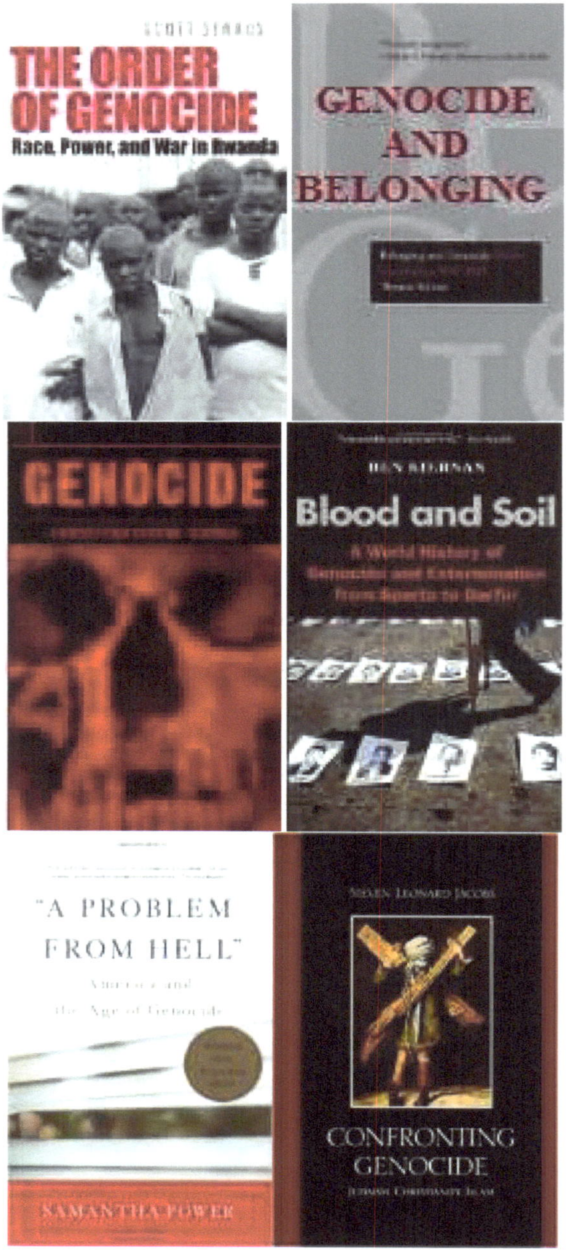
THE ORDER OF GENOCIDE
Race, Power, and War in Rwanda
GENOCIDE AND BELONGING
GENOCIDE
Blood and Soil
"A PROBLEM FROM HELL"
SAMANTHA POWER
CONFRONTING GENOCIDE

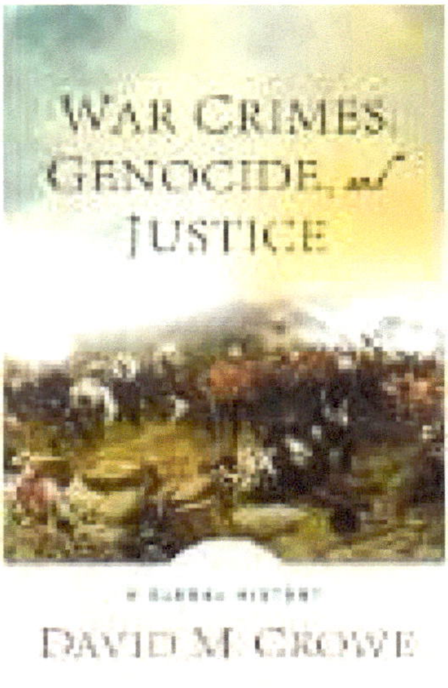
WAR CRIMES, GENOCIDE, and JUSTICE
DAVID M. CROWE

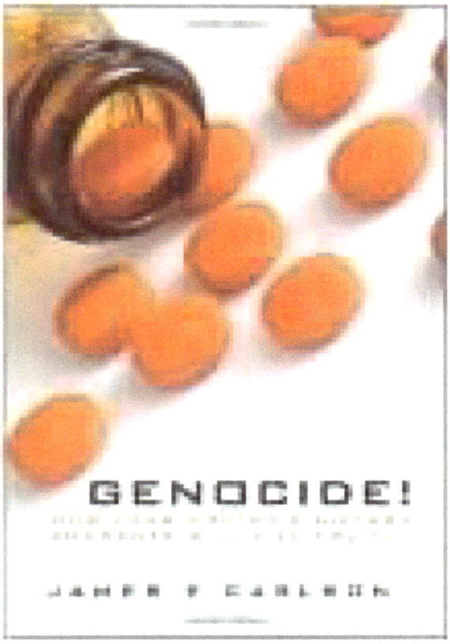
GENOCIDE!

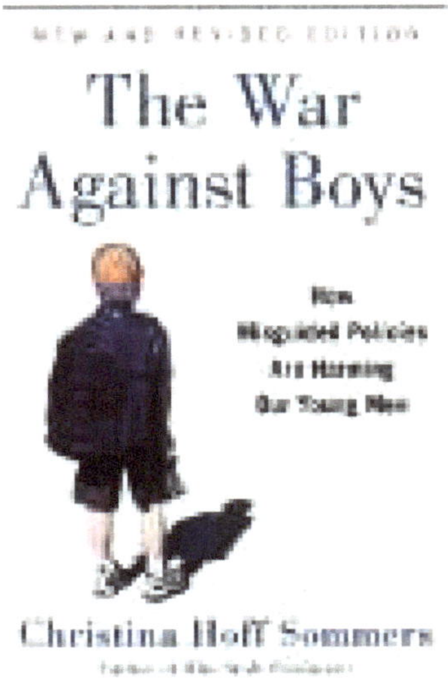
The War Against Boys
How Misguided Policies Are Harming Our Young Men
Christina Hoff Sommers

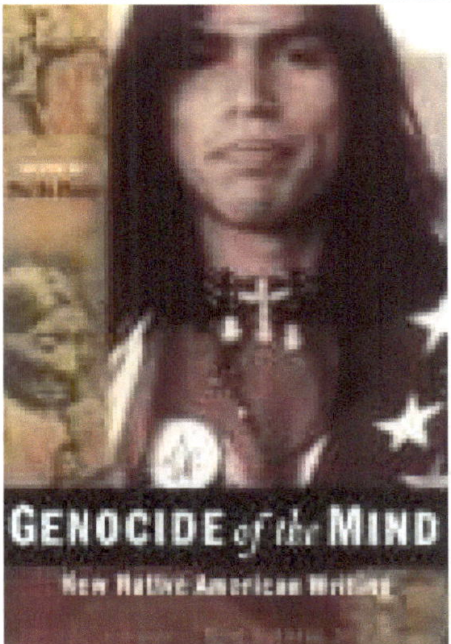
GENOCIDE of the MIND
New Native American Writing

The Nazis based their justification… on the simple concept of "LIFE UNWORTHY OF LIFE" (lebensunwert leben).

If you are going to cure a sickness anything is possible. The image of cure lends itself to the restorative myth of state violence and to the literal enactment of that myth…

In doubling, one part of the self ***disavows*** another part. What is repudiated is not reality itself – the individual Nazi doctor was aware of what he was doing via the Auschwitz self – but the **meaning** of that reality. The Nazi doctor knew that he selected, but did not interpret selections as murder. One level of disavowal, then, was the Auschwitz self's altering of the meaning of **anything** done by the Auschwitz self. Indeed disavowal was the life blood of the Auschwitz self.

Doubling can include elements considered characteristic of **psychopathic character impairment**.

Doubling may well be an important psychological mechanism for individuals living within any **criminal substructure**.

Generally speaking, doubling involves **five** characteristics:

1): A dialectic between two selves in terms of autonomy and connection.

2): Doubling follows a holistic principle. A psychic numbing in dissociation of the two parts of the self as well as toward victims.

3): Doubling has a life-death dimension.

4): Avoidance of guilt; the second self tends to be the one performing the dirty work.

5): Doubling involves both an unconscious dimension – taking place, as stated, largely outside awareness, - and a significant change in moral consciousness.

The SS doctor – deeply involved in the stark contradictions of the **schizophrenic condition… lay in the constructive medical work within a slaughterhouse**.

It becomes an **all-or-nothing matter**, **equally absolute** in its claim to truth and in its **rejection of alternate claims**.

The SS doctor – deeply involved in the stark contradictions of the **schizophrenic condition… lay in the constructive medical work within a slaughterhouse**.

Genocide is a response to collective fear of pollution and defilement… Purification tends to be associated with sacrificial victims, **whether in primitive or contemporary religious or secular terms**. Genocide can be understood as a quest to make sacrificial victims out of an entire people…

Medical materialism can overlay **symbol systems** that closely parallel those of **primitive purification rituals**… As it becomes total – the violent cure draws upon **all facets of the perpetrator's culture**.

The Nazis tapped **mythic relationships between healing and killing** that have had ancient expression in shamanism – (*horticultural by first returning to ancient Norse religion per Joseph Campbell*), religious purification, and human sacrifice, and evoked all three in ways that reveal more about their psychological motivations.

That genocidal threshold requires **prior ideological imagery** of imperative. One has to do this thing, see it through to the end, for the sake of **utopian vision** of national harmony, unity, wholeness.

One is always responsible for Faustian bargains – a responsibility in no way abrogated by the fact that such doubling takes place outside of awareness.

Generally speaking, they were more adept at feathering their own nests than at healing and usually their skill lay in killing rather than healing. Lifton quoting: **Kogon**, *Theory and Practice*, p. 150.

Genocide requires both a specific victim group and certain relationships to that group. ***Robert J. Lifton*** *The Nazi Doctors*

Fascism is not defined by the number of its victims, but by the way it kills them. Jean-Paul Sartre

(http://www.va.gov)

MENU

Office of Public Affairs

Richard J. Griffin

Deputy Inspector General

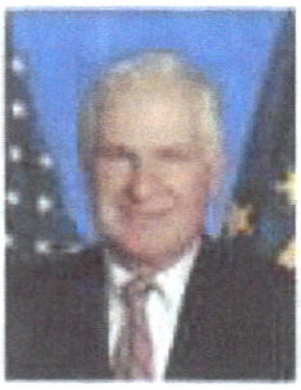

The Honorable Richard J. Griffin was appointed in November 2008 to the position of Deputy Inspector General, Department of VA. He is responsible for directing a nationwide staff of criminal investigators, auditors, health care inspectors, and support personnel. His office conducts independent oversight reviews to improve the economy, efficiency and effectiveness of VA programs, and to prevent and detect criminal activity, waste, abuse, and fraud. He previously served as VA Inspector General, November 1997 to June 2005, having been nominated by President Clinton in September 1997, and confirmed by the United States Senate in November 1997.

Mr. Griffin came to VA from the Department of Housing and Urban Development (HUD), Office of Inspector General, where he was the senior adviser to the Inspector General, March 2008 to November 2008, assisting him in managing all aspects of that organization's audits, inspections, investigations, congressional and public affairs, budget, and strategic planning.

Mr. Griffin was nominated by President George W. Bush in April 2005 and confirmed by the Senate in June 2005 to serve as Assistant Secretary for the Bureau of Diplomatic Security at Department of State, where he led a global workforce of 32,000 security and law enforcement professionals, June 2005 to November 2007. His office was responsible for ensuring the safe and secure conduct of U.S. diplomacy across the world. He concurrently served as Director of the Office of Foreign Missions, with the rank of Ambassador, where he managed reciprocity and immunity issues for foreign diplomats in the U.S.

Mr. Griffin previously served as Deputy Director at the U.S. Secret Service, where he was responsible for planning and directing all investigative, protective and administrative programs. He began his Secret Service career in 1971, as an agent in the Chicago office. Subsequent positions included: Assistant Special Agent in Charge of the Presidential Protective Division; Special Agent in Charge, Los Angeles, California; Deputy Assistant Director in the Office of Investigations; and Assistant Director for Protective Operations.

Mandated Report VA to CDC - Matteoli

During his career, he received a number of special achievement awards: Senior Executive Service Presidential Rank Award of Meritorious Executive in 1994 and 2011; and Exceptional Service Award of the Department of Veterans Affairs in 2005, for performance demonstrating the highest levels of integrity, leadership and executive excellence.

Mr. Griffin earned a bachelor's in economics in 1971, from Xavier University in Cincinnati, Ohio; in 1984, he received a master's in business administration from Marymount University in Arlington, Virginia. In May 2004, he received an honorary doctorate in Humane Letters from Marymount University. He is a 1963 graduate of the National War College.

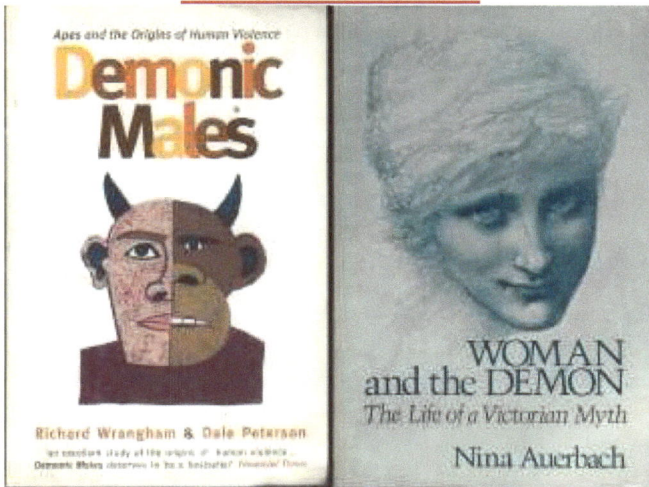

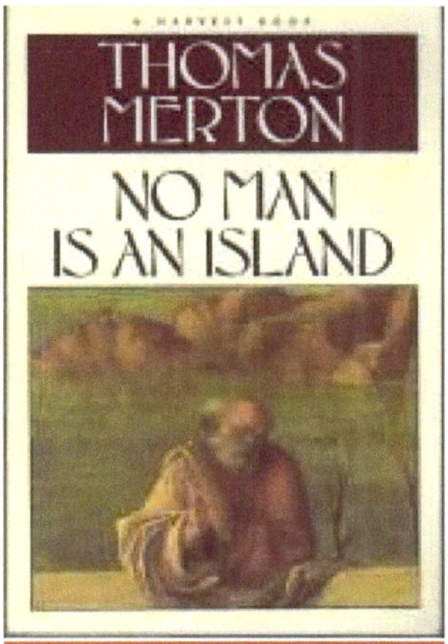

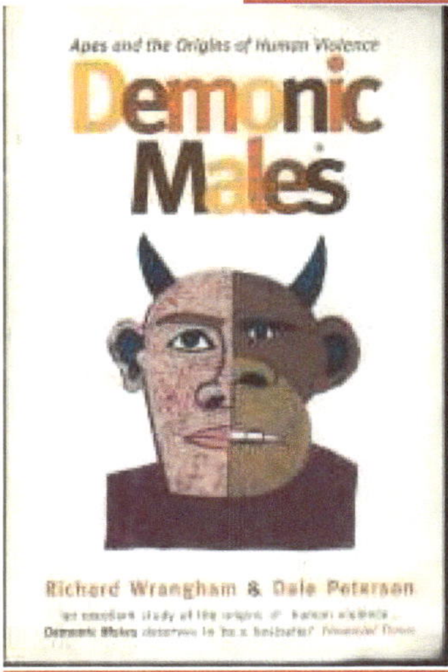

Veterans Affairs Still Has A Subpoena Out For The Names Of VA Whistleblowers

By GPD (http://www.veteranstoday.com/author/admin/) on July 9, 2014

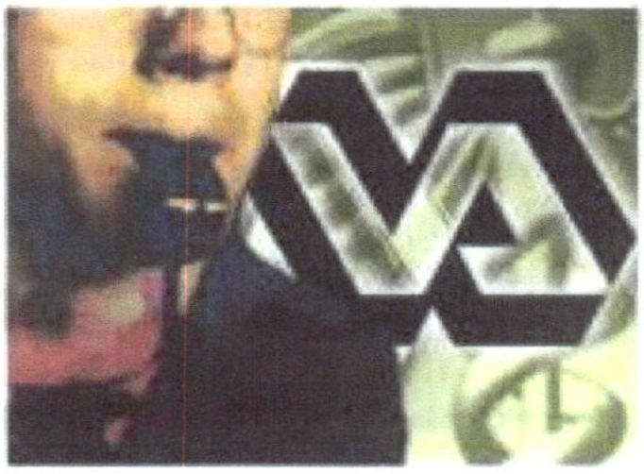

(http://www.veteranstoday.com/2014/07/09/veterans-affairs-still-has-a-subpoena-out-for-the-names-of-va-whistleblowers/va-whistleblower/)WASHINGTON — Former and current VA employees will tell congress at a hearing Tuesday that whistleblowing can entail severe retaliation from superiors at the VA, including reassignment to a windowless basement, separation from family and — in one case — a stress-induced heart attack.

Three VA doctors and a program administrator (http://www.ajc.com/news/news/atlanta-whistleblower to-testify-on-va-scandal/ngXtX/) are set to testify at Tuesday's House Veteran's Affairs Committee hearing (http://veterans.house.gov/hearing/va-whistleblowers-exposing-inadequate-service-provided-to-veterans-and-ensuring-appropriate), specifically focused on whistleblowers. All provided information on what they saw as inept practices inside the VA and say they faced retaliation, includin being placed on leave

The hearing should also provide illumination on the case of the VA's aggressive actions toward an outside veterans group that has called for whistleblowers to come forward.

In May, the Inspector General for the Veteran's Administration issued an extraordinary subpoena (http://washingtonexaminer.com/chilling-message-against-whistleblowers-feared-as-veterans-affairs-ig-presses-subpoena-against-watchdog/article/2549738) demanding a list of anonymous whistleblowers collected through a joint effort launched by the Project For Government Oversight, a watchdog group, and the Iraq and Afghanistan Veterans of America, one of the nation's most vocal advocates for veterans of post-9/11 conflicts. The groups built a special website (http://www.buzzfeed.com/evanmcsan/veterans-group-will-launch-whistleblower-project-after-va-ho) for VA employees and veterans to anonymously report problems with the way the federally-owned hospital network was delivering care to vets.

POGO and IAVA have collected around 800 names through the website and have pledged to keep them secret. The Inspector General's subpoena required POGO to hand them over so federal investigators can look into the claims. In an June letter (http://www.va.gov/OIG/pubs/statements/VA-IG-Response-to-Sen-Coburn-on-POGO.pdf) to members of congress, VA Inspector General Richard Griffin wrote that the subpoena was necessary because Griffin's team can't investigate claims of wrongdoing by IAVA and POGO unless they can independently verify the allegations themselves. Griffin pledged to keep the names secret and warned that unless he was able see the list himself, the complaints gathered by POGO and IAVA were "mere allegations."

CLICK TO READ FULL STORY >>>>> (http://www.buzzfeed.com/evanmcsan/veterans-affairs-still-has-a-subpoena-out-for-the-names-of-v)

The Fuhrer holds the cleansing of the medical profession far more important than, for example, that of the bureaucracy, since in his opinion the duty of the physician is or should be one of racial leadership. ***Martin Borman***

The directives coming from Berlin talk about 'special treatment' more and more often. I'd like to think that's not what you mean. ***Oskar Schindler****, Schindler's List*

It was the duty of these teams to segregate the prisoners of war who were candidates for execution... And to report to the office of the Gestapo. ***K. Lindeau****, Nuremburg Trials*

Hitler not only had the power of commander in chief in a political sense, but was also the highest ranking physician.
Victor von Weizsacker

To live means to kill. ***Ernst Junger***

He has the capacity to veer with every wind, or, stubbornly, to insert himself into some fantastically elaborated and irrational social institution only to perish with it... kill for shadowy ideas more ferociously than other creatures kill for food, then, in a generation or less, forget what bloody dream had oppressed him. ***Loren Eisley***

Not only will you break through the paralyzing difficulties of the time – you will break through time itself... and dare to be barbaric, twice barbaric indeed. ***Thomas Mann***

TWELVE OF THIRTEEN 20TH CENTURY GENOCIDES INVOLVE AGGRESSOR GENITAL DISMEMBERING SOCIETIES: LASTLY INCLUDING RAPE

YOU DECIDE ACADEMICALLY. THAT IS YOUR JOB.

Within USA including VA-CDC in Part

Religious Parochial into Medical Environment

Transgenerational Transmission of Trauma

Aestheticism – Sacred Pain

Fantasies Cemented by Age 16

John Douglas with Mark Olshaker

Paraphilia

Paraphilia is a condition characterized by abnormal sexual desires, typically involving extreme or dangerous activities.

CUTTING CLUB, ACORN SOCIETY, GILGAL SOCIETY

But then instead of doing it for medical purposes it was for killing… It was very much like a medical ceremony… They were so careful to keep the full precision of a medical process – but with the aim of killing. That what was so shocking. Auschwitz prisoner doctor.

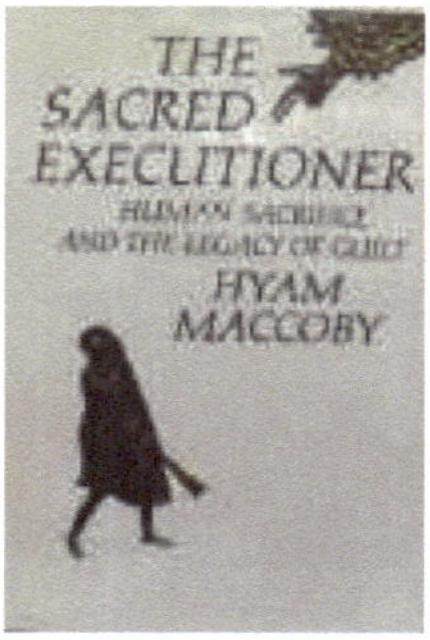

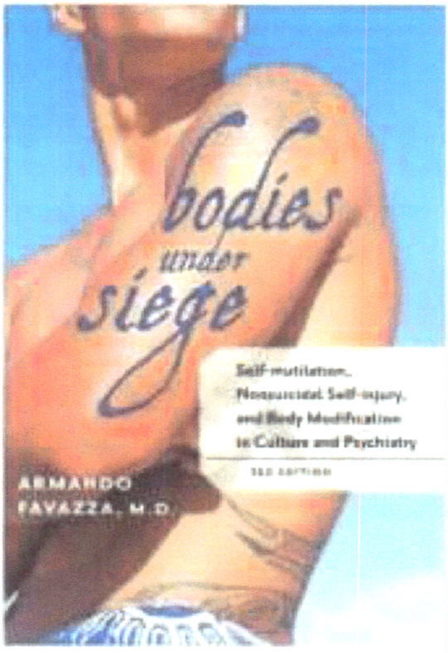

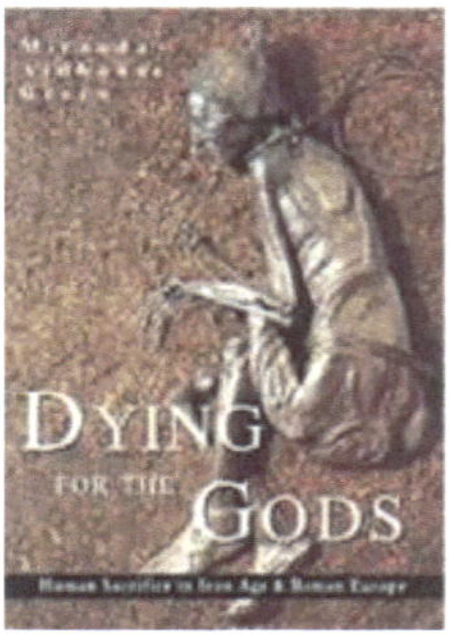

Self-Mortification is not the path to Enlightenment.

***Buddha*. Temple outside Pattaya Beach, Thailand**

Mandated Report VA to CDC - Matteoli

Read Picture Line as a Sentence

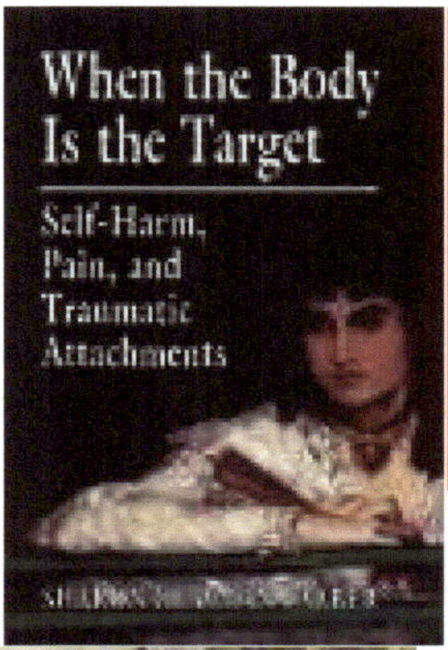

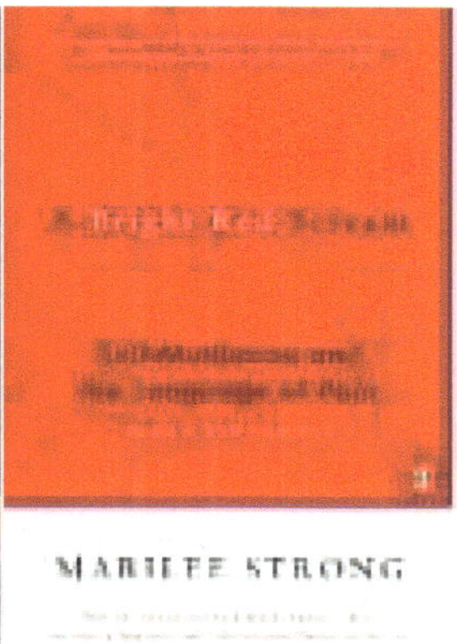

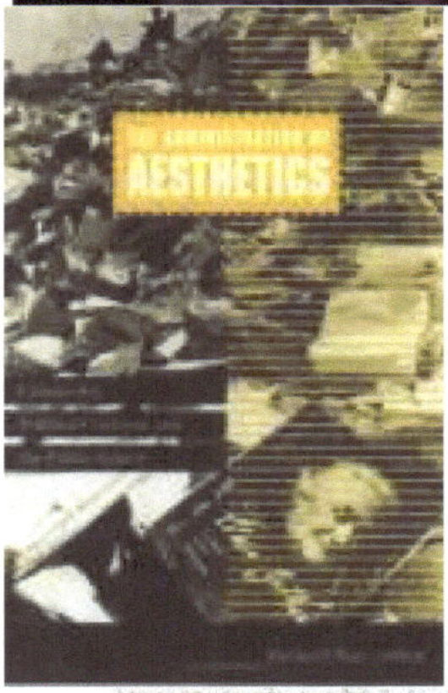

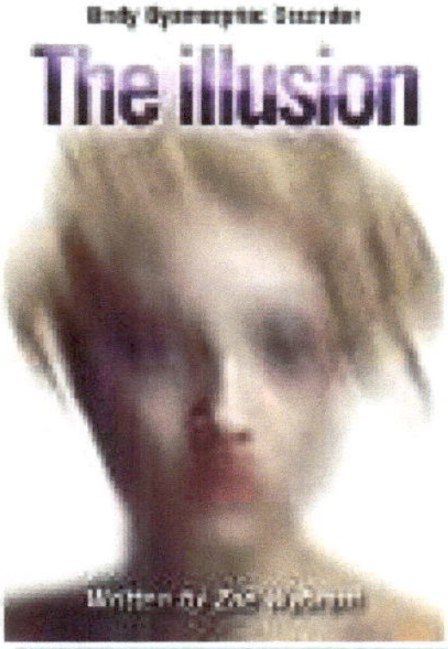

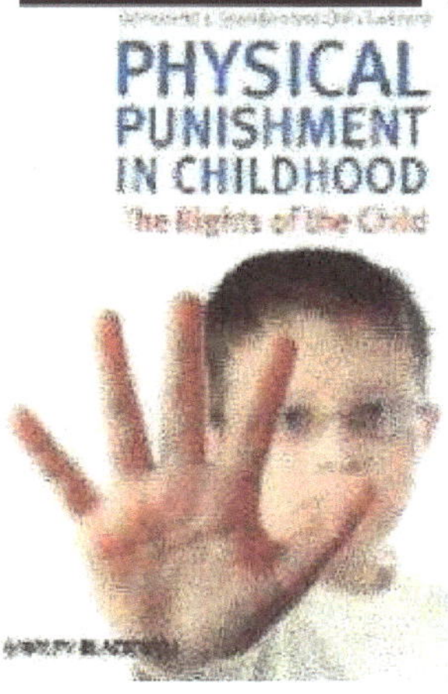

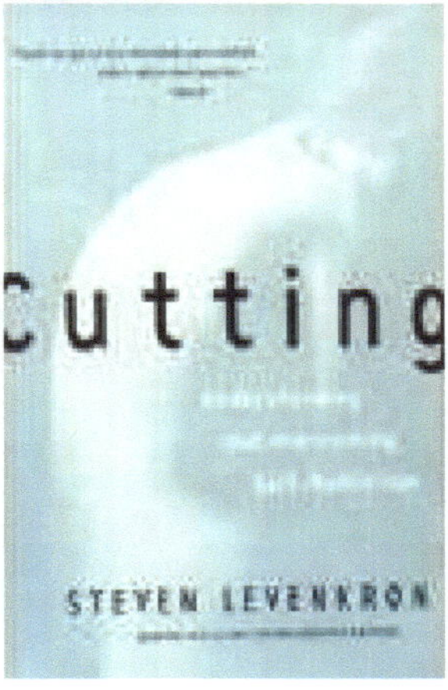

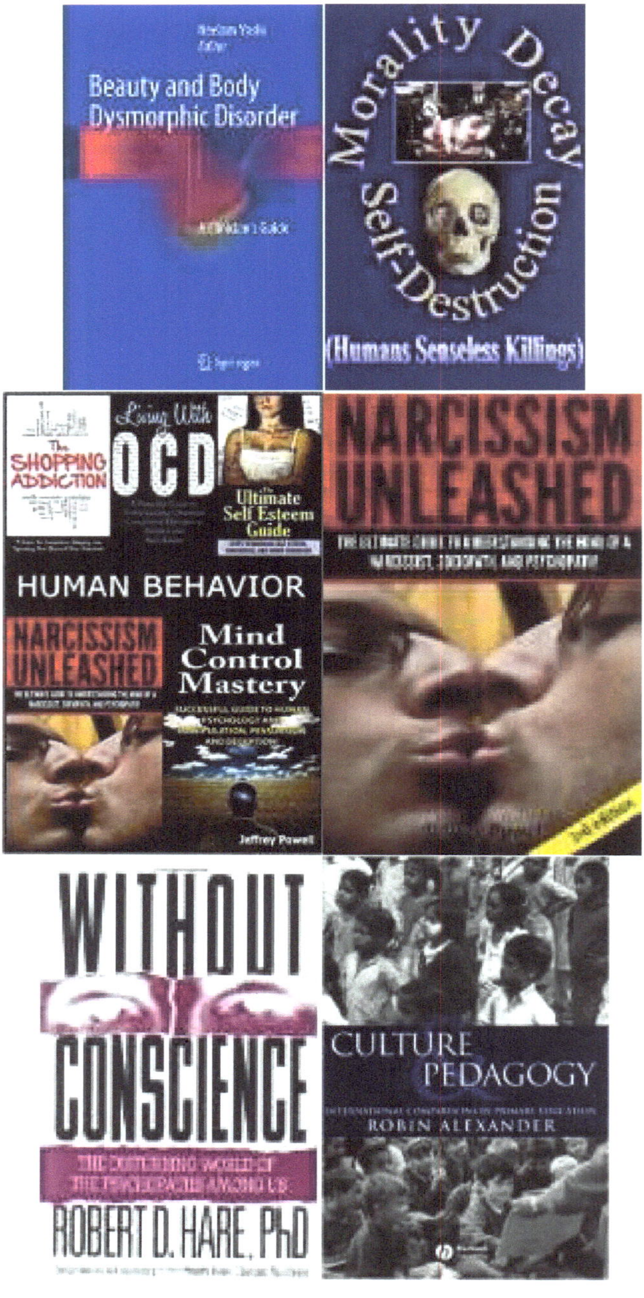
Beauty and Body Dysmorphic Disorder
Morality Decay
Self-Destruction
(Humans Senseless Killings)
The Shopping Addiction
Living With OCD
The Ultimate Self Esteem Guide
HUMAN BEHAVIOR
NARCISSISM UNLEASHED
Mind Control Mastery
Jeffrey Powell
NARCISSISM UNLEASHED
WITHOUT CONSCIENCE
THE DISTURBING WORLD OF THE PSYCHOPATHS AMONG US
ROBERT D. HARE, PhD
CULTURE PEDAGOGY
ROBIN ALEXANDER

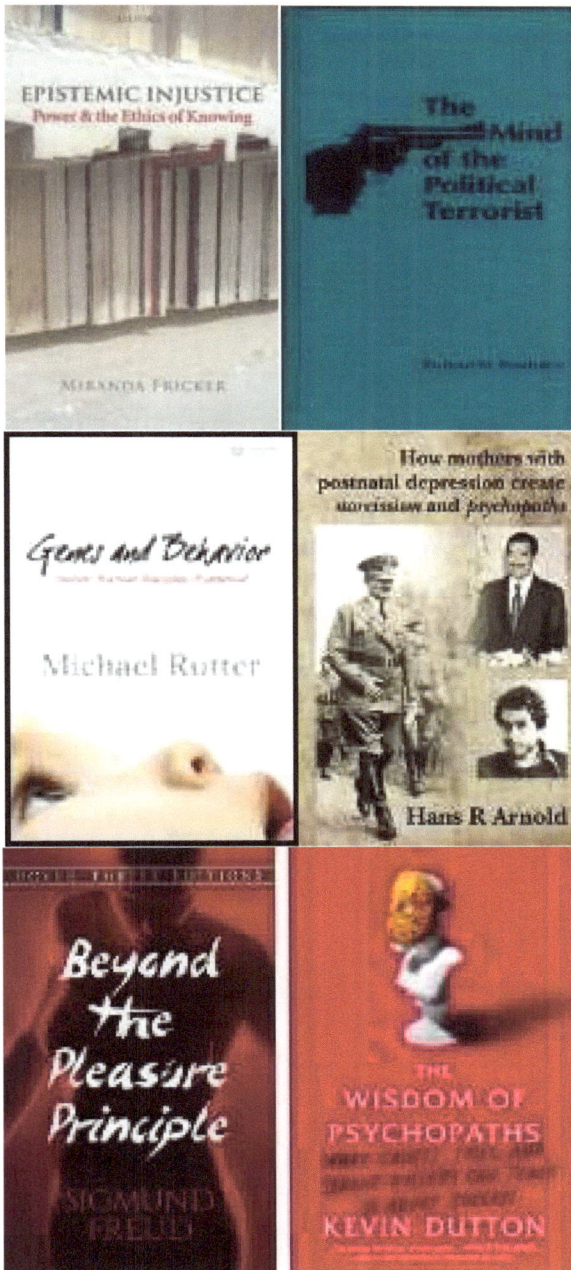

EPISTEMIC INJUSTICE
Power & the Ethics of Knowing
MIRANDA FRICKER

The Mind of the Political Terrorist

Genes and Behavior
Michael Rutter

How mothers with postnatal depression create narcissism and psychopaths
Hans R Arnold

Beyond the Pleasure Principle
SIGMUND FREUD

THE WISDOM OF PSYCHOPATHS
KEVIN DUTTON

UCSF<->VA
Johns Hopkins<->CDC

EXAMPLE BDSM CHILD PORNOGRAPHY FROM YOUTUBE

MANDATED REPORT FILED WITH DOJ

Joke Victim of this Doctor Counseled to Reporting

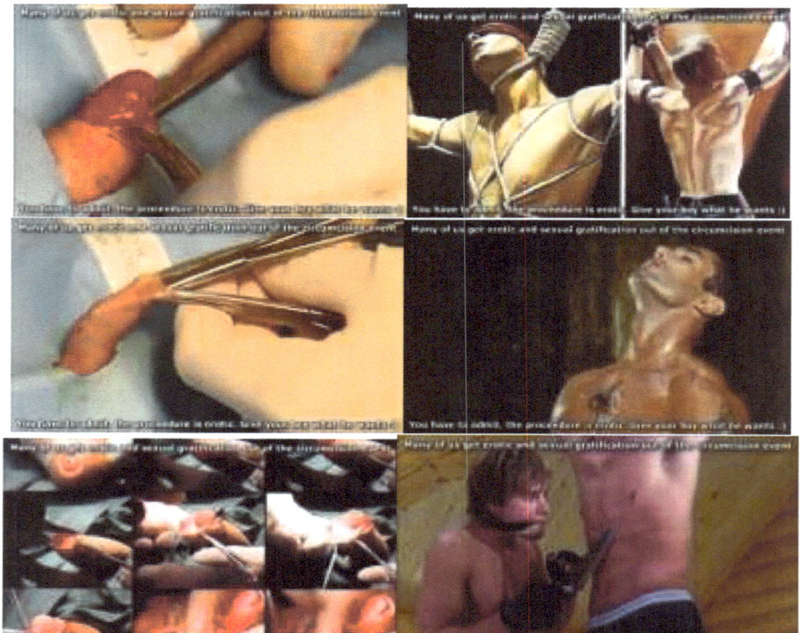

CUTTING CLUB, ACORN SOCIETY, GILGAL SOCIETY, CIRCLIST

FACT *V.* FICTION

THE VA IS A FINE ORGANIZATION THAT IS OVERWHELMED AND TAKEN OVER BY IMPROPRIETY. THE VA MUST BE CORRECTED NOT DESTROYED. PART OF THE VA'S CONCERNS ARE SHARED FROM THE DoD.

SOLUTIONS CAN MAINLY BE OVERCOME BY:
POLICIES, PROCEDURES AND ATTITUDES

THE VA NEEDS RESTRUCTURING WITH DoD:
Take care of Reservists, bring in Local Reserve Assets, Allow Tricare, Sell VA Hospitals for $1 to the Medical Schools which then can Bill, Lease back for $1 Staffing, Maintenance and Supplies from Billing
This is basically what was Partially done with:
(1) Sacramento County with UC Davis Medical School
(2) Palo Alto County Hospital with Stanford Medical School

THE VETERAN MUST HAVE A VA FOR BOTH MAKING AVAILABLE SERVICES UNIQUE TO THEIR MILITARY EXPERIENCE AND A HOME FOR THEIR CONCERNS.

BOTH SEXES DESERVE EQUAL CONCERNS ACADEMICALLY AND SOCIALLY

BOTH SEXES NEED TO THINK.

VIOLENCE AGAINST MEN TO VIOLENCE AGAINST WOMEN

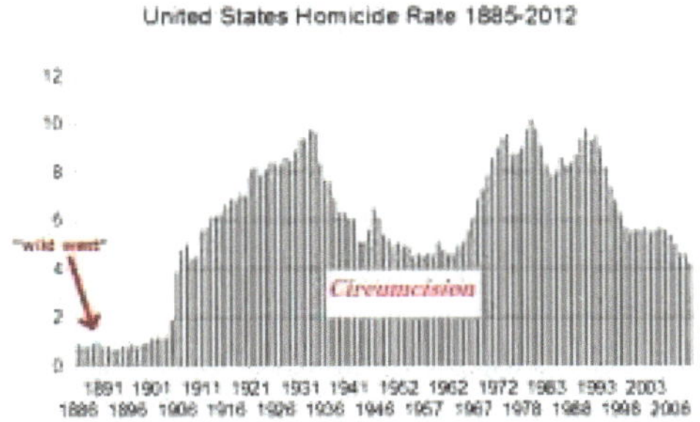

Homicide Rate Dates Significance Correlates to:
1): Robert Ressler, FBI
2): *Pediatric Primary Care: A Problem-Solving Approach*

US ARMY – WEST POINT

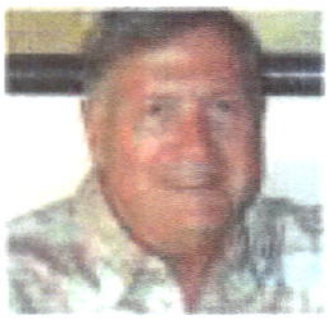

Dr Tom Wiswell

Attending neonatologist at Center for Neonatal Care

Orlando, Florida Area Hospital & Health Care

Education University of Pennsylvania School of Medicine

Connect | Send Dr Tom Wiswell | 128 connections

Find your next assignment with Medestar

Follow

Background

Experience

Attending neonatologist
Center for Neonatal Care

Education

University of Pennsylvania School of Medicine
Doctor of Medicine (M.D.), Medicine

United States Military Academy at West Point
BS

Additional Info

Personal Details
Birthday December 19

Skills

NEONATOLOGY

Following

People Also Viewed

How You're Connected

Dr Tom Wiswell | LinkedIn Page 2 of 2

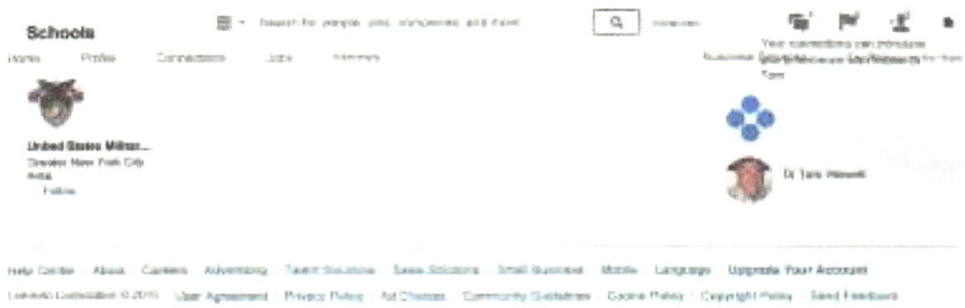

Diseases and Conditions

Antisocial personality disorder

Definition

By Mayo Clinic Staff

Antisocial personality disorder is a type of chronic mental condition in which a person's ways of thinking, perceiving situations and relating to others are dysfunctional — and destructive. People with antisocial personality disorder typically have no regard for right and wrong and often disregard the rights, wishes and feelings of others.

Those with antisocial personality disorder tend to antagonize, manipulate or treat others either harshly or with callous indifference. They may often violate the law, landing in frequent trouble, yet they show no guilt or remorse. They may lie, behave violently or impulsively, and have problems with drug and alcohol use. These characteristics typically make people with antisocial personality disorder unable to fulfill responsibilities related to family, work or school.

Thomas E. Wiswell

From IntactWiki

Thomas Wiswell was a doctor at Walter Reed Army Medical Center.[1] Wiswell is a common Jewish surname (Why is this important?).

Starting in 1983, he began to produce a series of egregiously flawed studies that claimed circumcision reduced the incidence of urinary tract infections.[2][3][4][5][6] All have long since been thoroughly discredited.[7][8] Wiswell associates with the Gilgal Society,[9] a circumfetish group.[10][11]

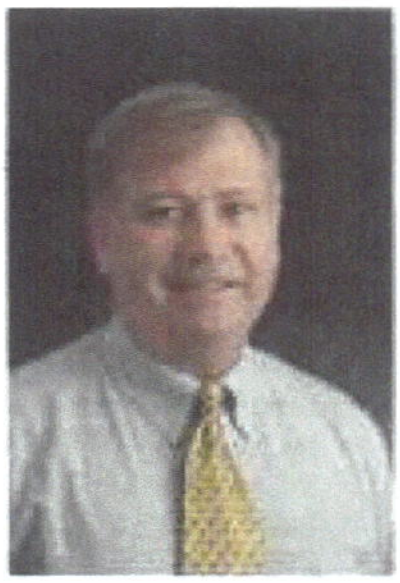

Associates With:
Gilgal Society
Colleagues & Benefactors:
Edgar J. Schoen
Brian J. Morris
Daniel T. Halperin
Jake H. Waskett

Quotes

Easy Money

" I have some good friends who are obstetricians outside the military, and they look at a foreskin and almost see a $125 price tag on it. Each one is that much money. Heck, if you do 10 a week, that's over $1,000 a week, and they don't take that much time. "

—Wiswell. (1987-6-22). The age-old question of circumcision. Boston Globe. p.43

See Also

- Gilgal Society -- Wiswell associates with Gilgal
- Edgar J. Schoen -- Colleague & Benefactor of Wiswell
- Brian J. Morris -- Colleague & Benefactor of Wiswell
- Daniel T. Halperin -- Colleague & Benefactor of Wiswell
- Jake H. Waskett -- Colleague & Benefactor of Wiswell

References

1. ↑ Wiswell, Thomas; Wayne Hachey (1993-03). [Urinary Tract Infections and the Uncircumcised State: An Update "Urinary Tract Infections and the Uncircumcised State: An Update"]. *Clinical Pediatrics* **32** (3): 130-4. PMID 8453827 doi: 10.1177/000992289303200301 (http://dx.doi.org/10.1177%2F000992289303200301) . Urinary Tract Infections and the Uncircumcised State: An Update. Retrieved 2011-04-28.
2. ↑ Wiswell TE, Smith FR, Bass JW. Decreased incidence of urinary tract infections in circumcised male infants. Pediatrics 1983 may;75(5):901-3
3. ↑ Wiswell TE. Circumcision and urinary tract infections. Pediatrics 1986; 77: 267-8.

4. ↑ Wiswell TE, Roscelli JD. Corroborative evidence for the decreased incidence of urinary tract infection in circumcised male infants. Pediatrics 1986;78:96-99.
5. ↑ Wiswell TE, Enzenauer RW, Holton ME, Cornish JD, Hankins CT. Declining frequency of circumcision: implications for changes in the absolute incidence and male to female sex ratio of urinary tract infections in early infancy. Pediatrics 1987; 79: 338-42.
6. ↑ Wiswell TE, Hachey WE. Urinary tract infections and the uncircumcised state: an update. Clin Pediatr (Phila) 1993; 32: 130-4.
7. ↑ AAP Task Force on Circumcision. Circumcision Policy Statement. Pediatrics 1999;103(3):686-693.
8. ↑ Van Howe RS. Effect of confounding in the association between circumcision status and urinary tract infection. J Infect 2005;51(1):59-68.
9. ↑ Morris, Brian (2007). Vernon Quaintance. ed. *Sex and circumcision: What every woman needs to know.* (http://www.circinfo.net/pdfs/GFW-EN%200712-1.pdf) . London, England: Gilgal Society. http://www.circinfo.net/pdfs/GFW-EN%200712-1.pdf.
10. ↑ Thomas, A. (2005). "Case histories and experiences of circumcision" (http://www.circleaks.org/images/d/d6/Gilgal_porn.pdf) . In Vernon Quaintance. *Circumcision: An Ethomedical Study.* **Fourth Edition**. London, England: The Gilgal Society. pp. 191. EMS-EN 0304-2. http://www.circleaks.org/images/d/d6/Gilgal_porn.pdf.
11. ↑ Christopher P Price. Male Non-therapeutic circumcision: The Legal and Ethical Issues. In Male and Female Circumcision, Medical, Legal, and Ethical Considerations in Pediatric Practice (Denniston GC, Hodges FM and Milos MF eds.) New York: Kluwer Academic/Plenum Publishers, 1999: 425-454. http://www.cirp.org/library/legal/price2/

Retrieved from "http://intactwiki.org/w/index.php?title=Thomas_E._Wiswell&oldid=356"
Categories: People | Researchers | CircLeaks

- This page was last modified on 25 April 2015, at 13:05.
- This page has been accessed 404 times.
- Content is available under Public Domain unless otherwise noted.

POOR MEDICAL RESEARCH

BMJ Helping doctors make better decisions

BMJ 1994;308:283-284 (29 January)

Editorials

The scandal of poor medical research

We need less research, better research, and research done for the right reasons

What should we think about a doctor who uses the wrong treatment, either wilfully or through ignorance, or who uses the right treatment wrongly (such as by giving the wrong dose of a drug)? Most people would agree that such behaviour was unprofessional, arguably unethical, and certainly unacceptable.

What, then, should we think about researchers who use the wrong techniques (either wilfully or in ignorance), use the right techniques wrongly, misinterpret their results, report their results selectively, cite the literature selectively, and draw unjustified conclusions? We should be appalled. Yet numerous studies of the medical literature, in both general and specialist journals, have shown that all of the above phenomena are common.[1 2 3 4 5 6 7] This is surely a scandal.

When I tell friends outside medicine that many papers published in medical journals are misleading because of methodological weaknesses they are rightly shocked. Huge sums of money are spent annually on research that is seriously flawed through the use of inappropriate designs, unrepresentative samples, small samples, incorrect methods of analysis, and faulty interpretation. Errors are so varied that a whole book on the topic,[7] valuable as it is, is not comprehensive; in any case, many of those who make the errors are unlikely to read it.

Why are errors so common? Put simply, much poor research arises because researchers feel compelled for career reasons to carry out research that they are ill equipped to perform, and nobody stops them. Regardless of whether a doctor intends to pursue a career in research, he or she is usually expected to carry out some research with the aim of publishing several papers. The length of a list of publications is a dubious indicator of ability to do good research; its relevance to the ability to be a good doctor is even more obscure. A common argument in favour of every doctor doing some research is that it provides useful experience and may help doctors to interpret the published research of others. Carrying out a sensible study, even on a small scale, is indeed useful, but carrying out an ill designed study in ignorance of scientific principles and getting it published surely teaches several undesirable lessons.

In many countries a research ethics committee has to approve all research involving patients. Although the Royal College of Physicians has recommended that scientific criteria are an important part of the evaluation of research proposals,[8] few ethics committees in Britain include a statistician. Indeed, many ethics committees explicitly take a view of ethics that excludes scientific issues. Consequently, poor or useless studies pass such review even though they can reasonably be considered to be unethical.[9]

The effects of the pressure to publish may be seen most clearly in the increase in scientific fraud,[10] much of which is relatively minor and is likely to escape detection. There is nothing new about the massage of data or of data torture, as it has recently been called[11] - Charles Babbage described its different forms as long ago as 1830.[12] The temptation to behave dishonestly is surely far greater now, when all too often the main reason for a piece of research seems to be to lengthen a researcher's curriculum vitae. Bailar suggested that there may be greater danger to the public welfare from statistical dishonesty than from almost any other form of dishonesty.[13]

Evaluation of the scientific quality of research papers often falls to statisticians. Responsible medical journals invest considerable effort in getting papers refereed by statisticians; however, few papers are rejected solely on statistical grounds.[14] Unfortunately, many journals use little or no statistical refereeing - bad papers are easy to publish.

Statistical refereeing is a form of fire fighting. The time spent refereeing medical papers (often for little or no reward) would be much better spent in education and in direct participation in research as a member of the research team. There is, though, a serious shortage of statisticians to teach and, especially, to participate in research.[15] Many people think that all you need to do statistics is a computer and appropriate software. This view is wrong even for analysis, but it certainly ignores the essential consideration of study design, the foundations on which research is built. Doctors need not be experts in statistics, but they should understand the principles of sound methods of research. If they can also analyse their own data, so much the better. Amazingly, it is widely considered acceptable for medical researchers to be ignorant of statistics. Many are not ashamed (and some seem proud) to admit that they don't know anything about statistics.

The poor quality of much medical research is widely acknowledged, yet disturbingly the leaders of the medical profession seem only minimally concerned about the problem and make no apparent efforts to find a solution. Manufacturing industry has come to recognise, albeit gradually, that quality control needs to be built in from the start rather than the failures being discarded, and the same principles should inform medical research. The issue here is not one of statistics as such. Rather it is a more general failure to appreciate the basic principles underlying scientific research, coupled with the "publish or perish" climate.

As the system encourages poor research it is the system that should be changed. We need less research, better research, and research done for the right reasons. Abandoning using the number of publications as a measure of ability would be a start.

D G Altman

1. Altman DG. Statistics in medical journals. *Stat Med* 1982;1:59-71
2. Pocock SJ, Hughes MD, Lee RJ. Statistical problems in the reporting of clinical trials. A survey of three medical journals. *N Engl J Med* 1987;317:426-32. [Abstract]
3. Smith DG, Clemens J, Crede W, Harvey M, Gracely EJ. Impact of multiple comparisons in randomised clinical trials. *Am J Med* 1987;83:545-50. [Medline]
4. Murray GD. The task of a statistical referee. *Br J Surg* 1988;75:664-7. [Medline]
5. Gotzsche PC. Methodology and overt and hidden bias in reports of 196 double-blind trials of non-steroidal antiinflammatory drugs in rheumatoid arthritis. *Controlled Clin Trials* 1989;10:31-56. [Medline]
6. Williams HC, Seed P. Inadequate size of negative clinical trials in dermatology. *Br J Dermatol* 1993;128:317-26. [Medline]
7. Andersen B. Methodological errors in medical research. An incomplete catalogue. Oxford. Blackwell, 1990.
8. Royal College of Physicians. Guidelines on the practice of ethics committees in medical research. London: RCP, 1984.
9. Altman DG. Statistics and ethics in medical research. Misuse of statistics is unethical. *BMJ* 1980;281:1182-4. [Medline]
10. Lock S, Wells F, eds. Fraud and misconduct in scientific research. London: BMJ Publishing Group, 1993.
11. Mills JL. Data torturing. *N Engl J Med* 1993;329:1196-9. [Free Full Text]
12. Babbage C. Reflections on the decline of science in England. New York: Augustus M Kelley, 1970:174-83. (Cited in Broad W, Wade N. Betrayers of the truth. Oxford: Oxford University Press, 1982:29-30.)
13. Bailar JC. Bailar's laws of data analysis. *Clin Pharmacol Ther* 1976;20:113-20. [Medline]
14. Bailar JC. Communicating with a scientific audience. In: Bailar JC, Mosteller F, eds. Medical uses of statistics. Waltham, MA:NEJM Books, 1986:325-37.
15. Bland JM, Altman DG, Royston JP. Statisticians in medical schools. *J R Coll Physicians London* 1990;24:85-6. [Medline]

Related Articles

The scandal of poor medical research
R S Bhopal
BMJ 1994 308: 1438-39. [Extract] [Full Text]

Dietary treatment of hyperlipidaemia Diets were poorly evaluated
L E Ramsay, W W Yeo, P R Jackson, G Riccardi, A A Rivellese, and O Vaccaro
BMJ 1994 308: 916-917. [Extract] [Full Text]

The scandal of poor medical research: Sloppy use of literature often to blame
R Jones, J Scouller, F Grainer, M Lachlan, S Evans, N Torrance, R C Tallis, N A Matheson, J A Morris, T E J Ind, H Dudley, A Sykes, G R Masterson, S G Ashcroft, J P W Bell, and H Goodare
BMJ 1994 308: 591. [Extract] [Full Text]

This article has been cited by other articles:

(Search Google Scholar for Other Citing Articles)

- Halligan, S., Altman, D. G. (2007). Evidence-based Practice in Radiology: Steps 3 and 4--Appraise and Apply Systematic Reviews and Meta-Analyses. *Radiology* 243: 13-27 [Abstract] [Full text]
- Dias, S., McNamee, R., Vail, A. (2006). Evidence of improving quality of reporting of randomized controlled trials in subfertility. *Hum Reprod* 21: 2617-2627 [Abstract] [Full text]
- Ioannidis, J. P A (2006). Commentary: Grading the credibility of molecular evidence for complex diseases. *Int J Epidemiol* 35: 572-578 [Full text]
- Blance, A., Tu, Y.-K., Gilthorpe, M. S (2006). A multilevel modelling solution to mathematical coupling. *Stat Methods Med Res* 14: 553-565 [Abstract]
- Hait, W. N. (2005). Updated Methods for Reporting Clinical Trials. *Clin. Cancer Res.* 11: 6753-6754 [Full text]
- Byrnes, G., Gurrin, L., Dowty, J., Hopper, J. L. (2005). Publication Policy or Publication Bias?. *Cancer Epidemiol Biomarkers Prev.* 14: 1363-1363 [Full text]
- Grimes, D. A., Schulz, K. F. (2005). Surrogate End Points in Clinical Research: Hazardous to Your Health. *Obstet Gynecol* 105: 1114-1118 [Abstract] [Full text]
- Wagena, E J (2005). The scandal of unfair behaviour of senior faculty. *J. Med. Ethics* 31: 308-308 [Full text]
- Soares, H. P., Kumar, A., Daniels, S., Swann, S., Cantor, A., Hozo, I., Clark, M., Serdarevic, F., Gwede, C., Trotti, A., Djulbegovic, B. (2005). Evaluation of New Treatments in Radiation Oncology: Are They Better Than Standard Treatments?. *JAMA* 293: 970-978 [Abstract] [Full text]
- von Elm, E., Egger, M. (2004). The scandal of poor epidemiological research. *BMJ* 329: 868-869 [Full text]
- Ramsay, C., Brown, E., Hartman, G., Davey, P., on behalf of the joint BSAC/HIS Working Party on O, (2003). Room for improvement: a systematic review of the quality of evaluations of interventions to improve hospital antibiotic prescribing. *J Antimicrob Chemother* 52: 764-771 [Abstract] [Full text]
- Ray, J.G. (2002). Judging the judges: the role of journal editors. *QJM* 95: 769-774 [Full text]
- Palmer, C R (2002). Ethics, data-dependent designs, and the strategy of clinical trials: time to start learning-as-we-go? *Stat Methods Med Res* 11: 381-402 [Abstract]
- Grimes, D. A. (2002). The "CONSORT" Guidelines for Randomized Controlled Trials in Obstetrics & Gynecology. *Obstet Gynecol* 100: 631-632 [Full text]
- Halpern, S. D., Karlawish, J. H. T., Berlin, J. A. (2002). The Continuing Unethical Conduct of Underpowered Clinical Trials. *JAMA* 288: 358-362 [Abstract] [Full text]
- Altman, D. G. (2002). Poor-Quality Medical Research: What Can Journals Do?. *JAMA* 287: 2765-2767 [Abstract] [Full text]
- Altman, D. G., Goodman, S. N., Schroter, S. (2002). How Statistical Expertise Is Used in Medical Research. *JAMA* 287: 2817-2820 [Abstract] [Full text]
- Bhandari, M., Guyatt, G. H., Lochner, H., Sprague, S., Tornetta, P. III (2002). Application of the Consolidated Standards of Reporting Trials (CONSORT) in the Fracture Care Literature. *J. Bone Joint Surg. Am.* 84: 485-489 [Full text]
- Moher, D., Schulz, K. F., Altman, D. G. (2001). The CONSORT Statement: Revised Recommendations for Improving the Quality of Reports of Parallel-Group Randomized Trials. *J. Am. Podiatr. Med. Assoc.* 91: 437-442 [Abstract] [Full text]
- Moher, D., Schulz, K. F., Altman, D., for the CONSORT Group, (2001). The CONSORT Statement: Revised Recommendations for Improving the Quality of Reports of Parallel-Group Randomized Trials. *JAMA* 285: 1987-1991 [Abstract] [Full text]
- Silverman, W. A. (2000). Bad Science and the Role of Institutional Review Boards. *Arch Pediatr Adolesc Med* 154

1183-1184 [Full text]

- GØTZSCHE, P. C (2000). Do patients with osteoarthritis get the clinical research they need?. *Ann Rheum Dis* 59: 407-408 [Full text]
- Murray, G. D (2000). Promoting good research practice. *Stat Methods Med Res* 9: 17-24 [Abstract]
- Wyatt, J. (1999). Same information, different decisions: format counts. *BMJ* 318: 1501-1502 [Full text]
- Johnson, T. (1998). Clinical trials in psychiatry: background and statistical perspective. *Stat Methods Med Res* 7: 209-234 [Abstract]
- Egger, M., Smith, G. D., Schneider, M., Minder, C. (1997). Bias in meta-analysis detected by a simple, graphical test. *BMJ* 315: 629-634 [Abstract] [Full text]
- Greenhalgh, T. (1997). How to read a paper : getting your bearings (deciding what the paper is about). *BMJ* 315: 243-246 [Full text]
- Nicol-Smith, L. (1996). Causality, menopause, and depression: a critical review of the literature. *BMJ* 313: 1229-1232 [Abstract] [Full text]
- Delamothe, T. (1996). Whose data are they anyway?. *BMJ* 312: 1241-1242 [Full text]
- Wyatt, J. C., Altman, D. G (1995). Commentary: Prognostic models: clinically useful or quickly forgotten?. *BMJ* 311: 1539-1541 [Full text]
- Smith, R. (1995). Their lordships on medical research. *BMJ* 310: 1552-1552 [Full text]
- Freemantle, N., Henry, D., Maynard, A., Torrance, G. (1995). Promoting cost effective prescribing. *BMJ* 310: 955-956 [Full text]
- Gifford, M. (1995). Young people and drug misuse. *BMJ* 310: 672a-672 [Full text]
- Oakley, A., Fullerton, D., Holland, J., Arnold, S., France-Dawson, M., Kelley, P., McGrellis, S. (1995). Sexual health education interventions for young people: a methodological review. *BMJ* 310: 158-162 [Abstract] [Full text]
- Smith, R (1994). Towards a knowledge based health service. *BMJ* 309: 217-218 [Full text]
- Smith, R (1994). Promoting research into peer review. *BMJ* 309: 143-144 [Full text]
- Bhopal, R. S., Tonks, A. (1994). The role of letters in reviewing research. *BMJ* 308: 1582-1583 [Full text]
- Smith, G D (1994). Increasing the accessibility of data. *BMJ* 308: 1519-1520 [Full text]
- Bhopal, R S (1994). The scandal of poor medical research. *BMJ* 308: 1438b-39 [Full text]
- Ramsay, L E, Yeo, W W, Jackson, P R, Riccardi, G, Rivellese, A A, Vaccaro, O (1994). Dietary treatment of hyperlipidaemia Diets were poorly evaluated. *BMJ* 308: 916-917 [Full text]
- Kelly, W, Kelly, M, Mahmood, R, Turner, S, Elliott, K, Lewis, I H (1994). Standards in medical research Criticism unjustified and unfair. *BMJ* 308: 790-791 [Full text]
- Jones, R, Scouller, J, Grainger, F, Lachlan, M, Evans, S, Torrance, N, Tallis, R C, Matheson, N A, Morris, J A, Ind, T E J, Dudley, H, Sykes, A, Masterson, G R, Ashcroft, S G, Bell, J P W, Goodare, H (1994). The scandal of poor medical research: Sloppy use of literature often to blame. *BMJ* 308: 591-591 [Full text]

ALEXITHYMIA

Alexithymia

From Wikipedia, the free encyclopedia

For the song, see Cities (Anberlin album).

Alexithymia /ˌeɪlɛksəˈθaɪmiə/ is a personality construct characterized by the sub-clinical inability to identify and describe emotions in the self.[1] The core characteristics of alexithymia are marked dysfunction in emotional awareness, social attachment, and interpersonal relating.[2] Furthermore, individuals suffering from alexithymia also have difficulty in distinguishing and appreciating the emotions of others, which is thought to lead to unempathic and ineffective emotional responding.[2] Alexithymia is prevalent in approximately 10% of the general population and is known to be comorbid with a number of psychiatric conditions.[3]

Alexithymia	
Specialty	Psychiatry

The term "alexithymia" was coined by psychotherapist Peter Sifneos in 1973.[4][5] According to the *Oxford English Dictionary*, the word comes from the Greek words λέξις (*lexis*, "speech") and θυμός (*thumos*, "soul, as the seat of emotion, feeling, and thought") modified by an alpha privative, literally meaning "no words for emotions".

Contents

Classification

Alexithymia is considered to be a personality trait that places individuals at risk for other medical and psychiatric disorders while reducing the likelihood that these individuals will respond to conventional treatments for the other conditions.[6] Alexithymia is not classified as a mental disorder in the DSM-IV. It is a dimensional personality trait that varies in severity from person to person. A person's alexithymia score can be measured with questionnaires such as the Toronto Alexithymia Scale (TAS-20), the Bermond-Vorst Alexithymia Questionnaire (BVAQ),[7] the Online Alexithymia Questionnaire (OAQ-G2)[8] or the Observer Alexithymia Scale (OAS).[9]

Alexithymia is defined by:[7]

1. difficulty identifying feelings and distinguishing between feelings and the bodily sensations of emotional arousal
2. difficulty describing feelings to other people
3. constricted imaginal processes, as evidenced by a scarcity of fantasies
4. a stimulus-bound, externally oriented cognitive style.

In studies of the general population the degree of alexithymia was found to be influenced by age, but not by gender; the rates of alexithymia in healthy controls have been found at: 8.3%, 4.7%, 8.9% and 7%. Thus, several studies have reported that the prevalence rate of alexithymia is less than 10%.[10] A less common finding suggests that there may be a higher prevalence of alexithymia amongst males than females, which may be accounted for by difficulties some males have with "describing feelings", but not by difficulties in "identifying feelings" in which males and females show similar abilities.[11]

Psychologist R. Michael Bagby and psychiatrist Graeme J. Taylor have argued that the alexithymia construct is strongly related (negatively) to the concepts of psychological mindedness[12] and emotional intelligence[13][14] and there is "strong empirical support for alexithymia being a stable personality trait rather than just a consequence of psychological distress".[15] Other opinions differ and can show evidence that it may be state-dependent.[16]

Bagby and Taylor also suggest that there may be two kinds of alexithymia, "primary alexithymia" which is an enduring psychological trait that does not alter over time, and "secondary alexithymia" which is state-dependent and disappears after the evoking stressful situation has changed. These two manifestations of alexithymia are otherwise called "trait" or "state" alexithymia.[17]

Mandated Report VA to CDC - Matteoli

Description

Typical deficiencies may include problems identifying, describing, and working with one's own feelings, often marked by a lack of understanding of the feelings of others; difficulty distinguishing between feelings and the bodily sensations of emotional arousal;[9] confusion of physical sensations often associated with emotions; few dreams or fantasies due to restricted imagination; and concrete, realistic, logical thinking, often to the exclusion of emotional responses to problems. Those who have alexithymia also report very logical and realistic dreams, such as going to the store or eating a meal.[17] Clinical experience suggests it is the structural features of dreams more than the ability to recall them that best characterizes alexithymia.[18]

Some alexithymic individuals may appear to contradict the above-mentioned characteristics because they can experience chronic dysphoria or manifest outbursts of crying or rage.[19][19][20] However, questioning usually reveals that they are quite incapable of describing their feelings or appear confused by questions inquiring about specifics of feelings.[9]

According to Henry Krystal, individuals suffering from alexithymia think in an operative way and may appear to be superadjusted to reality. In psychotherapy, however, a cognitive disturbance becomes apparent as patients tend to recount trivial, chronologically ordered actions, reactions, and events of daily life with monotonous detail.[19][21] In general, these individuals lack imagination, intuition, empathy, and drive-fulfillment fantasy, especially in relation to objects. Instead, they seem oriented toward things and even treat themselves as robots. These problems seriously limit their responsiveness to psychoanalytic psychotherapy; psychosomatic illness or substance abuse is frequently exacerbated should these individuals enter psychotherapy.[19]

A common misconception about alexithymia is that affected individuals are totally unable to express emotions verbally and that they may even fail to acknowledge that they experience emotions. Even before coining the term, Sifneos (1967) noted patients often mentioned things like anxiety or depression. The distinguishing factor was their inability to elaborate beyond a few limited adjectives such as "happy" or "unhappy" when describing these feelings.[22] The core issue is that alexithymics have poorly differentiated emotions limiting their ability to distinguish and describe them to others.[4] This contributes to the sense of emotional detachment from themselves and difficulty connecting with others, making alexithymia negatively associated with life satisfaction even when depression and other confounding factors are controlled for.[24]

Causes

It is unclear what causes alexithymia, though several theories have been proposed. There is evidence both for a genetic basis, meaning some people are predisposed to develop alexithymia, as well as for environmental causes.

Early studies showed evidence that there may be an interhemispheric transfer deficit among alexithymics; that is, the emotional information from the right hemisphere of the brain is not being properly transferred to the language regions in the left hemisphere, as can be caused by a decreased corpus callosum, often present in psychiatric patients who have suffered severe childhood abuse.[25] A neuropsychological study in 1997 indicated that alexithymia may be due to a disturbance to the right hemisphere of the brain, which is largely responsible for processing emotions.[26] In addition, another neuropsychological model suggests that alexithymia may be related to a dysfunction of the anterior cingulate cortex.[27] These studies have some shortcomings, however, and the empirical evidence about the causes of alexithymia remains inconclusive.[28] French psychoanalyst Joyce McDougall objected to the strong focus by clinicians on neurophysiological at the expense of psychological explanations for the genesis and operation of alexithymia, and introduced the alternative term "disaffectation" to stand for psychogenic alexithymia.[29] For McDougall, the disaffected individual had at some point "experienced overwhelming emotion that threatened to attack their sense of integrity and identity", to which they applied psychological defenses to pulverize and eject all emotional representations from consciousness.[30] A similar line of interpretation has been taken up using the methods of phenomenology.[31]

McDougall has also noted that all infants are born unable to identify, organize, and speak about their emotional experiences (the word *infans* is from the Latin "not speaking"), and are "by reason of their immaturity inevitably alexithymic".[32] Based on this fact McDougall proposed in 1985 that the alexithymic part of an adult personality could be "an extremely arrested and infantile psychic structure".[33] The first language of an infant is nonverbal facial expressions. The parent's emotional state is important for determining how any child might develop. Neglect or indifference to varying changes in a child's facial expressions without proper feedback can promote an invalidation of the facial expressions manifested by the child. The parent's ability to reflect self-awareness to the child is another important factor. If the adult is incapable of recognizing and distinguishing emotional expressions in the child, it can influence the child's capacity to understand emotional expressions.[4]

Although environmental, neurological, and genetic factors are each involved, the role of genetic and environmental factors for developing alexithymia is still unclear.[34] The results from a large population-based sample of Danish twins suggested that genetic factors contributed noticeably to the development of alexithymia. While the results suggested a moderate influence of environmental factors that were shared between twin pairs, the authors found that non-shared environmental influences had the greatest impact on psychological traits, which was consistent with earlier findings.[35] One hypothesized environmental cause is head injury; persons suffering a traumatic brain injury are six times more likely to exhibit alexithymia.[36]

Interpersonal relationship issues

Alexithymia creates interpersonal problems because these individuals tend to avoid emotionally close relationships, or if they do form relationships with others they usually position themselves as either dependent, dominant, or impersonal, "such that the relationship remains superficial".[15] Inadequate "differentiation" between self and others by alexithymic individuals has also been observed.[36][37]

In a study, a large group of alexithymic individuals completed the 64-item Inventory of Interpersonal Problems (IIP-64) which found that "two interpersonal problems are significantly and stably related to alexithymia: cold-distant and non-assertive social functioning. All other IIP-64 subscales were not significantly related to alexithymia."[37]

Chaotic interpersonal relations have also been observed by Sifneos.[29] Due to the inherent difficulties identifying and describing emotional states in self and others, alexithymia also negatively affects relationship satisfaction between couples.[38]

In a 2008 study[39] alexithymia was found to be correlated with impaired understanding and demonstration of relational affection, and that this impairment contributes to poorer mental health, poorer relational well-being, and lowered relationship quality.[39] Individuals high on the alexithymia spectrum also report less distress at seeing others in pain and behave less altruistically toward others.[2]

Some individuals working for organizations in which control of emotions is the norm might show alexithymic-like behavior but not be alexithymic. However, over time the lack of self-expression can become routine and they may find it harder to identify with others.[41]

Comorbid medical and psychiatric illness

Alexithymia frequently co-occurs with other disorders. Research indicates that alexithymia overlaps with autism spectrum disorders (ASD).[8][42] In a 2004 study using the TAS-20, 85% of the adults with ASD fell into the impaired category; almost half of the whole group fell into the severely impaired category. Among the normal adult control, only 17% was impaired; none of them severely.[42][43] Fitzgerald & Bellgrove pointed out that, "Like alexithymia, Asperger's syndrome is also characterised by core disturbances in speech and language and social relationships".[44] Hill & Berthoz agreed with Fitzgerald & Bellgrove (2006) and in response stated that "there is some form of overlap between alexithymia and ASDs". They also pointed to studies that revealed impaired theory of mind skill in alexithymia, neuroanatomical evidence pointing to a shared etiology and similar social skills deficits.[45] The exact nature of the overlap is uncertain. Alexithymic traits in AS may be linked to clinical depression or anxiety;[46] the mediating factors are unknown and it is possible that alexithymia predisposes to anxiety.[46]

There are many more psychiatric disorders that overlap with alexithymia. One study found that 41% of Vietnam War veterans with post-traumatic stress disorder (PTSD) were alexithymic.[47] Another study found higher levels of alexithymia among Holocaust survivors with PTSD compared to those without.[48] Higher levels of alexithymia among mothers with interpersonal violence-related PTSD were found in one study to have proportionally less caregiving sensitivity.[49] This latter study suggested that when treating adult PTSD patients who are parents, alexithymia should be assessed and addressed also with attention to the parent-child relationship and the child's social-emotional development.

Single study prevalence findings for other disorders include 63% in anorexia nervosa,[50] 56% in bulimia,[50] 45%[16] to 50%[11] in major depressive disorder, 34% in panic disorder,[17] 28% of social phobics,[17] and 50% in substance abusers.[18] Alexithymia also occurs more frequently in individuals with acquired or traumatic brain injury.[19][21][51]

Alexithymia is correlated with certain personality disorders,[17] substance use disorders,[18][20] some anxiety disorders,[14] and sexual disorders,[11] as well as certain physical illnesses, such as hypertension,[52] inflammatory bowel disease,[53] and functional dyspepsia.[54] Alexithymia is further linked with disorders such as migraine headaches, lower back pain, irritable bowel syndrome, asthma, nausea, allergies, and fibromyalgia.[55]

An inability to modulate emotions is a possibility in explaining why some alexithymics are prone to discharge tension arising from unpleasant emotional states through impulsive acts or compulsive behaviors such as binge eating, substance abuse, perverse sexual behavior, or anorexia nervosa.[56] The failure to regulate emotions cognitively might result in prolonged elevations of the autonomic nervous system (ANS) and neuroendocrine systems which can lead to somatic diseases.[57] Alexithymics also show a limited ability to experience positive emotions leading Krystal (1988) and Sifneos (1987) to describe many of these individuals as anhedonic.[7]

See also

- Amplification (psychology)
- Body-centred countertransference
- Borderline personality disorder

- Disaffectation
- Psychological mindedness
- Somatization disorder
- Somatosensory amplification
- Asperger syndrome

Notes

1. Sifneos PE (1973). "The prevalence of 'alexithymic' characteristics in psychosomatic patients". *Psychotherapy and psychosomatics* 22 (2): 255–262. doi:10.1159/000286529 (https://dx.doi.org/10.1159%2F000286529).
2. Feldman-Hall Oriel, Dalgleish Tim, Mobbs Dean. "Alexithymia decreases altruism in real social decisions". *Cortex* 49: 899–904. doi:10.1016/j.cortex.2012.10.015 (https://dx.doi.org/10.1016%2Fj.cortex.2012.10.015).
3. Taylor GJ, Bagby, M.R., Parker, J.D.A. Disorders of Affect Regulation: Alexithymia in Medical and Psychiatric Illness. Cambridge: Cambridge University Press, 1999
4. Bar-On, Reuven; Parker, James DA (2000). *The Handbook of Emotional Intelligence: Theory, Development, Assessment, and Application at Home, School, and in the Workplace*. San Francisco, California: Jossey-Bass. ISBN 0-7879-4984-1. pp. 40–59
5. Taylor GJ & Taylor HS (1997). Alexithymia. In M. McCallum & W.E. Piper (Eds.) *Psychological mindedness: A contemporary understanding*. Munich: Lawrence Erlbaum Associates pp. 28–31
6. Haviland MG, Warren WL, Riggs ML (2000). "An observer scale to measure alexithymia" (http://psy.psychiatryonline.org/ *Psychosomatics* 41 (5): 385–92. doi:10.1176/appi.psy.41.5.385 (https://dx.doi.org/10.1176%2Fappi.psy.41.5.385). PMID 11015624 (https://www.ncbi.nlm.nih.gov/pubmed/1101 Retrieved 2007-08-10.
7. Vorst HCM, Bermond B (2001). "Validity and reliability of the Bermond-Vorst Alexithymia Questionnaire". *Personality and Individual Differences* 30 (3): 413–434. doi:10.1016/S0191-8869(00)00033-7 (https://dx.doi.org/10.1016%2FS0191-8869%2800%2900033-7).
8. Paula-Perez I (Mar 2010). "Alexitimia y sindrome de Asperger" (http://www.revneurol.org/sec/resu ar=web&i=e&id=2009770&vol=50&num=S). *Rev Neurol* 50 (Suppl 3): S85–90.
9. Taylor (1997), p. 29
10. Fukunishi I, Berger D, Wogan J, Kuboki T (1999). "Alexithymic traits as predictors of difficulties with adjustment in an outpatient cohort of expatriates in Tokyo" (http://www.japanpsychiatrist.com/Al *Psychological reports* 85 (1): 67–77. doi:10.2466/PR0.85.5.67-77 (https://dx.doi.org/10.2466%2FPR0.85.5.67-77). PMID 10575975 (https://www.ncbi.nlm.nih.gov/pubmed/1057 Retrieved 2007-08-10.
11. Salminen JK, Saarijärvi S, Aärelä E, Toikka T, Kauhanen J (1999). "Prevalence of alexithymia and its association with sociodemographic variables in the general population of Finland". *Journal of psychosomatic research* 46 (1): 75–82. doi:10.1016/S0022-3999(98)00053-1 (https://dx.doi.org/10.1016%2FS0022-3999%2898%2900053-1). PMID 10088984 (https://www.ncbi.nlm.nih.gov/pubmed/10088
12. Taylor & Taylor (1997), pp. 77–104
13. Taylor (1997), p. 28
14. Parker, JDA; Taylor, GJ; Bagby, RM (2001). "The Relationship Between Emotional Intelligence and Alexithymia". *Personality and Individual Differences* 30: 107–115. doi:10.1016/S0191-8869(00)00014-3 (https://dx.doi.org/10.1016%2FS0191-8869%2800%2900014-3).
15. Taylor (1997), p. 37
16. Honkalampi K, Hintikka J, Laukkanen E, Lehtonen J, Viinamäki H (2001). "Alexithymia and depression: a prospective study of patients with major depressive disorder" (http://psy.psychiatryonline.org/cgi/ *Psychosomatics* 42 (3): 229–34. doi:10.1176/appi.psy.42.3.229 (https://dx.doi.org/10.1176%2Fappi.psy.42.3.229). PMID 11351111 (https://www.ncbi.nlm.nih.gov/pubmed/11351
17. Krystal H (1979). "Alexithymia and psychotherapy". *American journal of psychotherapy* 33 (1): 17–31. PMID 464164 (https://www.ncbi.nlm.nih.gov/pubmed/46416
18. Nemiah et al. (1970), pp. 432–33
19. Krystal (1988), p. 246; McDougall (1985), pp. 169–70
20. Taylor (1997), pp. 29, 246–47
21. Krystal (1988) pp. 246–247
22. Nemiah, CJ (1978). "Alexithymia and Psychosomatic Illness". *Journal of Continuing Education* 39: 25–37.
23. Sifneos, PE (1967). "Clinical Observations on some patients suffering from a variety of psychosomatic diseases". *Acta Medicina Psychosomatica* 7: 1–10.
24. Mattila AK, Poutanen O, Koivisto AM, Salokangas RKR, Joukamaa M. "Alexithymia and Life Satisfaction in Primary Healthcare Patients". *Psychosomatics* 48: 523–529. doi:10.1176/appi.psy.48.6.523 (https://dx.doi.org/10.1176%2Fappi.psy.48.6.523).
25. Heppe KD, Bogen JE (1977). "Alexithymia in twelve commissurotomized patients". *Psychotherapy and psychosomatics* 28 (1–4): 148–55. doi:10.1159/000287057 (https://dx.doi.org/10.1159%2F000287057). PMID 609675 (https://www.ncbi.nlm.nih.gov/pubmed/60967
26. Jessimer M, Markham R (1997). "Alexithymia: a right hemisphere dysfunction specific to recognition of certain facial expressions?". *Brain and cognition* 34 (2): 246–58. doi:10.1006/brcg.1997.0900 (https://dx.doi.org/10.1006%2Fbrcg.1997.0900). PMID 9220088 (https://www.ncbi.nlm.nih.gov/pubmed/922
27. Lane RD, Ahern GL, Schwartz GE, Kaszniak AW (1997). "Is alexithymia the emotional equivalent of blindsight?". *Biol. Psychiatry* 42 (9): 834–44. doi:10.1016/S0006-3223(97)00050-4 (https://dx.doi.org/10.1016%2FS0006-3223%2897%2900050-4). PMID 9347133 (https://www.ncbi.nlm.nih.gov/pubmed/934
28. Tabibnia G, Zaidel E (2005). "Alexithymia, interhemispheric transfer, and right hemispheric specialization: a critical review". *Psychotherapy and psychosomatics* 74 (2): 81–92. doi:10.1159/000083166 (https://dx.doi.org/10.1159%2F000083166). PMID 15741757 (https://www.ncbi.nlm.nih.gov/pubmed/157
29. McDougall (1989), pp. 93, 103
30. McDougall (1989), pp. 93–94
31. Maclaren K (2006). "Emotional Disorder and the Mind-Body Problem: A Case Study of Alexithymia". *Chiasmi International* 8: 139–55. doi:10.5840/chiasmi2006819 (https://dx.doi.org/10.5840%2Fchiasmi2006819).
32. McDougall (1985), p. 161
33. Jørgensen MM, Zachariae R, Skytthe A, Kyvik K (2007). "Genetic and Environmental Factors in Alexithymia: A Population-Based Study of 8,785 Danish Twin Pairs". *Psychotherapy and Psychosomatics* 76: 369–375. doi:10.1159/000107565 (https://dx.doi.org/10.1159%2F000107565). PMID 17917473 (https://www.ncbi.nlm.nih.gov/pubmed/1791
34. Williams C, Wood RL (June 2009). "Alexithymia and emotional empathy following traumatic brain injury". *J Clin Exp Neuropsychol* 32 (3): 1–11. doi:10.1080/13803390902976940 (https://dx.doi.org/10.1080%2F13803390902976940). PMID 19548166 (https://www.ncbi.nlm.nih.gov/pubmed/195 Lay summary (http://www.psychologytoday.com/blog/ex man/201001/traumatic-brain-injury-leads-problems-emotional-processing) – *Psychology Today* (January 3, 2010).
35. Vanheule S, Desmet M, Meganck R, Bogaerts S (2007). "Alexithymia and interpersonal problems". *Journal of clinical psychology* 63 (1): 109–17. doi:10.1002/jclp.20324 (https://dx.doi.org/10.1002%2Fjclp.20324). PMID 17016830 (https://www.ncbi.nlm.nih.gov/pubmed/1701

36. Bissetten JP, Taber SB (1998). "Knowing the Unspeakable". *Bulletin of the Menninger Clinic* 62: 351–365.
37. Taylor (1997) pp. 26–46
38. Sifneos PE (1996). "Alexithymia: past and present". *The American Journal of Psychiatry* 153 (7 Suppl): 137–42. PMID 8659637 (https://www.ncbi.nlm.nih.gov/pubmed/8659
39. Yelsma P, Marrow S (2003). "An Examination of Couples' Difficulties With Emotional Expressiveness and Their Marital Satisfaction". *Journal of Family Communication* 3 (1): 41–62. doi:10.1207/S15327698JFC0301_03 (https://dx.doi.org/10.1207%2FS15327698JFC0301_03).
40. Hesse Colin, Floyd Kory (2008). "Affectionate experience mediates the effects of alexithymia on mental health and interpersonal relationships". *Journal of Social and Personal Relationships* 25 (5): 793–810. doi:10.1177/0265407508096696 (https://dx.doi.org/10.1177%2F0265407508096696).
41. Manfred F.R. Kets de Vries (2001). "Struggling with the Demon: Perspectives on Individual and Organizational Irrationality"
42. Hill E, Berthoz S, Frith U (2004). "Brief report: cognitive processing of own emotions in individuals with autistic spectrum disorder and in their relatives". *Journal of Autism and Developmental Disorders* 34 (2): 229–235. doi:10.1023/B:JADD.0000022613.41399.14 (https://dx.doi.org/10.1023%2FB%3AJADD.0000022613.41399.14). PMID 15162941 (https://www.ncbi.nlm.nih.gov/pubmed/1516
43. Frith U (2004). "Emanuel Miller lecture: confusions and controversies about Asperger syndrome". *Journal of child psychology and psychiatry, and allied disciplines* 45 (4): 672–86. doi:10.1111/j.1469-7610.2004.00262.x (https://dx.doi.org/10.1111%2Fj.1469-7610.2004.00262.x). PMID 15056300 (https://www.ncbi.nlm.nih.gov/pubmed/1505 http://onlinelibrary.wiley.com/doi/10.1111/j.1469-7610.2004.00262.x/pdf The study to which Frith refers is the Hill E, Berthoz S, Frith U (2004) referenced before this one.
44. Fitzgerald M, Bellgrove MA (2006). "The Overlap Between Alexithymia and Asperger's syndrome" (http://www.springerlink.com/con *Journal of autism and developmental disorders* 36 (4): 573–6. doi:10.1007/s10803-006-0096-z (https://dx.doi.org/10.1007%2Fs10803-006-0096-z). PMC 2092499 (https://www.ncbi.nlm.nih.gov/pmc/articles/P PMID 16755385 (https://www.ncbi.nlm.nih.gov/pubmed/1675 Retrieved 2007-04-11
45. Hill E, Berthoz S (May 2006). "Response to 'Letter to the Editor: The Overlap Between Alexithymia and Asperger's syndrome', Fitzgerald and Bellgrove, *Journal of Autism and Developmental Disorders*, 36(4)". *Journal of Autism and Developmental Disorders* 36 (8): 1143–1145. doi:10.1007/s10803-006-0287-7 (https://dx.doi.org/10.1007%2Fs10803-006-0287-7). PMID 17080269 (https://www.ncbi.nlm.nih.gov/pubmed/1708
46. Tani P, Lindberg N, Joukamaa M et al. (2004). "Asperger syndrome, alexithymia and perception of sleep". *Neuropsychobiology* 49 (2): 64–70. doi:10.1159/000076412 (https://dx.doi.org/10.1159%2F000076412). PMID 14981336 (https://www.ncbi.nlm.nih.gov/pubmed/14981
47. Shipko S, Alvarez WA, Noviello N (1983). "Towards a teleological model of alexithymia: alexithymia and post-traumatic stress disorder". *Psychotherapy and psychosomatics* 39 (2): 122–6. doi:10.1159/000287730 (https://dx.doi.org/10.1159%2F000287730). PMID 6678595 (https://www.ncbi.nlm.nih.gov/pubmed/6678
48. Yehuda R, Steiner A, Kahana B, Binder-Brynes K, Southwick SM, Zemelman S, Giller EL (1997). "Alexithymia in Holocaust survivors with and without PTSD". *J Trauma Stress* 10 (1): 93–100.
49. Schechter DS, Suardi F, Manini A, Cordero MI, Sancho Rossignol A, Gex-Fabry Merminod G, Moser DA, Rusconi Serpa S. "How do maternal PTSD and alexithymia interact to impact maternal behavior?" *Child Psychiatry and Human Development*
50. Cochrane CE, Brewerton TD, Wilson DB, Hodges EL (1993). "Alexithymia in the eating disorders". *The International Journal of Eating Disorders* 14 (2): 219–22. doi:10.1002/1098-108X(199309)14:2<219::AID-EAT2260140212>3.0.CO;2-G (https://dx.doi.org/10.1002%2F1098-108X%28199309%2914%3A2%3C219%3A%3AAID-EAT2260140212%3E3.0.CO%3B2-G). PMID 8401555 (https://www.ncbi.nlm.nih.gov/pubmed/84015
51. The Relationship between Alexithymia and General Symptoms of Patients with Depressive Disorders. Kim JH, Lee SJ, Rim HD, Kim HW, Bae GY, Chang SM. Psychiatry Investig. 2008 Sep; 5(3):179-85. Epub 2008 Sep 30. http://www.ncbi.nlm.nih.gov/pmc/articles/PM
52. Cox BJ, Swinson RP, Shulman ID, Bourdeau D (1995). "Alexithymia in panic disorder and social phobia". *Comprehensive Psychiatry* 36 (3): 195–8. doi:10.1016/0010-440X(95)90081-6 (https://dx.doi.org/10.1016%2F0010-440X%2895%2990081-6). PMID 7648842 (https://www.ncbi.nlm.nih.gov/pubmed/76488
53. Taylor GJ, Parker JD, Bagby RM (1990). "A preliminary investigation of alexithymia in men with psychoactive substance dependence". *The American Journal of Psychiatry* 147 (9): 1228–30. PMID 2386256 (https://www.ncbi.nlm.nih.gov/pubmed/23862
54. Williams C, Wood RL (March 2010). "Alexithymia and emotional empathy following traumatic brain injury". *J Clin Exp Neuropsychol* 32 (3): 259–67. doi:10.1080/13803390902976940 (https://dx.doi.org/10.1080%2F13803390902976940). PMID 19548166 (https://www.ncbi.nlm.nih.gov/pubmed/195
55. Koponen S, Taiminen T, Honkalampi K, et al. (2005). "Alexithymia after traumatic brain injury: its relation to magnetic resonance imaging findings and psychiatric disorders". *Psychosom Med* 67 (5): 807–12. doi:10.1097/01.psy.0000181278.92249.e5 (https://dx.doi.org/10.1097%2F01.psy.0000181278.92249.e5). PMID 16204442 (https://www.ncbi.nlm.nih.gov/pubmed/1620
56. Becerra R, Amos A, Jongenelis S (July 2002). "Organic alexithymia: a study of acquired emotional blindness". *Brain Inj* 16 (7): 633–45. doi:10.1080/02699050110119817 (https://dx.doi.org/10.1080%2F02699050110119817). PMID 12119081 (https://www.ncbi.nlm.nih.gov/pubmed/121
57. Schizotypal, dependent and avoidant disorders are particularly indicated. See Taylor (1997), pp. 162–165
58. Li CS, Sinha R (1 March 2006). "Alexithymia and stress-induced brain activation in cocaine-dependent men and women" (https://www.ncbi.nlm.nih.gov/pmc *Journal of psychiatry & neuroscience : JPN* 31 (2): 115–21. PMC 1413961 (https://www.ncbi.nlm.nih.gov/pmc/articles/ PMID 16575427 (https://www.ncbi.nlm.nih.gov/pubmed/165
59. Lumley MA, Downey K, Stettner L, Wehmer F, Pomerleau OF (1994). "Alexithymia and negative affect: relationship to cigarette smoking, nicotine dependence, and smoking cessation". *Psychotherapy and psychosomatics* 61 (3–4): 156–62. doi:10.1159/000288884 (https://dx.doi.org/10.1159%2F000288884). PMID 8066152 (https://www.ncbi.nlm.nih.gov/pubmed/8066
60. Jones BA (1984). "Panic attacks with panic masked by alexithymia" (http://psy.psychiatryonline.org 959). *Psychosomatics* 25 (11): 858–9. doi:10.1016/S0033-3182(84)72947-1 (https://dx.doi.org/10.1016%2FS0033-3182%2884%2972947-1). PMID 6505131 (https://www.ncbi.nlm.nih.gov/pubmed/6505 Retrieved 2006-12-17
61. Michetti PM, Rossi R, Bonanno D, Tiesi A, Simonelli C (2006). "Male sexuality and regulation of emotions: a study on the association between alexithymia and erectile dysfunction (ED)" (http://www.nature.com/ijir/journal/v1 *Int. J. Impot. Res.* 18 (2): 170–4. doi:10.1038/sj.ijir.3901386 (https://dx.doi.org/10.1038%2Fsj.ijir.3901386). PMID 16151475 (https://www.ncbi.nlm.nih.gov/pubmed/161 Retrieved 2007-02-02

62. Jula A, Salminen JK, Saarijärvi S (1 April 1999). "Alexithymia: a facet of essential hypertension" (http://hyper.ahajournals.org/cg Hypertension 33 (4): 1057–61. doi:10.1161/01.HYP.33.4.1057 (https://dx.doi.org/10.1161%2F01.HYP.33.4.1057). PMID 10205248 (https://www.ncbi.nlm.nih.gov/pubmed/1020 Retrieved 2006-12-17
63. Verissimo R, Mota-Cardoso R, Taylor G (1998). "Relationships between alexithymia, emotional control, and quality of life in patients with inflammatory bowel disease" Psychotherapy and psychosomatics 67 (2): 75–80. doi:10.1159/000012263 (https://dx.doi.org/10.1159%2F000012263). PMID 9556198 (https://www.ncbi.nlm.nih.gov/pubmed/95561
64. Jones MP, Schettler A, Olden K, Crowell MD (2004). "Alexithymia and somatosensory amplification in functional dyspepsia" (http://psy.psychiatryonline.org/c Psychosomatics 45 (6): 508–16. doi:10.1176/appi.psy.45.6.508 (https://dx.doi.org/10.1176%2Fappi.psy.45.6.508). PMID 15546828 (https://www.ncbi.nlm.nih.gov/pubmed/155 Retrieved 2006-12-17
65. Taylor (1997), pp. 216–240
66. Taylor (1997), pp. 31

References

- Krystal, H (1988). *Integration and Self Healing: Affect, Trauma, Alexithymia*. Hillsdale, NJ: The Analytic Press. ISBN 0-88163-070-5.
- Linden W, Wen F, Paulhaus DL (1994). Measuring alexithymia: reliability, validity, and prevalence. In: J. Butcher, C. Spielberger (Eds.). *Advances in Personality Assessment*. Hillsdale, NJ: Lawrence Erlbaum Associates.
- McDougall, J (1989). *Theaters of the Body: A Psychoanalytic Approach to Psychosomatic Illness*, Norton.
- McDougall, J (1985). *Theaters of the Mind: Truth and Illusion on the Psychoanalytic Stage*. New York: Basic Books. ISBN 0-946960-70-4.
- Nemiah JC, Freyberger H, Sifneos PE. "Alexithymia: A View of the Psychosomatic Process" in O.W. Hill (1970) (ed), *Modern Trends in Psychosomatic Medicine*, Vol 2.
- Taylor, Graeme J; Bagby, R. Michael; Parker, James DA (1997). *Disorders of Affect Regulation: Alexithymia in Medical and Psychiatric Illness*. Cambridge: Cambridge University Press. ISBN 0-521-45610-X.

External links

- Emotional Intelligence (https://www.dmoz.org/Science/Social_Sciences/Psychology/Intelligence/Emotional_Intelligence/) at DMOZ

Look up alexithymia in Wiktionary, the free dictionary.

Retrieved from "https://en.wikipedia.org/w/index.php?title=Alexithymia&oldid=678598782"

Categories: Agnosia | Cognition | Neuropsychology | Personality traits | Symptoms and signs: Cognition, perception, emotional state and behaviour

- This page was last modified on 30 August 2015, at 11:58.

CIRCUMCISION IS THE HUMAN TOTEM POLE

Totemism is a religious as well as a social system. On its religious side it consists of the relations of mutual respect and consideration between a person and his totem, and on its social it is composed of obligations of the members of the clan towards each other and toward other tribes. In the latter history of totemism these two sides show a tendency to part company; the social system often survives the religious and conversely remnants of totemism remain in the religion of countries in which the social system based on totemism disappeared. In the present state of our ignorance about the origin of totemism we cannot say with certainty how these two sides were originally combined.

Sigmund Freud

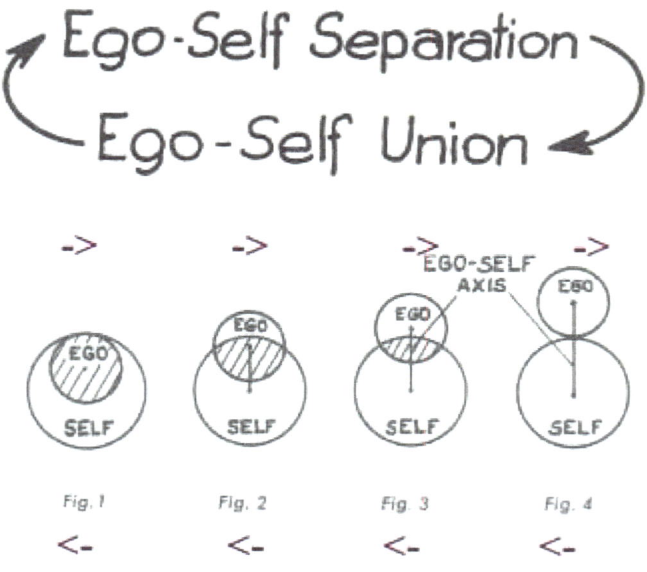
Ego-Self Separation
Ego-Self Union
EGO-SELF
AXIS
EGO
SELF
EGO
SELF
EGO
SELF
EGO
SELF
Fig. 1
Fig. 2
Fig. 3
Fig. 4

Dismemberers are in the Highest Rated Evil

On The Scale Of Evil, Where Do Murderers Rate?
by NPR STAFF
IMPULSIVE MURDERERS
SEMI-PSYCHOPATHS
PSYCHOPATHS
1 2 3 4 5 6 7 8 9 10 11 12 13 14 15 16 17 18 19 20 21 22
Roll over the blocks above to learn more about the 22 gradations of evil identified by Dr. Michael Stone. Scroll down to see who made the grade

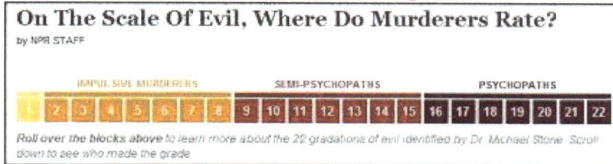

Highest Level #22: Psychopathic Torture-Murderers

Defined by a primary motivation to inflict prolonged, diabolical torture. Most are male serial killers. Dismemberments are a Signature indicating a Lust Crime. Circumcision servants apply.

Most of these guys have no burn-out point.
John Douglas with Mark Olshaker, *Mind Hunter*.

SELF-DEIFICATION

The serial killer who strangles and allows revival before the actual killing is telling the victim they have the power of Life and Death over the victim's existence, thus Self-Deification in/with Society.

ATTENUATED HOMICIDE

The act of causing a Death Act that is Attenuated whose intent is not to cause actual death and is the common motif in ritual.

MISUSE OF STATISTICS IN FALSE STUDIES

Carl Jung in *The Undiscovered Self* observed:[97]

In this broad band of unconsciousness, which is immune to conscious criticism and control, we stand defenseless, open to all kinds of influences and psychic inflections. As with all dangers, we can guard against the risk of psychic inflection only when we know what is attacking us, and how, where and when the attack will come. Since self-knowledge is a matter of getting to know the individual facts, theories help very little in this respect. For the more a theory lays claim to universal validity, the less capable it is of doing justice to the individual facts. Any theory based on experience is necessarily "statistical;" that is to say, it formulates an ideal average" which abolishes all exceptions at either end of the scale and replaces them by an abstract mean. This means is quite valid, though it need not necessarily occur in reality...

The statistical method shows the facts in the light of the ideal average but does not give us a picture of their empirical reality. While reflecting an indisputable aspect of reality, it can falsify the actual truth in a most misleading way. This is particularly true of theories which are based on statistics. The distinctive thing about real facts, however, is their individuality. Not to put too fine a point on it, one could say that the real picture consists of nothing but exceptions to the rule, and that, in consequence, absolute reality has predominately the character of irregularity.

THE TRIPARTITE NATURE OF EGO

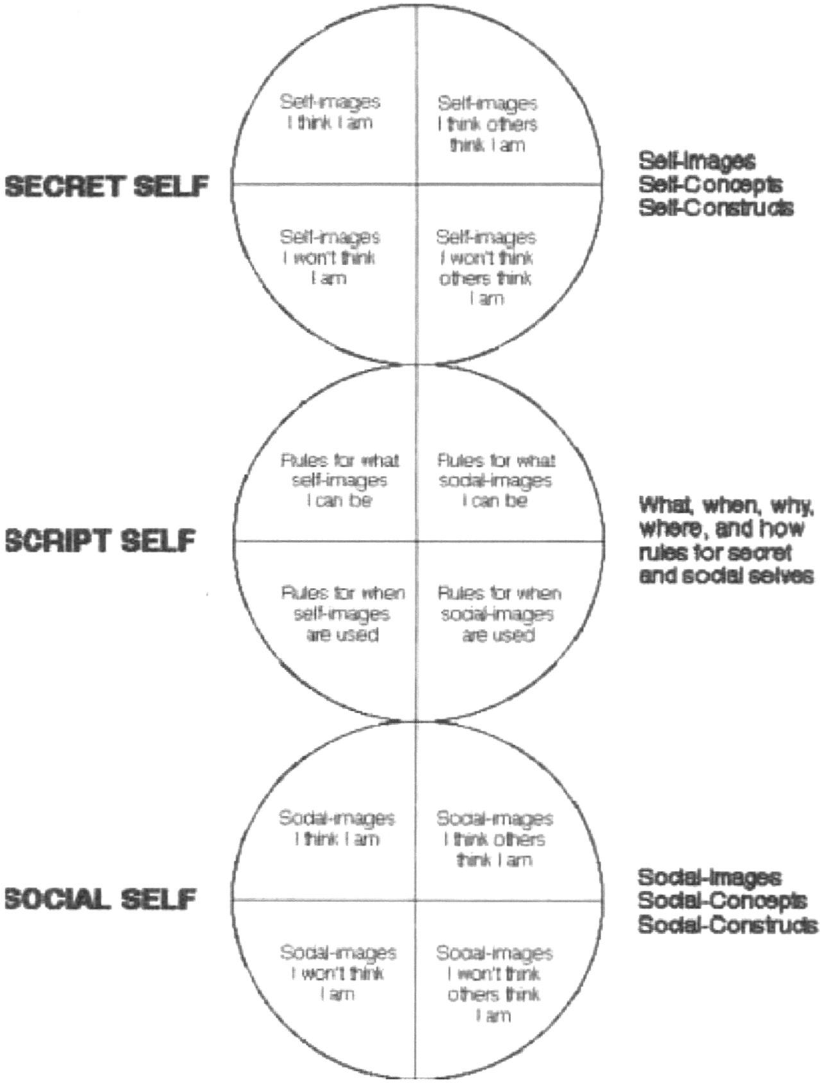
SECRET SELF
Self-images I think I am
Self-images I think others think I am
Self-images I won't think I am
Self-images I won't think others think I am
Self-Images
Self-Concepts
Self-Constructs
SCRIPT SELF
Rules for what self-images I can be
Rules for what social-images I can be
Rules for when self-images are used
Rules for when social-images are used
What, when, why, where, and how rules for secret and social selves
SOCIAL SELF
Social-images I think I am
Social-images I think others think I am
Social-images I won't think I am
Social-images I won't think others think I am
Social-Images
Social-Concepts
Social-Constructs

THE TRIPARTITE STRUCTURE OF EGO

Discover *Ego* to learn **how to** understand, overcome, and **uproot your ego**.

EGO: Ego is based on three classes of thought. The first type of thought is considered to be your permanent self. The second type of thought is considered to be your active self. And the third type of thought is considered to be your product self.

These three thoughts are the actual makings of ego--not mere descriptions of the imagined activities of self as in, for instance, psychodynamic theory (superego, ego, id).

The "I" is the result of having a thought about identity and identifying with that thought as if it were identity itself.

NAMES: It helps to name these three thoughts that form the structure of ego differently both to bring out different aspects and to offer different ways for you to relate to and experience the information.

GLOBAL THOUGHT	SPECIFIC NOW	SPECIFIC PAST OR FUTURE
First Thought	**Second Thought**	**Third Thought**
Permanent Self	Active Self	Changing Self
Eternal Self	Present Self	Past/Future Self
Judge	Judgment	Judged
Experiencer	Experiencing	Experience
Observer	Performer	Observed
Recorder	Recording	Recorded
Chooser	Actor	Action
Knower	Doer	Be-er
Witness	Cause	Effect
Designer	Programmer	Program
Boss	Worker	Product
Desire	Pursuit	Object
Start	Becoming	End
Actual	Striving	Ideal Future
Defective	Condemning	Damned Past
What-is	Developing	Should-be
Thinker	Thinking	Thought

PSYCHIC

MEDICAL ETHICS:
Johnson, Seigler, Winslade, *Clinical Ethics*.[B: 9-10]

MEDICAL PATERNALISM:

One of the most common ethical issues raised by the principle of respect for autonomy is paternalism. The term refers to the practice of overriding or ignoring a person's preferences in order to benefit them or enhance their welfare. In essence, it consists in the judgment that beneficence takes priority over paternalism. Today, while still common it is considered ethically suspect.

PATIENT PREFERENCE:

In all medical treatment, the preferences of the patient, based on the patient's own values and his or hers personal assessment of the benefits and burdens, are ethically relevant. In every clinical case, the questions must be raised: what are the patient's goals? What does the patient want? The systematic review of this topic requires further questions. Has the patient been provided sufficient information? Does the patient comprehend? Is the patient consenting voluntarily? Has the patient been coerced?

ANXIETIES:
Little, *Transference Neurosis & Transference Psychosis*.[A: 1]

NEUROTIC ANXIETY:

Neurotic Anxiety has to do with separation from an object perceived as a whole and separate from you, problems with sexual identity, loss of one's body

PSYCHOTIC ANXIETY:

Psychotic Anxiety has to do with questions of survival or annihilation, the question of separation from something of which you are a part (or which is a part of you), and problems with identity.

COGNITIVE DISSONANCE:

The mental stress or discomfort experienced by an individual who holds two or more contradictory beliefs, ideas, or values at the same time, or is confronted by new information that conflicts with existing beliefs, ideas, or values.

Avoidance of Cognitive Dissonance may be applied through: 1) Constructive Displacement for the positive. 2) Doubling for the negative structural and social. 3) Dismissive Cognition for the psychopathic negative.

DIFFUSION OF RESPONSIBILITY:
Bystander Effect; Attribution: Darby and Latane

A socio-psychological phenomenon whereby a person is less likely to take responsibility for an action or inaction when others are present. Considered a form of attribution, the individual assumes others are either responsible for taking action or have already done so. The phenomenon tends to occur in groups of people above a certain critical size and when responsibility is not explicitly assigned. It rarely occurs when the person is alone and diffusion increases with groups of three or more.

FEAR CONDITIONING:
Fear by Osmosis; see: Parable of the 5 Monkeys

Fear Conditioning is a behavioral paradigm in which organisms learn to predict averse events. It is a form of learning in which averse stimulus (e.g. electrical shock) is associated with a particular neutral context (e.g. a room) or neutral stimulus (e.g. a tone), resulting in the expression of fear responses to the originally neutral stimulus or context. This can be done with paring the neutral stimulus with an averse stimulus (e.g. shock, loud noise, or unpleasant odor). Eventually, the neutral stimulus alone can elicit the state of fear. In the vocabulary of classical conditioning, the neutral stimulus or context is the "conditional stimulus" (CS) the averse stimulus is the "unconditional stimulus" (US), and the fear is the "conditional response," (CR).

MODUS OPERENDI and SIGNATURE:
Douglas and Olshaker, *Mind Hunter*.[A: 5]

MODUS OPERENDI (MO) (Learned Behavior, Union Need)

MO is what the perpetrator does to commit the crime. It is dynamic – that is, it can change. Change is induced with success to ensure further success with refinement in predator safety and security.

SIGNATURE (Static, Criminal *Ritual*):

What the perpetrator has to do for fulfillment. Never changes.

PASSIVE INITIATION:

Having someone else perform on act for you.

TRANSFERENCE OF AGGRESSION: (definition: TRANSFERENCE):

The deliberate displacement of one's unresolved conflicts, dependencies, and aggressions onto a substitute object.

CODEPENDENT THINKING

Codependent Thinking involves 9 modes of thinking that are involved in and lead to dysfunctional relationships:[26]

BLACK AND WHITE THINKING
is any negative thing that happens gets turned into a Sweeping Generality.[27]

NEGATIVE FOCUS
is always thinking a glass is half empty, not half full. The other extreme is focusing on the positive to deny feelings.[28]

MAGICAL THINKING
is often in ritual to replace reality and a way of creating a self-fulfilling prophesy.[29]

STARRING IN A SOAP OPERA
involves blowing tings out of proportion. Users become the King or Queen of Tragedy. They are *trauma dramas*. Intensity of dramatic scenes in conflict are common themes. Individual overindulgence predominates.[30]

SELF-DISCOUNT
includes the inability to receive, or to admit to our own positive qualities.[31]

EMOTIONAL REASONING
is from feeling by believing that we feel is who we are, without separating the inner Child's feelings and Adult feeling in the present.[32]

SHOULDS,
musts, and *have tos*, come from authority figures. Adults do not have *shoulds* – Adults have choices.[33]

SELF-LABELING
identifies our perceived shortcomings and imperfections by not accepting one's humanity.[34]

PERSONALIZING THE BLAME
is blaming oneself as personally and totally responsible for happenstance, and how someone else feels. Conversely, it is blaming other people, or fate, to one's attitudes and behavior that may have contributed to a problem.[35]

A DEVELOPMENTAL PATHWAY OF SOCIAL PATHOLOGY

CULTURE BOUND SYNDROME
A local pattern of aberrant behavior with troubling experiences. They do not become accepted social behaviors and considered a type of sickness in that society. Such behavior may be from *schadenfreude*, (German: schaden=damage; freunde=joy) a feeling of enjoyment that comes from seeing or hearing about others troubles. Socially and as well to the self, *schadenfreude* may extend to Culture Specific Syndromes.

CULTURE SPECIFIC SYNDROME
A form of disturbed specific to a cultural system. Culture Specific Syndromes are considered normal behavior in that society. They may spread to other cultures from contact through Cultural Imperialism.

SHARED PSYCHOTIC DISORDER (Folie Imposee to Folie a Deux to Folie a Plusieurs)
A delusion imposed on a person from a close relationship with another who already has a Psychotic Disorder with prominent delusions. The delusion in the second person is similar to the delusion of the person who already has a delusion and termed *Induced Delusional Disorder* (Folie Imposee).

Shared Psychotic Disorder may develop in families (Folie en Famille). Family closeness may exist in group including social groups in work relationships. Extreme socialization creates Folie a Plusieurs).

Left untreated Shared Psychotic Disorder becomes chronic and pervasive. Sometimes Major Sadism develops.

RETURNING TO KEVIN FITZMAURICE
TRIPARTATE NATURE OF THE EGO: Part I

Fitz Maurice explains that the ego has only five actions with many variations:[36-38]

1. Seek death and destruction
2. Cover death and destruction with darkness
3. Cover death and destruction with names of good
4. Cover calling evil good (#3) with darkness
5. Cover death and destruction with victim role

Maurice then explains these as ego responses to threat or disturbance from:

1. Pain, hurt, shame, loss of face, humiliation
2. Fear of ego pain
3. Anger, fighting
4. Anxiety, avoidance, fear, escapism, flight

FREUD: THANATOS

Importance of Fitz Maurice is that the focus of ego functions is within Freud's *Thanatos* commonly known as the Death Wish as opposed to the Pleasure Principle which resides in our survival instinct through Eros and may apply to deep seated id manifestations within Veterans Affairs. Eros and Thanatos appear to represent the Light-life aspect of existence whose opposite side of this concept's coin is Dark-death.[39-41] Aspects of the definition include:

Psychiatry

1. A desire for self-destruction, often accompanied by feelings of depression, hopelessness and self-reproach.
2. The desire, often unconscious, for the death of another person, such as a parent, toward whom one has unconscious hostility.
3. A suicidal urge thought to drive certain people to put themselves consistently dangerous situations.
4. *Psychology (in Freudian psychology)* the desire for self-annihilation. See also *Thanatos*.
5. (*Classical Myth & Legend*) the Greek personification of death: son of Nyx , goddess of night and Erebos, god of darkness and his twin brother Hypnos, sleep. Siblings included: Geras – old age; Oizys – suffering; Moros – doom; Apate – deception; Momus – blame; Eris – strife; Nemesis – retribution and even Charon the ferryman who transported newly deceased across the rivers Styx and Acheron into Hades. Roman counterpart: Mors.

Thantalos, by using WWI as an example, allowed Freud to explain man's desire for murder and destruction including the fact that the death-drive is stronger than the life-drive.

Repetition Compulsion is closely bound to Thanatos and the need to repeat traumatic events in order to deal with and give a sense of control over them. Repetition Compulsion is an aspect of *Maslow's Self-actualization Hierarchy of Needs*. The sense of self-actualization, thus living at the top of the ladder, requires psychic reinforcement and successful Patterns of Behavior will be repeated. The drive for psychic fulfillment in Criminology is termed a *ritual*.[43-54]

EDINGER'S SELF DEIFICATION FROM THE EGO-SELF RELATIONSHIP[6]
CREATING A HOSPITAL-RELIGIOUS SUBCULTURE: MENDELSHON:[7]

The hospital is the church
Doctors are the priests
Nurses are the nuns
Medications are the sacraments
X-rays and surgery are the rituals
Questioning or disobedience equates to heresy

All this within the schizophrenic condition Lifton termed Doubling in *The Nazi Doctors: Medical Killing and the Psychology of Genocide*, Basic Books, 1986 where he stated the thing they thought they were doing was as "constructive work in a slaughterhouse." See: pp. 210 and 418, 420-424 and 488.

ACCOUNTABILITY

The approach of demons to individuals may be commonly classed in three ways: Oppression, Obsession, and Possession.
John A. MacMillan. *Encounter with Darkness.*

It's deja-vu all over again. Yogi Berra.

RES IPSA LOQUITUR: The thing speaks for itself

ALTRUISTIC ETHOS: a postured form of argument or discussion to enhance a belief or position as it relates to humanity in general

SELECTIVE ETHOS: a postured form of argument or discussion to enhance a belief or position that usually separates one person or group of persons from another person or group of persons usually via perceived innate differences between them, and often contains deceptions from altruistic posturing with subsequent actions in Situation Ethics, which is a fallacy

BABELIAN IMPERATIVE: **1.** The act of deceiving through use of a euphemism. **2.** The use of language in deception through obfuscation.

BERNAYS EFFECT: the improper and successful manipulation of an individual, group or the general public for power, control, and authority or financial gain; *see*: Eddy Bernays: Logical Fallacies (Power of Words), Persuasion Analysis, Propaganda Techniques, Public Relations

DELIBERATE DIFFERENCE: setting apart an individual or identifiable group, either expressly or by mute sanction, for different laws, equality, equity, actions, or inactions toward

DELIBERATE INDIFFERENCE: Deliberate Indifference is the conscious or reckless disregard of the consequences of one's acts or omissions. Deliberate Difference entails something more than negligence, but is satisfied by something less than acts or omissions for the very purpose of causing harm or with knowledge that harm will result.[B: 16]

DISMISSIVE COGNITION: The psychopathic ability to put aside all Cognitive Dissonance, often through Malignant Narcissism, by Dissociation of the humanity of others giving ability in criminality.

DISSOCIATE: **1.** To separate from association or union with another: DISCONNECT **2.** DISUNITE

DISSOCIATION (Criminal): criminal dissociation involves the separation of humanity of another individual to object status therefore a psychological lessening of the humanity of another that may lead to criminal behavior.

DISSOCIATION: **1.** The act or process of dissociating: the state of being dissociated **b.** the separation of idea or activity from the mainstream of consciousness or of behavior esp. as a mechanism of ego defense **2.** Psychiatry **a.** A psychological defense mechanism in which specific, anxiety producing thoughts, emotions, or physical separations are separated from the rest of the psyche **b.** The separation of a group of mental processes or ideas from the rest of the personality, so that they lead an independent existence,

DISSONANCE: **1.** Lack of agreement; *specif*: inconsistency between the beliefs one holds or one's actions and one's beliefs: DISCORD

DISSONANT: **1.** Marked by dissonance: DISCORDANT **2.** INCONGRUOUS **3.** Harmonically unresolved – dissonantly *adv*

DOMESTICATED VIOLENCE: socialized and/or acculturated use of violence in Transference of Aggression personally and/or interpersonally often detrimental to self and others in ritualistic behavior
DOUBLING: Doubling is the division of the self into two functioning selves, so that a part-self acts as the entire self. From Mandated Report:[B: 98]

COLLECTIVE GUILT: guilt of a collective group whether valid or not

IATROGENIC PATHOPHYSIOLOGY: pathophysiology caused by agency usu. As a result from a physician, or another, acting as a health care provider

MALIGNANT HERO SYNDROME: a person or group of persons who falsely and often maliciously create a crisis then miraculously rush in to the problem they in a self-glorification

MUNCHAUSEN COMPLEX: involves Munchausen Syndrome and Munchausen Syndrome by Proxy inclusive to social use often involving a type of self-glorification. *see*: Factitious Disorder

MUNCHAUSEN SYNDROME IN SOCIAL AGENCY: the agency relationship between the person with a primary agency as a parent or in a care giver relationship as the "principle," with a person who accepts secondary agency, usu. a doctor or shaman, that creates an act of abuse

COLLECTIVE MUNCHAUSEN SYNDROME IN SOCIAL AGENCY: the occurrence of Munchausen Syndrome in Social Agency with a group of any kind, in part, family, society, or culture

MUNCHAUSEN SYNDROME IN COLLECTIVE TRANSMISSION (MSICT): is a delusional transmission of a condition or simulation of a disease taken to clinical significance whether to a person or another person or group of persons. It is the transference of alleged identity to a personal relationship, family, community, society, or culture. It operates by deliberate transmission from one generation to subsequent generations of unresolved conflicts, dependencies, and aggressions onto a substitute body or body part abject as well as heirs

MUNCHAUSEN SYNDROME IN SOCIAL TRANSFERENCE (MSIST): is the identity transference of the self into a social group that practices forms of Munchausen behavior

MUNCHAUSEN SYNDROME FOR PROFIT: is the fabrication of disease or exacerbation of an existing medical condition or simulation of disease often with a Specialized Agent as an attorney or other special interest group, to gain sympathy from others and/or society for financial gain; *see*: Quid Pro Quo, Bribery

COLLECTIVE MUNCHAUSEN SYNDROME FOR PROFIT: occurs with group activity, with the motive for profit, that involves the abuse of a child or any other person

SOCIALIZED STALKING: organized improper social behavior directed toward an individual or group

TRANSGENETATIONAL MUNCHAUSEN SYNDROME (TMS): is generational abuse in family and/or social groups and a step toward acculturation

TRANSFERRED COLLECTIVE GUILT: 1. the transference of guilt onto an identifiable group from the actions of another or others 2. applied collective guilt by substitution through denial, deception, and deferral

TRANSFERRED GUILT: 1. the transference of guilt onto an identifiable group from the actions of another or others. 2. applied collective guilt by substitution through denial, deception, and deferral

TRANSFERRED REPRESENTATION: a transference of identity of an object, a person or objectified body part imparting new meaning that may create an altered meaning or focus of attention whether consciously or unconsciously directed

EDINGER'S SELF DEIFICATION FROM THE EGO-SELF RELATIONSHIP[6]
CREATING A HOSPITAL-RELIGIOUS SUBCULTURE: MENDELSHON:[7]

The hospital is the church
Doctors are the priests
Nurses are the nuns
Medications are the sacraments
X-rays and surgery are the rituals
Questioning or disobedience equates to heresy

All this within the schizophrenic condition Lifton termed Doubling in *The Nazi Doctors: Medical Killing and the Psychology of Genocide*, Basic Books, 1986 where he stated the thing they thought they were doing was as "constructive work in a slaughterhouse." See: pp. 210 and 418, 420-424 and 488.

A DEVELOPMENTAL PATHWAY OF SOCIAL PATHOLOGY

CULTURE BOUND SYNDROME

A local pattern of aberrant behavior with troubling experiences. They do not become accepted social behaviors and considered a type of sickness in that society. Such behavior may be from *schadenfreude*, (German: schaden=damage; freunde=joy) a feeling of enjoyment that comes from seeing or hearing about others troubles. Socially and as well to the self, *schadenfreude* may extend to Culture Specific Syndromes.

CULTURE SPECIFIC SYNDROME

A form of disturbed specific to a cultural system. Culture Specific Syndromes are considered normal behavior in that society. They may spread to other cultures from contact through Cultural Imperialism.

SHARED PSYCHOTIC DISORDER (Folie Imposee to Folie a Deux to Folie a Plusieurs)

A delusion imposed on a person from a close relationship with another who already has a Psychotic Disorder with prominent delusions. The delusion in the second person is similar to the delusion of the person who already has a delusion and termed *Induced Delusional Disorder* (Folie Imposee).

Shared Psychotic Disorder may develop in families (Folie en Famille). Family closeness may exist in group including social groups in work relationships. Extreme socialization creates Folie a Plusieurs).

Left untreated Shared Psychotic Disorder becomes chronic and pervasive. Sometimes Major Sadism develops.

<u>ON MENGELE</u>: He was capable of being so kind to the children, to have them become fond of him, to bring them sugar, to think of small details in their daily lives, and to do things we would genuinely admire… And then, next to that,… the crematoria smoke, and these children, tomorrow or in a half-hour, he is going to send them there. Well, that is where the anomaly lay. Auschwitz prison doctor.

Social Psychology concentrates on any and all aspects of human behavior. It involves our relationships to other persons, groups, social institutions, and to society as a whole. This includes clinical-social behavior.[60] Summaries:

ASSOCIATION

Psychosocial growth and development implies association with other individuals. Much of a person's mental content comes from others including beliefs, standards, values and ideals. Customs are powerful. And institutions of power, control, and authority with their laws in government, religion, social mores and ceremony are somewhat static because *prestige* lies in *precedent*, which is to say a type of *antiquity*. Thus a person's experiences are connected in subordination to the group's leading principles. But, leading principles evolve over time through *suggestive* interaction and are not static, uniform, or final. Stasis, uniformity, and finality attach themselves to closed scientific systems like mathematics but the open system of the human mind does not restrict pursuits like language, literature or religion.[61]

ACTS

Social acts or behavior, whether collective or individual, often have the purpose of influencing and controlling others. *Acts*, as surgery, that modify objects are *technical acts*. *Acts* that elicit pleasure or avoid pain are *hedonistic acts*. *Esthetic acts* are those that give meaning to an object (veteran). Besides the final outcome, that object becomes the *social token*. Tokens are used in all rituals by the Ritual Agent, whether the Ritual Agent is an individual or the culture itself. Tokens are often taken by criminals in similar manner to a sports trophy to be used to relive the successful experience.[62]

ACCULTURATION

A change in an original culture from contact with another culture or many cultures. This is different from *assimilation*, where different groups come together to form a new way of life. *Acculturation* deals with survival, resistance, modification, adaptation, and destruction of the old culture. *Diffusion* is adopting another culture's practice independent of population movement.[63]

CULTURAL APPROPRIATION

Occurs when a culture adopts an introduced behavior.[64]

CULTURAL IMPERIALISM

The phenomenon of an incoming group forcing new practices in their adopted culture.[65]

SOCIALIZATION

Socialization of new employee into the existing culture is *enculturation*. *Enculturation* is established through communal reinforcement by repeating the values and norms of the society to the new employee regardless of the lack of evidence to support society's, VA's, position. *Introjection* occurs when such behaviors become unconsciously accepted in the new employee's personality. *Introjection* is *internalization* of identification with parental figures, supervisors, and other aspects of the person's known world. Introjection is often accompanied with coping defense mechanisms and are forms of denial, self-deception, and deferral and are, as well, essential in *ritual*.[66]

Thomas WI, "The Relation of the Medicine Man to the Origin of the Profession," *Decennial Publications of the University of Chicago*, First Series, 4(1903): 241-256,

GROUP DYNAMICS

Involves behavior to current happenings. This behavior differs according to the individual's response to the local group. To achieve a new agreement the barriers of prejudices, expectations, ideology, theology, and control must be overcome. This can give rise to *social constructionism* which creates a perceived reality. The new reality birthed in social constructionism is an invention of the culture that eventually appears obvious and as natural knowledge. This then establishes a *consensus reality* that is the reality the group or culture wishes to believe.[68-69]

PEER PRESSURE

Peer Pressure then imposes the group norm on individuals and requires people to conform. Peer Pressure works when *opinion leaders* prevail.[70]

GROUPTHINK

Is when people intentionally go along with what they think is the group's opinion. *Groupthink* leads to improper and non-logical decisions. It uses the need of people to belong with others. Symptoms of *groupthink* include:[71]

1. illusion with invulnerability from unity
2. unquestioned belief
3. group rationalization
4. stereotyping opponents
5. self-censorship
6. direct pressure to conform
7. self-appointed guardians

COMMUNAL BEHAVIOR

Community reinforces *collective behavior* by instilling *fear*. *Collective Hysteria*, at times, is imbedded to ignite social change as well as maintain social stasis.[72]

STRUCTURATION

Structuration is repeating leader positions with implied *special knowledge* who set rules for others to live by. These people are acting as the *social agent* in an effort to change people's behavior. This *agency* is also used by the social agent to *repress*.[73-74]

INSTITUTIONALIZATION

The overall successful result is *institutionalization*. Success expands (as perceived VA Oakland with VA Phoenix appear to have collaborated in criminal behavior, possibly as well the Radiologist in VA LA).[75] *Cultural Imperialism* is set.

SOCIAL NORM

Once a Social Norm is established it becomes easily enforceable. Violations of norms are punished., even if only through social shunning. Violators are thought to be eccentric and alternatives are not acknowledged.[76]

MORES

Mores are strongly held norms and customs and customs, similar to social norms, that increase the ability to isolate detractors from society.[77]

FOLKWAY

The endpoint is to establish and maintain a folkway that are strictly reinforced.[78]

MEME

A *meme*, introduced by Dawkins in *The Selfish Gene*, is the pathway of cultural practice and may be thought of as a *social gene*. It is an element of culture or system of behavior that may be considered to be passed from one individual to another by non-genetic means. A successful *meme* is a part of cultural tradition. It may be a tune, an idea or catch-phrase that remains in people's memories and capable of rapid evolution into society. As genes, *memes* are passed on through the *meme pool* being transmitted from brain to brain which, in a broad sense, can be called *learning* or *imitation*.[79]

PROGRESSION OF SOCIAL MOVEMENTS

Social Movements may be positive or negative according to a person's personal ethics. *Mobilization* toward a new social reality is generated when current social procedures are deemed improper and it is thought a new social order will provide an improved social experience. *Rebellion* and *changes* produced from mobilization create a new social tendency. The following 3 systems work in unison in the creation Social Movements:[80-82]

1. A *social situation* usually starts with an idealized purpose. Advocates of that ideal work together to create a new social system. Examples can include governments, economic systems or religions.
2. The *social act* puts the social purpose into effect.
3. *Social tendency* evolves from the perception of the social act as the proper way to behave. Then it becomes static behavior until a new social situation enters to correct any problems created by the original social situation, act or tendency.

SOCIAL ORDER

Social order refers to a set of interlocking social structures, social institutions and social practices that conserve, maintain and enforce group defined *normal* ways of behaving and relating that are considered essential control and order in the society. The *social order is forced* on the individual. *Social sublimation* occurs with conformity to and psychological acceptance of the *social ideal*. With cognizance a positive reaction occurs with acceptance of the social ideal and *social value* system are met. A negative occurs with unacceptance and will be met with a corresponding negative to *maintain stability*. *Social defense* occurs if the negative originates from outside the *social order*.[83]

SOCIAL OBJECT

The VA's *Social Object* is the veteran.[84-85]

OBJECT PERSON

An *object person* is someone who has been dehumanized due to an attribute or physical quality they possess. The object person will accept whatever happens if it does not conflict with their concept of the *social purpose*. If the person objects then psychological inner conflict occurs. The perpetrator, the *ritual agent or parental figure*, is likewise conflicted when the victim's doubt attempts the perpetrator's desired action. This inhibits the *original social act* and the perpetrator must then resort to making *claims* and *arguments* in support of his *social ideal* as a counter moral force to inhibit the *object person's* moral protestations. Or, the perpetrating *social force* may impose *repression*. Repression creates opposing social values that must eventually be resolved. *Moral standards* are part of social values that, when improper, are often held by *manipulative arguments* that restrict contradiction.[86]

REFLECTED SELF IMAGE

How does the victim, here the veteran, feel about himself or herself after being forced to submit to improper VA practices? The inner, internalized, *Reflected Self Image* of the veteran is altered due to the overwhelming power of the VA's *social forces*. The prevailing *social personality*, through a Social Agent's self-image, has essentially told him or her they must submit or be shunned as when Dr. Daniel in Ukiah told the staff, two of which I worked with at Indian Health before their VA employment, that I was not to be medically appointed. But if the person removes himself from the overpowering social process, if possible, and uses logical, objective thought, it will lead him to end the social subjugation. When this happens the social body in identity crisis must necessarily take steps to maintain itself hopefully with the correction of impropriety.[87-88]

DEPENDENCE

Dependence also means that other people are opportunities by others *imposing* their conceptual way of life, *imago vivendi*, onto others. That can be used personally and socially for one's selfish gratification and fulfillment. This leads to conflict when needs, wants desires and perception among individuals or groups differ. When successful, social movements overwhelm individual choice, free will and human rights.[89]

INTERDEPENDENCE

Interdependence entails personal and societal responsibilities. We subsist through the monetary *reward* our *occupations* provide. They are not simply jobs; they carry significant *responsibilities*. The question we must ask is whether the occupation's *service* or *contribution* to society is more beneficial, mischievous or harmful.[90]

ASSERTIONS – OFFICIAL POSITIONS

To be an acceptable member of a group a person needs to conform to certain codes of conduct termed *cohort codes*. For this the social organization adopts *official positions*. Official positions of impropriety are *justified* through manipulative *advise* and *decisions* from self and/or social *authority figures*.[91]

GROUP-FANTASY

Lloyd DeMause's *Foundations of Psychohistory* documents social abuse, often generational, by illustrating 3 causes: 1): the unified group; 2): the effect of the group's abuse on the individual; and, 3): the individual's subsequent responses back to the group. *Group-Fantasy*:[92-94]

A group-fantasy, then, is produced by a collection of social alters as an agreement by groups of people to pool their traumas into a delusional social construction. Social alters have 4 main characteristics:

1. separate neural memory modules that are repositories for traumatic events and accompany feelings frozen in time.

2. organized into dynamic structures containing a different set of goals, values and defenses than the main self that help prevent the traumas and resulting despair from overwhelming one's life.

3. split off by a senseless wall of denial, depersonalization, discontinuity of affect and disownership of responsibility that is maintained in collusion with others in society who have similar alters to deny; and

4. communicated, elaborated and acted out in group-fantasies embedded in political, religious and ***social institutions.***

They [the SS doctors] did their work just as someone goes to an office goes about his work. They were gentlemen who came and went, who supervised and were relaxed, sometimes smiling, sometimes joking, but never unhappy. They were witty if they felt like it. Personally I did not get the impression that they were much affected by what was going on- nor shocked. It went on for years. It was not just one day. **Auschwitz prisoner doctor**

MASCULINE SERVANCY to the HUMAN FEMALE GODDESS

Mistress of the Two Trees

From Bovine and Full Human Sacrifices of either sex, though the vast majority are to the male, the Garden of Eden is a multiple Jungian Tetrad within feminine theology as a Paradigm Shift away from all Mythic Expression and used therefrom a complete cessation of both Full and Partial Sacrifice. YET, a sacrifice of some kind will be demanded and to fit differently as a veil of the Taboo. *Eve IS the Tree of Life and Death.*

Locus of Power and **Locus of Control – Social Primal Wound**

1): Buckley and Gottleib explained women in small tribal associations will synchronize their menstruation which then determines social cycles.

2): Mayan women bled the prepuce and fertilized Mother Earth with it.

3): Reah Tannahill stated: *The mystical significance of **all** blood has to be remembered when the subject of menstruation crops up, as it increasingly does today in discussions on the relative status of the sexes.*

Exodus 4:25-26 "Surely you are a bridegroom of blood <u>to</u> me."

Re is the feminine bleeding counterpart onto masculine Ra

What does it mean? It means the blood which fell from the phallus of Re.

Egyptian Book of the Dead, *The Papyrus of Ani.*

Circumcision – Social Tribal Wound – Sacred Pain

Re: Circumcision: As an act of incestuous nature (CG Jung, de Mause, Kitahara) in a Dismemberment Lust Crime with Passive Initiation, Slater mentioned in *The Glory of Hera* that circumcision of either sex is a bridge back to the womb – **Thantos** for Resurrection, and away from – Rebirth from the womb, as a Life/Death/Life event. The tissue is then given to the mother as her incestuous token. Some societies include cannibalism to incorporate the powers of the opposite sex.

Re: Circumcision; (7) The fourth, and most important, is that which relates to the provision thus made for prolificness; for it is said that the seminal fluid proceeds in its path easily, neither being at all scattered, nor flowing on its passage into what may be called the bags of the prepuce.

Josephus, *The Special Laws, I*

Cutting Club

From IntactWiki

Groups such as the **Cutting Club**, the Gilgal Society, and the Acorn Society openly admit to a morbid fascination with circumcision to the point of sado-masochistic fetish. These groups advertise that doctors are among their members. There are those on the Internet who discuss the erotic stimulation they experience by watching other males being circumcised, swap fiction and about it, and trade in videotapes of actual circumcisions.[1]

Members & Associates:

Vernon Quaintance

Brian J. Morris

Jake H. Waskett

Related Organizations:

Gilgal Society

Circlist

Acorn Society

References

1. ↑ Christopher P Price. Male Non-therapeutic circumcision: The Legal and Ethical Issues. In Male and Female Circumcision, Medical, Legal, and Ethical Considerations in Pediatric Practice (Denniston GC, Hodges FM and Milos MF eds.) New York: Kluwer Academic/Plenum Publishers, 1999: 425-454. http://www.cirp.org/library/legal/price2/

Retrieved from "http://intactwiki.org/w/index.php?title=Cutting_Club&oldid=264"
Categories: Organizations | CircLeaks

- This page was last modified on 23 April 2015, at 20:23.
- This page has been accessed 492 times.
- Content is available under Public Domain unless otherwise noted.

Acorn Society

From IntactWiki

Groups such as the **Acorn Society**, the Gilgal Society, and the Cutting Club openly admit to a morbid fascination with circumcision to the point of sado-masochistic fetish. These groups advertise that doctors are among their members. There are those on the Internet who discuss the erotic stimulation they experience by watching other males being circumcised, swap fiction and about it, and trade in videotapes of actual circumcisions.[1]

Acorn Society

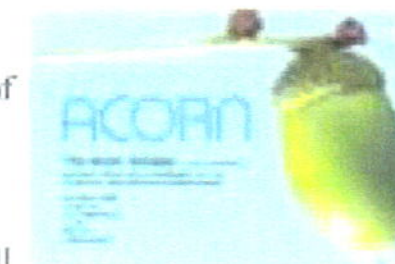

Acorn refers to the exposed glans.

Members & Associates:

Vernon Quaintance

Brian J. Morris

Jake H. Waskett

Related Organizations:

Gilgal Society

Circlist

Cutting Club

Story

Article for Acorn Society Magazine

> " I got myself a regular girlfriend [...] I asked her if she thought I ought to be circumcised. She considered this to be a very good idea.
>
> The next time my friend and I were together I told him that I had decided that I wanted to be circumcised. [...] Fortunately, as a member of the Acorn Society he was able to ask for other members' recommendations.
>
> [...] a Jewish doctor who charged £200. All the reports on this doctor were good and so we decided to go to him.
>
> Eventually I went to see the doctor at his North London surgery at the end of November 1994. I had a long discussion with him and he examined my foreskin and frenulum. He agreed to perform a circumcision under local anaesthetic and we agreed a fee of £200.
>
> I told the doctor that I wanted my frenulum removed and a fairly tight circumcision [...] I undressed completely and got onto the couch [...]

> Meanwhile, my friend set up a video camera which the doctor had agreed we could use to record the operation so that my girlfriend could later see it.
>
> The doctor was soon clamping my foreskin and determining exactly where he was going to place the cut. [...] One quick stroke of the scalpel along the side of the forceps removed my foreskin for ever. [...] The frenulum was quite tough and the doctor had to use both scissors and scalpel to cut through it.
>
> Despite all his efforts with the cautery device, the doctor could not completely stop me from bleeding where the skin had been removed.
>
> [...] my friend put away the video camera.
>
> I would recommend circumcision to anyone [...] I hope that these notes will be helpful to anyone still trying to make up their mind. "
>
> —Gilgal Society. Quaintance, V. (2001, September). *One man's account of his adult circumcision.* (http://www.circinfo.com/an_account.html)

References

1. ↑ Christopher P Price. Male Non-therapeutic circumcision: The Legal and Ethical Issues. In Male and Female Circumcision, Medical, Legal, and Ethical Considerations in Pediatric Practice (Denniston GC, Hodges FM and Milos MF eds.) New York: Kluwer Academic/Plenum Publishers, 1999: 425-454. http://www.cirp.org/library/legal/price2/

Additional Sources

- Quaintance, V. (2001, September). One man's account of his adult circumcision. *Acorn Society Magazine*.

Retrieved from "http://intactwiki.org/w/index.php?title=Acorn_Society&oldid=226"
Categories: Organizations | CircLeaks

- This page was last modified on 22 April 2015, at 22:18.
- This page has been accessed 562 times.
- Content is available under Public Domain unless otherwise noted.

Gilgal Society

From IntactWiki

Notice: Please see Vernon G. Quaintance for the latest information regarding the creator of the Gilgal Society. Quaintance was recently arrested for child pornography, was exposed as a child molester, and more.

Gilgal Society

The Gilgal Society

Logo is a snake trail from burning foreskins (biblical)

Owner:

Vernon Quaintance

Members & Associates:

Bertram Auvert

Robert C. Bailey

Daniel Halperin

Brian J. Morris

Edgar J. Schoen

Howard J. Stang

Jake H. Waskett

Thomas E. Wiswell

Related Organizations:

Circlist

Cutting Club

The Gilgal Society is a UK-based not-for-profit organization administered by (Circlist moderator) Vernon Quaintance.[3] Gilgal is Hebrew for "hill of foreskins." [4]

Groups such as the **Gilgal Society**, the Acorn Society, and the Cutting Club openly admit to a morbid fascination with circumcision to the point of sado-masochistic fetish. These groups advertise that doctors are among their members. There are those on the Internet who discuss the erotic stimulation they experience by watching other males being circumcised, swap fiction and about it, and trade in videotapes of actual circumcisions.[5]

Contents

- 1 Some Members and Associates of Gilgal Include [6]
- 2 Gilgal Porn
  - 2.1 Stories
  - 2.2 Videos
- 3 Circumcision Helpdesk - Gilgal Society Rebranded
- 4 See Also
- 5 References

Some Members and Associates of Gilgal Include [6]

Many of these people are the authors of the most recent pro-circumcision papers published in various medical journals (these works are used to push for circumcision in the media and through government organizations). Click their names for more information.

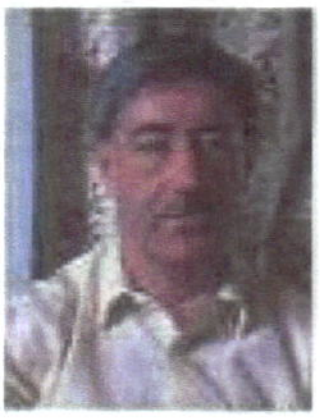

Vernon Quaintance (1997)[1] head of the Gilgal Society

- **Bertram Auvert**, MD, PhD
- **Robert C. Bailey**, Ph.D
- **Stefan Bailis**, MA
- **Xavier Castellsagué**, MD PhD
- Mike Cormier
- Guy Cox, DPhil
- Jane Gelbaum, RN NCAM
- **Daniel Halperin**, PhD
- Dawn Harvey, MA
- Sam Kunin, MD
- **Brian J. Morris**, PhD
- **Edgar J. Schoen**, MD
- Roger Short, AM FRS ScD
- **Howard J. Stang**, MD
- **Jake H. Waskett**
- Helen Weiss, PhD
- Robin Willcourt, MD
- **Thomas E. Wiswell**, MD

A quick search for these names in PubMed reveals that these are the most common "researchers" and editors of the latest circumcision to prevent HIV research, which is being funded the American government, and the World Bank.

Gilgal Porn

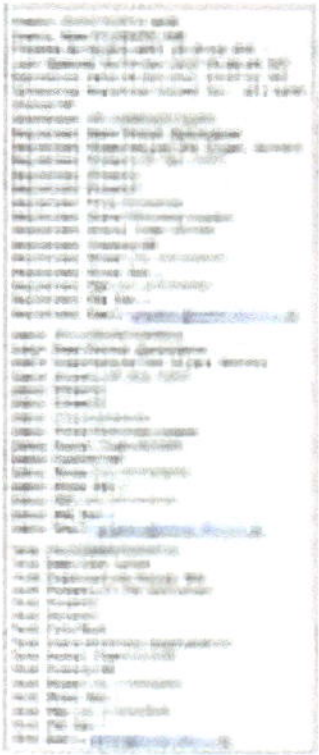

gilgalsoc.org is registered to Vernon Quaintance [9]

Stories

The Gilgal Society published a book (http://www.circleaks.org/images/d/d6/Gilgal_porn.pdf) containing stories eroticizing the circumcision of minors.

Published by The Gilgal Society

> He had not reached puberty but soon would: a few hairs were starting to grow at the base of his penis. Neil was then asked to lie on the couch for the penis to be photographed ...the doctor tested the fit of two sizes of Gomco Clamp bell. During this procedure Neil erected, but was not embarrassed by it and made no attempt to hide it.
>
> Mark came in next and again dropped his trousers readily. He had reached puberty and was quite well developed ... Its like an elephants trunk was the doctors comment, to which Mark heartily agreed. ... Photographs of his penis were taken...
>
> He had realised after sex education lessons at school that he had a problem.
>
> ...the boys were given plenty of wine to relax them ...the discussion was about the sex lives of the boys and their school friends. The doctor asked how often the boys wanked... The doctor showed the boys his microscope and asked if they had ever seen sperm under one. ... He suggested to Mark that if he wanted to, **he could have a quiet wank whilst Neil was being circumcised**... This was eagerly accepted. ... He lay back with his eyes closed and just let the doctor get on
>
> He returned to the surgery and put on his underpants (tight jockey briefs). His penis was guided up against his abdomen... Photographs had been taken...
>
> We all returned to the lounge where Mark was watching TV, having had his quiet wank. ...the doctor put some of Marks semen on a slide and put it under the microscope on high power. Each of us looked at the live sperm swimming vigorously around in the semen.
>
> ...there is hope that the circumcision will give him the confidence to overcome his shyness [bed wetting]
>
> The boys also looked at the book and noted a number of horrors which they would be spared now that they were circumcised.
>
> On this occasion there were three boys to be circumcised, two of them brothers aged 8 and 10. The doctor had planned to take the younger one first... ...did not need circumcision, but it was being done for uniformity with his brother
>
> He went down fighting and, because he had just been screaming, appeared to stop breathing. This worried his father, but the doctor said it was quite normal...
>
> [his] foreskin was long... ...it needed to come off.
>
> After lunch we had a five-year-old to do ... Robert has shown his off to his school-friends. I hope some of them ask their parents if they can have their penis circumcised too
>
> — *Acknowledgements to VQ* [Vernon Quaintance]

Case histories and experiences of circumcision, *Circumcision: An Ethnomedical Study* (p. 191), Gilgal Society (http://www.circleaks.org/images/d/d6/Gilgal_porn.pdf) [10]

Videos

Gilgal Circumcision Porn Book

Gilgal offers a circumcision VHS tape that you can order from their website. It is "unlabelled to allow your own discretion on labeling". [11]

Circumcision Helpdesk - Gilgal Society Rebranded

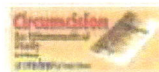

As of July 14th of 2014, date of the beginning of Vernon Quaintance's trial on charges of child sex abuse, the Gilgal Society's website has gone blank. However, upon verifying the Circumcision Information Resource Centre (another website by Vernon Quaintance which was "sponsored by the Gilgal Society"), we found that it is now sponsored by "The Circumcision Helpdesk."

The Circumcision Helpdesk website is also owned by Vernon Quaintance since 2003, and now contains the information previously presented by the Gilgal Society.

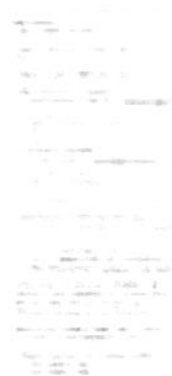

infocirc.com is also registered to Vernon Quaintance on behalf of The Gilgal Society. According to the main page "The International Circumcision Information Reference Centre is sponsored by The Gilgal Society"[9]

See Also

- Vernon Quaintance – Creator of the Gilgal Society
- Brian J. Morris – Member of the Gilgal Society
- Bertran Auvert – Associates with the Gilgal Society.
- Robert C. Bailey – Associates with the Gilgal Society
- Daniel T. Halperin – Associates with the Gilgal Society
- Brian J. Morris – Associates with the Gilgal Society.
- Jake H. Waskett – Associates with the Gilgal Society
- Thomas E. Wiswell – Associates with the Gilgal Society
- Circlist – Related group
- Acorn Society – Related group
- Cutting Club – Related group

References

Note: If a link is broken, you will find a PDF archive link directly behind it (under the same reference number).

1. ↑ Quaintance, Vernon. "Qreunion" (http://web.archive.org/web/20001026044806/www.martinq.dircon.co.uk/Qreunion/photos/Quaintance_Vernon.jpg). http://web.archive.org/web/20001026044806/www.martinq.dircon.co.uk/Qreunion/photos/Quaintance_Vernon.jpg. Retrieved 2011-03-09.
2. ↑ "WhoIs Record For GilgalSoc.org" (http://whois.domaintools.com/gilgalsoc.org). Domain Tools. http://whois.domaintools.com/gilgalsoc.org. Retrieved 2011-03-09.
3. ↑ "WHOIS information for gilgalsoc.org" (http://www.whois.net/whois/gilgalsoc.org). WhoIS.net. http://www.whois.net/whois/gilgalsoc.org. Retrieved 2011-04-27.
4. ↑ "Gilgal" (http://en.wikipedia.org/wiki/Gilgal). Wikipedia. http://en.wikipedia.org/wiki/Gilgal. Retrieved 2011-04-27.
5. ↑ Christopher P Price. Male Non-therapeutic circumcision: The Legal and Ethical Issues. In Male and Female Circumcision, Medical, Legal, and Ethical Considerations in Pediatric Practice (Denniston GC, Hodges FM and Milos MF eds.) New York: Kluwer Academic/Plenum Publishers, 1999: 425-454. http://www.cirp.org/library/legal/price2/
6. ↑ Morris, Brian (2007). Vernon Quaintance. ed. *Sex and circumcision. What every woman needs to know.* (http://www.circinfo.net/pdfs/GFW-EN%200712-1.pdf). London, England: Gilgal Society. http://www.circinfo.net/pdfs/GFW-EN%200712-1.pdf
7. ↑ Thomas, A. (2005). "Case histories and experiences of circumcision" (http://www.circleaks.org/images/d/d6/Gilgal_porn.pdf). In Vernon Quaintance. *Circumcision: An Ethnomedical Study*. **Fourth Edition.** London, England: The Gilgal Society. pp. 191 EMS-EN 0304-2. http://www.circleaks.org/images/d/d6/Gilgal_porn.pdf.
8. ↑ Shaw, Tony. "Circumcision, an ethnomedical study: A review by Tony Shaw" (http://www.gilgalsoc.org/b_reviews/ethnomed.html). *Gilgal Society*. Gilgal Society. http://www.gilgalsoc.org/b_reviews/ethnomed.html. Retrieved 2011-02-28.
9. ↑ "WhoIs Record For InFocirc.com" (http://whois.domaintools.com/infocirc.com). Domain Tools. http://whois.domaintools.com/infocirc.com. Retrieved 2011-03-09.
10. ↑ Quaintance, Vernon. "Adult Circumcision Video" (http://www.gilgalsoc.org/publications/acv.html). Gilgal Society. http://www.gilgalsoc.org/publications/acv.html. Retrieved 2011-03-11. Archive: File:Gilgal Video.pdf

Retrieved from "http://intactwiki.org/w/index.php?title=Gilgal_Society&oldid=280"
Categories: Organizations | CircLeaks

- This page was last modified on 23 April 2015, at 21:36.
- This page has been accessed 988 times.
- Content is available under Public Domain unless otherwise noted.

Circlist - IntactWiki Page 1 of 7

Circlist

From IntactWiki

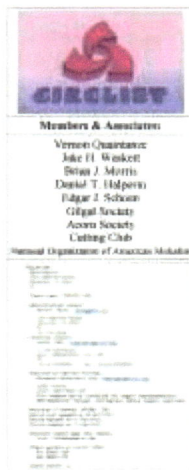

Members & Associates

Vernon Quaintance
Jake H. Waskett
Brian J. Morris
Daniel T. Halperin
Edgar J. Schoen
Gilgal Society
Acorn Society
Cutting Club
National Organization of American Mohalim

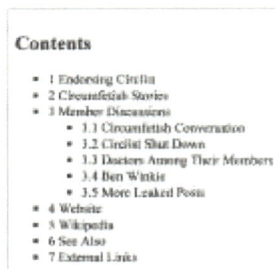

Circlist is a website and discussion group for men who sexually fantasize about performing and receiving circumcisions,[1] often on small children.[2] A few well known Circlist members include Vernon Quaintance[3] and Jake Waskett.[4][5] Professor Brian J. Morris, doctor Edgar J. Schoen, and researcher Daniel T. Halperin also associate with Circlist.[6][7]

Groups such as Circlist, the Gilgal Society, the Acorn Society, and the Cutting Club openly admit to a morbid fascination with circumcision to the point of sado-masochistic fetish. These groups advertise that doctors are among their members. There are those on the Internet who discuss the erotic stimulation they experience by watching other males being circumcised, swap fiction and about it, and trade in videotapes of actual circumcisions.[8]

Contents

- 1 Endorsing Circlist
- 2 Circumfetish Stories
- 3 Member Discussions
  - 3.1 Circumfetish Conversation
  - 3.2 Circlist Shut Down
  - 3.3 Doctors Among Their Members
  - 3.4 Ben Winkie
  - 3.5 More Leaked Posts
- 4 Website
- 5 Wikipedia
- 6 See Also
- 7 External Links

http://www.intactwiki.org/wiki/Circlist 8/25/2015

Mandated Report VA to CDC - Matteoli

- 8 References

Endorsing Circlist

Circlist Endorsers:

- Daniel T. Halperin (HIV/AIDS researcher)[9]
- National Organization of American Mohalim[10]
- Brian J. Morris[11]
- Jake H. Waskett[12]
- Vernon Quaintance[13]
- Edgar J. Schoen[14]

Circumfetish Stories

Circlist Story: *Circumcision Slut*

[illegible]

Circlist Story: *Circ Nurse*

[illegible]

Mandated Report VA to CDC - Matteoli

Circlist Story: *Wife Gives Husband Erotic Circ*

" commenting on how beautiful young William was. [...] He was a handsome baby, but that took an experienced eye to appreciate. [...] Mary got up to change his diaper. [...] Beth had even admitted that her future husband was uncircumcised when they first met. She had shocked Mary by proudly announcing that she had circumcised him herself a month and a half before the wedding. [...] Well, Beth went on, I discussed the idea one night with Tom before we had sex. I had been stroking his penis gently for several minutes and he was horny as hell. We had discussed circumcision many times before, and Tom knew I was very much in favor of it. While Tom was not as pro-circumcision as I was, he was curious about it as well. He confessed that he had wondered all his life what it would be like to have a circumcised penis. He had masturbated as a child and young adult fantasizing about being circumcised against his will. Not really fighting it, just being told that it was going to happen, and not being able to stop it. [...] the role playing of him submitting to me and letting me circumcise him had become a major and enjoyable part of our sex play. [...] "Will you video tape the operation so I can see it sometime?" You bet! Tom and I had planned to do that anyway. Beth and Tom had made the Tara Clamp a regular part of their sex play. Beth would place the clamp over Tom's glans, pull his thick foreskin up over the cone and partially close the clamp. Beth would put just enough pressure on the two locking arms that Tom could feel the clamp pinching his prepuce. [...] Beth had bought him a special pair of black silk under shorts for tonight's ritual. [...] Tom knew perfectly well what was about to happen, and he had been semi erect all the drive home from work. [...] Beth was secretly ecstatic because she knew this was the last time she'd ever do this for Tom with his foreskin intact. [...] Beth enjoyed sex with Tom very much. Soon, she'd enjoy it infinitely more, she thought to herself. [...] Looking into Tom's eye's, she said, "Are you ready"? Tom simply nodded that he was. Beth moved the video camera, which was on a tripod, over to where it would be able to record everything she did. [...] Beth grabbed the tip of Tom's foreskin in each hand and pulled the foreskin forward as far up over the clamp as possible. [...] Beth examined how much skin would be removed after clamping. She wanted Tom cut fairly tight, with little or no foreskin bunching up behind his glans when he was flaccid. [...] Beth managed to get what she felt was the correct amount of foreskin in front of the clamping jaws. [...] Beth was startled to hear the clamp "click" shut. [...] Exciting, it was for her to be the instrument of ridding her future husband of his foreskin. Beth left the clamp in place for fifteen minutes before reaching for the disposable knife. [...] He said to Beth, "Go ahead baby. Circumcise me!" With that Beth pushed down with the knife and felt it cut into the thick layer of skin. [...] Beth continued cutting around the clamp. [...] she described to Tom the feelings she was having exploring his new circumcised organ. [...] All this activity had made Beth extremely horny! "

—Circlist [illegible]

Member Discussions

Happy Circlist Member

" Hi! I've just spent the last week going over your website in detail. I must say how wonderful it is... full of important content and actually amusing at the same time. "

—Circlist [illegible]

FROM: Bodjarrell...

TO: Jake H. Waskett (at Circlist Yahoo Group)

" I was cut at birth but I have lots of excess skin. Actually, when I'm sitting, the skin fully covers my penis head. I'd like to get cut again, but I'd like to make it an erotic experience with either a female doctor or at least I'd like to have one or two female nurses do the prep. Any suggestions? "

- Yahoo Circlist, Message #27849, 2000 Dec 29th

How many circumcisions has a Circlist member had?

0 circumcisions	13, or 14.13 % of total responses
1 circumcisions	43, or 46.74 % of total responses
2 circumcisions	27, or 29.35 % of total responses
3 circumcisions	5, or 5.43 % of total responses
4 circumcisions	2, or 2.17 % of total responses
5 circumcisions	0
6 circumcisions	2, or 2.17 % of total responses
7 circumcisions	0

—Yahoo Circlist, Message [illegible], 2003 Nov [illegible]

Promoting "The Rough-Head Club"

- The rough-head club is for circumcised men, and for uncircumcised men who permanently leave their foreskins in the retracted position to experience the rough-head feeling. Though we shouldn't have to do this because EVERY man should be circumcised at birth to experience the proven sexual and medical benefits. So uncut men, strip 'em back and get that famous head-rub.

—Circlist http://webcache.googleusercontent.com/search?q=cache:[illegible]:www.circlist.org/[illegible].html

Erotic Circumcision

- First learned of circ at 6. Best friend had to have it done for phimosis. He showed it with pride. Even at that age I found it erotic! From then I wanted to have a penis that looked like that, but it was many, many years before I plucked up the courage to have my desire fulfilled.

—Yahoo Circlist, Message [illegible], 2003 Oct [illegible]

Circumfetish Conversation

FROM: Circumsi[illegible]@hotmail...

TO: Jake H. Waskett (at Circlist Yahoo Group)

- Some of us who do get erotic and sexual gratification out of not only the finished product, but also the procedure itself. The act of becoming a man is just as important as the bare head he shows.

—Yahoo Circlist, Message [illegible], 2003 Nov

FROM: [illegible]@hotmail...

TO: Jake H. Waskett (at Circlist Yahoo Group)

I'm with Circumstar on this one. Having a cut dick is important, but how you

" gay it is also of interest. "

—Yahoo Circlist. Message [illegible], 2003 Nov.

FROM: [illegible] (John S.)

TO: John H. Winkett (at Circlist Yahoo Group)

" As for the fact that some people find the rite of circumcision erotic, some do. The fact that it involves a surgical procedure on the penis, which permanently alters its appearance — has feelings (which understandably may cause erotic feelings in some men. "

—Yahoo Circlist. Message [illegible], 2003 Nov.

Circlist Shut Down

FROM: [illegible]

TO: Circlist

" Hi David, Vernon and fellow CIRCLISTers!

Congratulations on getting the group re-established with what I hope will be a much more open-minded host – though like the rest, I'm at a loss to imagine what they thought we were doing wrong! :-(

Richard "

—Google Circlist. 2003 May 27th (http://[illegible]Winkett_2003-05-24.pdf)

Doctors Among Their Members

FROM: David Cornell, M.D.

TO: Circlist

" Hi David and Vernon

Good luck with establishing the new group. I would say you have your work cut out for you.

Regards,
David Cornell, M.D., FACS "

—Google Circlist Jun 4 2003 8:59pm (http://[illegible]Winkett_2003-05-24.pdf)

Ben Winkie

" Circlist has always permitted, and will continue to permit, circumcision related fetish/sexual postings/materials, straight, gay or otherwise. Individuals may use Circlist to make contact with one another, including for sexual purposes. The list is not just a medical interest list, but rather all things circumcision, including circ-fetish, sexual info, medical info and a place to meet up with fellow circumcision enthusiasts and proponents. "

—Ben Winkie. (2003, June) *International Circumcision Symposium*, Washington, D.C. (http://www.circumstitions.com/Glossary2.html)

Mandated Report VA to CDC - Matteoli

More Leaked Posts

Member banned for disagreeing with forced circ fetish

Old enough to appreciate a circumcision experience.

Circlist post rated 5 stars

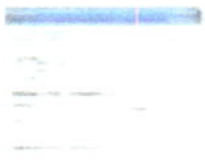

The Jehn Gallery

Projection

Circumcision makes it all better

Mandatory circumcision

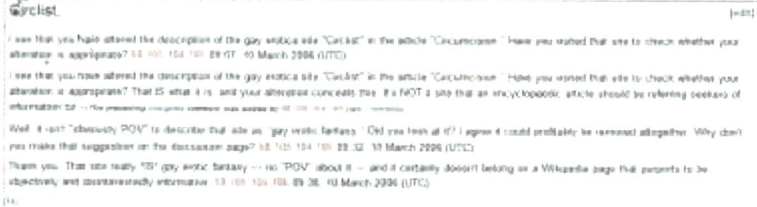

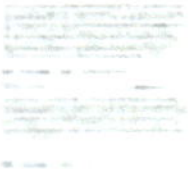

Circumcise Europe, quickly

Remove ALL skin (including shaft skin!)

Website

On the links page, a list of newsgroups is listed as follows:[11]

- misc.kids
- misc.kids.health
- misc.kids.pregnancy
- alt.male.hygiene
- alt.circumcision

Wikipedia

What happened to the Circlist Wikipedia article:

Circlist [edit]

I see that you have altered the description of the gay erotica site "Circlist" in the article "Circumcision." Have you visited that site to check whether your alteration is appropriate? 68.105.154.186 09:07, 10 March 2006 (UTC)

I see that you have altered the description of the gay erotica site "Circlist" in the article "Circumcision." Have you visited that site to check whether your alteration is appropriate? That IS what it is, and your alteration conceals this. It's NOT a site that an encyclopaedic article should be referring seekers of information to! —The preceding unsigned comment was added by 68.105.154.186 (talk • contribs).

Well, it isn't "obviously POV" to describe that site as "gay erotic fantasy." Did you look at it? I agree it could profitably be removed altogether. Why don't you make that suggestion on the discussion page? 68.105.154.186 09:32, 10 March 2006 (UTC)

Thank you. That site really "IS" gay erotic fantasy — no "POV" about it — and it certainly doesn't belong on a Wikipedia page that purports to be objectively and dispassionately informative. 68.105.154.186 09:38, 10 March 2006 (UTC)

[12]

See Also

- Gilgal Society – Associated circumfetish group.

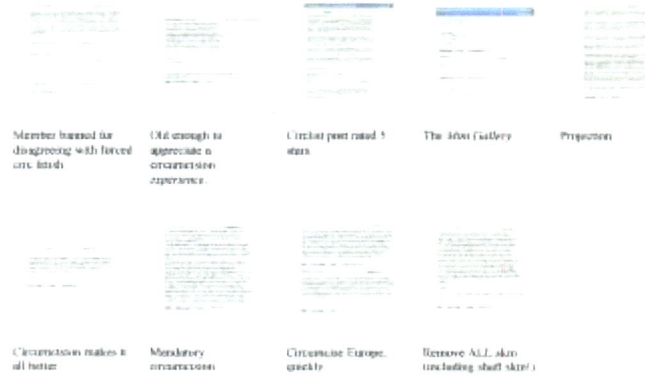

- Acorn Society -- Associated circumfetish group.
- Cutting Club -- Associated circumfetish group.
- Vernon Quaintance -- Moderator of Circlist.
- Jake H. Waskett -- Proud member of Circlist.
- Brian J. Morris -- Endorses Circlist.
- Daniel T. Halperin -- Endorses Circlist.
- Edgar J. Schoen -- Endorses Circlist.
- Circumfetish -- What drives someone to become a Circlist member.

External Links

- Circlist Stories (http://classic-web.archive.org/web/20010610100735/circlist.org/emasculatehat.html) -- Pornographic circumfetish stories published by Circlist.
- Daniel T. Halperin (http://www.circumcisioninformation.com/halperin_inverview1.htm) -- Pro-circumcision HIV/AIDS researcher Endorsing Circlist.
- National Organization of American Mohalim (http://www.beritmila.org/Resources/articles.htm) -- Endorsing Circlist.

References

1. † Ben Winkie. (2005, June) *International Circumcisual Symposium*, Washington, D.C (http://www.circumstitions.com/Glossary2.html)
2. † Thomas, A. (2005). "Case histories and experiences of circumcision" (http://www.circleaks.org/images/d/d6/Gilgal_porn.pdf) . In Vernon Quaintance. *Circumcision: An Ethnomedical Study*. **Fourth Edition**. London, England: The Gilgal Society. pp. 191. EMS-EN 0304-2. http://www.circleaks.org/images/d/d6/Gilgal_porn.pdf
3. † Yahoo Circlist. Message #26333, 2003 July 30th
4. † Yahoo Circlist. Message numbers: 26279, 26333, 27182, 27370, 27399, 27849, 27363, 27383, 27424, 27642, 28047 & 31662.
5. † Google Circlist. Message: 2005 May 24th 12:06pm
6. † Morris, Brian J. (2007-08-29). "Circumcision Websites & Online Discussion Groups" (http://circleaks.org/images/3/31/Web.archive.org-web-20070829145507-circinfo.net-circumcision_websites_online_discussion_groups.html-1.pdf) . circinfo.net. http://circleaks.org/images/3/31/Web.archive.org-web-20070829145507-circinfo.net-circumcision_websites_online_discussion_groups.html-1.pdf. Retrieved 2011-03-06. Archive: http://web.archive.org/web/20070829145507/circinfo.net/circumcision_websites_online_discussion_groups.html
7. † "The Great Circumcision Debate with Daniel Halperin, PhD" (http://www.circumcisioninformation.com/halperin_inverview1.htm) . http://www.circumcisioninformation.com/halperin_inverview1.htm. Retrieved 2011-04-27.
8. † Christopher P Price. Male Non-therapeutic circumcision: The Legal and Ethical Issues. In Male and Female Circumcision, Medical, Legal, and Ethical Considerations in Pediatric Practice (Denniston GC, Hodges FM and Milos MF eds.) New York: Kluwer Academic/Plenum Publishers, 1999: 425-454. http://www.cirp.org/library/legal/price2/
9. † "The Great Circumcision Debate with Daniel Halperin, PhD" (http://www.circumcisioninformation.com/halperin_inverview1.htm) . http://www.circumcisioninformation.com/halperin_inverview1.htm. Retrieved 2011-04-14.
10. † "Berit Mila Program of Reform Judaism" (http://www.beritmila.org/Resources/articles.htm) . National Organization of American Mohalim. http://www.beritmila.org/Resources/articles.htm. Retrieved 2011-03-11. Archive: File:National Organization of American Mohalim.pdf
11. † Morris, Brian J. (2007-08-29). "Circumcision Websites & Online Discussion Groups" (http://circleaks.org/images/3/31/Web.archive.org-web-20070829145507-circinfo.net-circumcision_websites_online_discussion_groups.html-1.pdf) . circinfo.net. http://circleaks.org/images/3/31/Web.archive.org-web-20070829145507-circinfo.net-circumcision_websites_online_discussion_groups.html-1.pdf. Retrieved 2011-03-06. Archive: http://web.archive.org/web/20070829145507/circinfo.net/circumcision_websites_online_discussion_groups.html
12. † Google Circlist. Message, 2005 May 24th 12:06pm (more here)
13. † Yahoo Circlist. Message #26333, 2003 July 30th (more here)
14. † Schoen, E. (2006, April 22). *My recent circ pubs* [Online Forum Comment]. Retrieved from http://health.groups.yahoo.com/group/MCIRC/message/16 Archive: http://circleaks.org/images/1/1f/MCIRC_-_Msg_16.pdf
15. † "Circumcision Resources" (http://replay.waybackmachine.org/20020220124910/http://circlist.org/cresources.html) . Circlist. 2002-02-20. http://replay.waybackmachine.org/20020220124910/http://circlist.org/cresources.html. Retrieved 2011-04-02.
16. † "User talk:Fuzzie" (http://en.wikipedia.org/wiki/User_talk:Fuzzie#Circlist) . Wikipedia. 2006-03-10. http://en.wikipedia.org/wiki/User_talk:Fuzzie#Circlist. Retrieved 2011-04-02.

Retrieved from "http://intactwiki.org/w/index.php?title=Circlist&oldid=255"
Categories: Organizations | CircLeaks

- This page was last modified on 23 April 2015, at 20:13.
- This page has been accessed 1,821 times.
- Content is available under Public Domain unless otherwise noted.

Vernon G. Quaintance

From IntactWiki
(Redirected from Vernon Quaintance)

Notice: Recently, Vernon Quaintance was arrested on charges of child pornography. The page you are viewing is likely (at least partially) responsible for the tip-off that lead to this arrest (although this is currently unconfirmed, it's almost certain). See the section labeled Arrested for Child Pornography for more information. If you work in a field of law, please note that incriminating evidence on this article is vastly more inclusive and incriminating since Quaintance's arrest, and is currently being added to on an almost daily basis as new information comes in. You will find many connections to Quaintance here that warrant further investigation. Please support Circleaks by promoting the site to help further the cause.

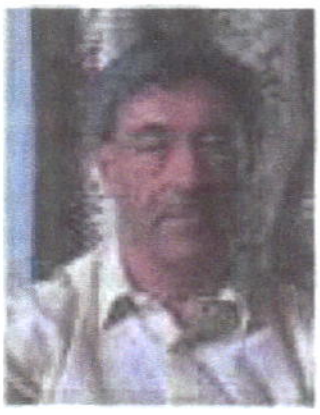

Convicted of:
Possession of child pornography
Owner Of:
Gilgal Society
Member Of:
Circlist
Acorn Society
Benefactors:
Jake H. Waskett
Brian J. Morris
Bertran Auvert
Robert C. Bailey
Daniel Halperin
Thomas E. Wiswell
Edgar J. Schoen

Vernon Geoffrey Quaintance[1] is a 69-year-old pedophile[2][3][4] and photographer[3] who recently ran a children's computer club.[2] It is alleged that he molested altar boys in his church,[4] who were from Henley Gardens, Upper Norwood, England.[4] He was employed as a sacristan and server for the Order of Malta's Mass (Roman Catholicism).[4] Quaintance is a Circlist moderator (a private group that shares child circumcision pornography),[6] head of the Gilgal Society (another private group that shares circumcision pornography),[7] a member of the Acorn Society,[8] owner of infocirc.com,[9] gilgalsociety.org,[10] and a writer of erotic circumcision porn (including graphic descriptions of circumcising young boys while others masturbate).[11] On April 11th 2011, Quaintance was arrested after having been caught with a hoard of child porn.[1] Quaintance is friends with Jake Waskett (top ranking Wikipedia circumcision editor, and a member of the circumfetish group Circlist)[12] and has worked closely with circumcision proponent Brian J. Morris.[13][14] Quaintance is also connected to many pro-circumcision doctors, and even a great deal of the prominent "circumcision to prevent HIV" researchers that are published in academic journals.[11][14] Quaintance is a retired telephone engineer.[?]

There are those on the Internet who discuss the erotic stimulation they experience by watching other males being circumcised, swap fiction about it, and trade in videotapes of actual circumcisions.[15] Quaintance is one of these individuals.[16][17] Some call them Circumfetishists.[18]

Contents

- 1 Gilgal Society
  - 1.1 Gilgal Porn
    - 1.1.1 Stories
    - 1.1.2 Videos
  - 1.2 Gilgal Society rebranded
- 2 Arrests for Child Pornography and Sexual Offences Against Children
  - 2.1 2011 Arrest
    - 2.1.1 Judge's Response
    - 2.1.2 Response From Neighbors
    - 2.1.3 Release
  - 2.2 2013 Arrest
  - 2.3 2014 Trial
  - 2.4 2014 Sentence
- 3 Ran a Children's Group

Gilgal Society

The Gilgal Society (headed by Quaintance) is a UK-based not-for-profit organization administered by Quaintance.[19] Gilgal is Hebrew for "hill of foreskins."[20]

Logo is a smoke trail from burning foreskins (biblical).

Groups such as the Gilgal Society, the Acorn Society, and the Cutting Club openly admit to a morbid fascination with circumcision to the point of sado-masochistic fetish. These groups advertise that doctors are among their members.[21]

Some Members and Associates of Gilgal include Bertran Auvert, Robert C. Bailey, Stefan Baliis, Xavier Castellsagué, Mike Cormier, Guy Cox, Ilene Gelbaum, Daniel Halperin, Dawn Harvey, Sam Kunin, Brian J. Morris, Edgar J. Schoen, Roger Short, Howard J. Stang, Jake H. Waskett, Helen Weiss, Robin Willcourt, and Thomas E. Wiswell.[22] A quick search for these names in PubMed (http://www.ncbi.nlm.nih.gov/pubmed/) reveals that many of these are the most common *researchers* and editors of the latest circumcision to prevent HIV research, which is being funded the American government, and the World Bank.

Gilgal Porn

Stories

Published by The Gilgal Society

> He had not reached puberty but soon would: a few hairs were starting to grow at the base of his penis. Neil was then asked to lie on the couch for the penis to be photographed. ...the doctor tested the fit of two sizes of Gomco Clamp bell. During this procedure Neil erected, but was not embarrassed by it and made no attempt to hide it.
>
> Mark came in next and again dropped his trousers readily. He had reached puberty and was quite well developed. ... Its like an elephants trunk was the doctors comment, to which Mark heartily agreed. ... Photographs of his penis were taken...
>
> He had realised after sex education lessons at school that he had a problem
>
> ...the boys were given plenty of wine to relax them. ...the discussion was about the sex lives of the boys and their school friends. The doctor asked how often the boys wanked. ... The doctor showed the boys his microscope and asked if they had ever seen sperm under one. ... He suggested to Mark that if he wanted to, he could have a **quiet wank whilst Neil was being circumcised**... This was eagerly accepted. ... He lay back with his eyes closed and just let the doctor get on.
>
> He returned to the surgery and put on his underpants (tight jockey briefs). His penis was guided up against his abdomen... Photographs had been taken...

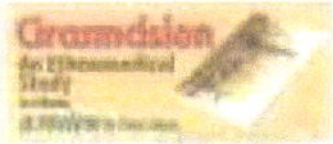

Gilgal Circumcision Porn Book

> We all returned to the lounge where Mark was watching TV, having had his quiet wank. ...the doctor put some of Marks semen on a slide and put it under the microscope on high power. Each of us looked at the live sperm swimming vigorously around in the semen.
>
> ...there is hope that the circumcision will give him the confidence to overcome his enuresis (bed wetting)
>
> The boys also looked at the book and noted a number of horrors which they would be spared now that they were circumcised
>
> On this occasion there were three boys to be circumcised, two of them brothers aged 8 and 10. The doctor had planned to take the younger one first... ...did not need circumcision, but it was being done for uniformity with his brother
>
> He went down fighting and, because he had just been screaming, appeared to stop breathing. This worried his father, but the doctor said it was quite normal...
>
> [illegible] foreskin was long... ...it needed to come off
>
> After lunch we had a five-year-old to do... . Robert has shown his off to his school-friends. I hope some of them ask their parents if they can have their penis circumcised too.
>
> — *Acknowledgement to VQ* (Vernon Quaintance)

Case histories and experiences of circumcision. *Circumcision: An Ethnomedical Study* (p. [illegible]). Gilgal Society (http://www.[illegible]) [23][24]

Videos

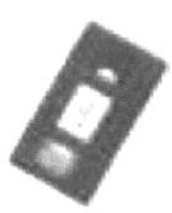

image from a Gilgal Society webpage.[25]

Gilgal offers a circumcision VHS tape that you can order from their website. It is "unlabelled to allow your own discretion on labeling".[25] Quaintance has additionally been caught by local officials with at least 3 VHS tapes that include 7-9 hours of child pornography [1]

Gilgal Society rebranded

As of July 14th of 2014, the Gilgal Society's website has gone blank. However, upon verifying the Circumcision Information Resource Centre (another website by Vernon Quaintance which was "Sponsored by the Gilgal Society"), we found that it is now sponsored by "The Circumcision Helpdesk."

The Circumcision Helpdesk website is also owned by Vernon Quaintance since 2003, and now contains the information previously presented by the Gilgal Society

Arrests for Child Pornography and Sexual Offences Against Children

2012 Arrest

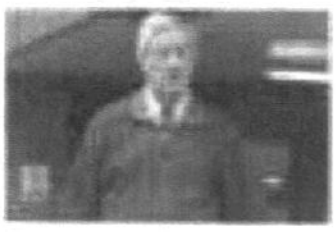

Quaintance at the courthouse, after getting caught with 7-9 hours of child pornography [14]

Police raided Quaintance's home in Henley Gardens, Upper Norwood, after receiving a tip-off.[7] The wiki page you are currently reading on CircLeaks may have lead to his arrest. Quaintance was caught with a hoard of child porn, located in a box in his office. They found three video cassettes with nine-hours worth of clips showing boys as young as 11 engaging in sex acts. The videos seized included graphic footage of child abuse ranked at the second-highest level of severity. The children in these tapes were estimated to be between the ages of 11 and 17 years. Quaintance claims to have been celibate for his entire life. Quaintance admitted three counts of possession of indecent photographs of a child.[9]

Judge's Response

Judge Nicholas-Lumine Smith told him: "You said you had watched the videos but claimed to have got no sexual enjoyment. I'm afraid I very much doubt that since you retained them." But he said Quaintance's willingness to address his problems meant he could suspend his prison sentence.[3]

Response From Neighbors

Residents in Hunley Gardens, where Quaintance is known as the respected head of the local community association, were shocked to hear of his conviction. One neighbour, who did not want to be named, said: "I know he is a very religious man and is committed to the church."[42]

Release

Quaintance was recently given a 40-week suspended sentence for possessing child pornography.[2]

The following image is from Court News UK, on April 17th 2012.[21]

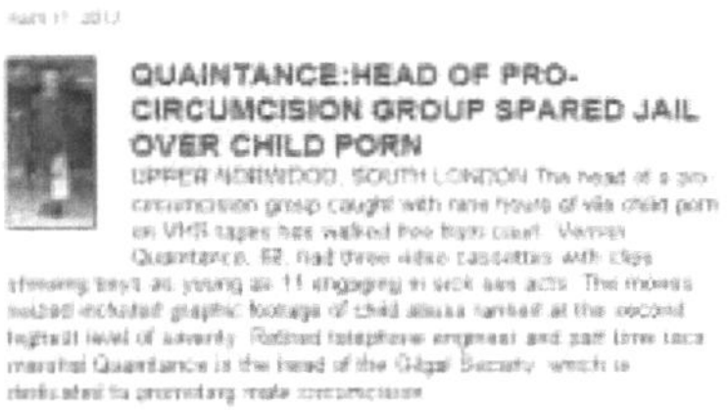
April 17, 2012

QUAINTANCE:HEAD OF PRO-CIRCUMCISION GROUP SPARED JAIL OVER CHILD PORN

UPPER NORWOOD, SOUTH LONDON The head of a pro-circumcision group caught with nine hours of vile child porn on VHS tapes has walked free from court. Vernon Quaintance, 68, had three video cassettes with clips showing boys as young as 11 engaging in sick sex acts. The movies seized included graphic footage of child abuse ranked at the second highest level of severity. Retired telephone engineer and part time race marshal Quaintance is the head of the Gilgal Society, which is dedicated to promoting male circumcision.

2013 Arrest

According to a news report in The Tablet, an international Catholic Weekly, "Vernon Quaintance, of Upper Norwood, south-east London, has been charged with one count of indecent assault against a 10-year-old boy in 1966, the same offence against an 11-year-old in 1976, and a single count of sexual assault against a boy aged 11. He is further accused of three counts of inciting a boy aged under 16 to commit an act of gross indecency. Charges against him also include the possession of1,285 indecent images of children."[47]

2014 Trial

On July 16th, 2014, Quaintance pleaded guilty to nine sex offences including those against boys as young as 11 he had met in the 1960s and 70s, as follows: five counts of indecency with a child between 1966 and 1976 and four counts of possession of indecent images. An additional count of sexual assault alleged to have taken place in 2011 on a child was left to lie on file.

Judge Anthony Leonard QC adjourned sentencing until September. Quaintance was released on conditional bail, with the requirement to have no unsupervised contact with anyone under 18.[18]

2014 Sentence

On October 3rd, 2014, Vernon Quaintance was sentenced to two years and four months in prision for targeting young boys and asking them to expose themselves under the pretense of inspecting whether or not they were circumcised. Judge Anthony Leonard QC said Quaintance used his interest in the surgical procedure to look at young boys. The judge took into consideration that this offending did not carried over into Quaintance's later years, and his less than perfect health, to offer some allowance.[54]

Ran a Children's Group

Quaintance is a former chairman of Croydon Computer Club, who also started a free computer group for children.[3]

A Child Molester By Age 33

In an online book written by Mike Harper, the author remembers back at 11 years old of a much older Vernon Quaintance (in 1977-1979) pulling young Harper's foreskin back to imitate a circumcised penis while parked in a car. He also remembers Quaintance telling a circumcision joke, and an attempt to show young Harper Quaintance's penis [31]

Chapter 7: Let me take you by the hand. (Part 1)

Towards Norbury Central

> [...] my nemesis, Vernon Quaintance [...] ran the computer demonstrations there and never went back.

—Harper, M. (2010). Little Mikey H - A Norbury Lad. *Towards Norbury Central* (http://www.authonomy.com/books/20510/little-mickey-h-a-norbury-lad/read-book/?chapterid=194970) Archive (http://circleaks.org/images/a/a6/Little-mickey-h-take-you-by-the-hand.pdf)

Chapter 12: In the presence of the Lord.

Altar Boy

> We usually served on the altar with the same group of boys, some of whom normally served at other services but would occasionally join us. [...] Vernon Quaintance (brother of Veronica who had driven Gill and me part of the way to the school coach stop many years before) [...]
>
> Generally the older boys/men would be awarded these privileges [Ringing the consecration bell and other activities]. Once one had been an altar boy for a considerable while, one would be inducted into the guild of altar servers, the Archconfraternity of St Stephen [...]
>
> My altarboyship has one particularly grim memory, one that left an extremely unpleasant (though fortunately not literally) taste in the mouth. No one except Vernon Quaintance and me know the full facts (until now!) though some may have an inkling of what might have happened based on a later similar occurrence.
>
> As an altar server, Vernon, who was much older than most of us, maybe in his late twenties or early thirties, and only beaten by Mr Cowie in terms of age, possessed a most solemn and holy air on the altar and strongly disapproved of any of us younger boys messing about. This air of solemnity was enhanced by a long face and aquiline nose, though on opening his mouth, one could see stretches of rotten teeth.
>
> One Saturday morning when I was perhaps eleven years old, Vernon called at our house enquiring if I would like to go out for a drive that afternoon. Clearly held in respect by my parents, they could see nothing wrong with me going for a drive with Vernon and neither could I. And so, that afternoon, perhaps around 3pm, Vernon picked me up in his purple Austin Allegro and drove in the general direction of Box Hill in Surrey. After some time during which amongst other things, he commented on the metal 'Scorpio' ring (signifying my astrological persuasion – not that it meant anything to me, I just thought that it looked 'cool') that I frequently wore, the conversation turned slightly seedier.
>
> Having pulled over into a secluded car park somewhere in the woods near Box Hill, he told me a joke about two soldiers square-bashing (i.e. drill on a barracks square). I don't recall the exact nature of the joke but the punch line involved some confusion between castration and circumcision. He then asked me if I knew what a circumcision was, to which I replied 'No'. He then explained what it was. It sounds dumb to say it but somehow, he made it seem ok for me to show him my willy, and seemed interested in determining how far I could pull my foreskin back, even gently trying to do so himself. Being only a young boy, I could hardly do so, but he said that if I kept trying, I would soon be able to. He then asked if I wanted to see an example of a circumcision, which I understood to mean that he wanted to show me his willy.

Having already realized that this was not appearing to be as innocent a car ride as it had at first seemed, but until that point not being able to see an easy way out, I blurted out that I had told my Mum that I would be going to confession that day and so, had to get back. Fortunately, perhaps due to the mention of church, he didn't pursue the issue and drove me back to St Barts where confession was still in progress late on that Saturday afternoon.

I didn't tell anyone what had happened, but I felt horrified, sickened and used and if I have made you uncomfortable, dear reader, I hope you may have a notion of how I felt about this for quite a while. Having realized what a creep Vernon was, when he popped round some weeks later and asked whether I wanted to go out for another drive, I quickly declined with the excuse that I was going into Croydon that afternoon. A few weeks later still, he tried again, and hawking the same excuse, I think he finally got the message and never bothered me again.

Some thoughts and questions arise from this whole sordid issue:

- Firstly, why me? Or was I simply one of a long string of boys that Vernon duped? Based on later evidence, almost certainly…
- Secondly, it surprises me that children (and indeed their parents) can be duped in this way. I'm fairly bright but still succumbed to Vernon's persuasion. Therefore I am inclined to think that generally, children implicitly trust adults, especially those who are involved with the church, and do not expect to be taken advantage of. Adults who prey on this trust should be punished.
- Thirdly, when I declined his further invitations, was he worried that I would shop him to the police? For how long would he have desisted, before being tempted again?
- Fourthly, did he feel guilty after these events? Did he go home and toss himself off or kneel down and flagellate himself to excise his guilt?
- Fifthly and simply, what kick do paedophiles get out of messing with young children?

A few years later, I understand that Vernon was shopped to the police by the parents of Anthony Vassallo, a younger altar boy. I guess that this information became generally public. Following this, Vernon no longer served on the altar but could be seen sitting near the front of the pews as unsmilingly solemn and devout as ever. That must have been an interesting interview, when he would have had to relinquish his status, perhaps having to admit that he was a perv. I guess that Mum and Dad and probably some/most/all of my siblings became aware of his fall from grace too and the reasons for it, but none of them ever raised the subject with me. If they did know, they must have been scared of what they might hear or else perhaps they felt that I was dealing with it in my own way, which I eventually did. If my parents did know, or suspect, then they let me down. They should have raised it with me to make sure I was okay. Who wouldn't want to protect their child from something like this? While I didn't let it get to me too much, I felt sick at the time for being taken advantage of. As the years passed, it affected me less and less as time went on until by the time I reached my late teens, I had put it down to experience. It certainly contributed to my withdrawal from the church, that there could be such unchristianness in a person who was perceived by all of us to be one of the most devout.

There are lots of things that can mess children up and this sequence of events haunted me for a long time, during which I didn't feel I could tell anybody. Nowadays, it seems all too regular that paedophiles are being outed by their victims, but I bet that there are many, many, many cases that never come to light. I hate to imagine that this could happen to my own children and that they would not feel able to tell me.

As a coda to this episode, it should be noted that some years after, Vernon could be found in the local library teaching rudimentary computing to…wait for it…children! I guess that this would have been before the 'Sex Offenders Register' was inaugurated, but I do wonder how many of this new source of young flesh he managed to work his way through before he was again caught, if he ever was. I would like to think that if I saw him again, performing any similar role, that I could shop him to the authorities (probably anonymously so that I wouldn't have to potentially face him in court) and ruin his career and his life as he could have ruined mine. I don't know if he is still following his sordid urges, but if he is, I hope the young children that he is grooming have the good sense to stick razor blades up their bottom

> Frankly in my opinion, any grown man found guilty of messing about with young children should have their tackle whipped off. Very plain and simple. Removing a dog's gonads curbs its sexual urges, but dogs don't menace young children (at least not sexually), so a stronger punishment/deterrent is required for us intelligent beings. Quite simply, grown men who should be able to exercise some restraint should lose both their dick and balls. Painfully? Maybe, if they have been particularly evil, but at least remove their desire to prey on youngsters. [...]

—Harper, M. (2010). Little Mikey II - A Norbury Lad. *Altar Boy*. (http://www.authonomy.com/books/20510/little-mickey-ii-a-norbury-lad/read-book/?chapterid=194978) Archive (http://circleaks.org/images/0/82/Little-mickey-ii-a-norbury-lad-r.pdf)

Chapter 15: have you seen the writing on the wall? (Part 3)

Fourth Year – 4.3 (Sep 1979 – Jul 1980)

> [...] Sometime towards the latter part of the school year, a second strange incident with paedophilic overtones occurred. As with the Vernon Quaintance incident, this has never been mentioned to anyone else. UNTIL NOW!!! [...]
>
> As with Vernon Quaintance five years earlier, the way the suggestion was couched made it appear an acceptable thing to do at the time. [...]
>
> Given how the law has tightened around paedophiles or 'kiddy- fiddlers' as they are colloquially known, men such as Vernon Quaintance and Chris Wilshire who put themselves in such risky positions must be running scared that one day they may be caught and damned for eternity. But knowing the risks [...] many paedos commit offences again and again. Is it the element of risk that provides that extra frisson of excitement over which they can furiously masturbate after the event?
>
> The final questions with Chris Wilshire are, as with Vernon, how many other boys did he try this risky trick on and how many other adults are there in authority that use their position in this way, but never get caught? [...] I can't imagine that I was the only boy that this happened to, and in a school of 192 boys in each year – perhaps 1000 boys in total, he would have been able to cherry- pick those amongst us who he thought would not blab.
>
> [...] I don't hold Chris Wilshire in the same contempt as I held Vernon [...]

—Harper, M. (2010). Little Mikey II - A Norbury Lad. *Fourth Year*. (http://www.authonomy.com/books/20510/little-mickey-ii-a-norbury-lad/read-book/?chapterid=194982) Archive 3 (http://circleaks.org/images/b/b7/Little-mickey-ii-writing-on-the-wall.pdf)

Work in the Church

Quaintance was employed as a sacristan and server for the Order of Malta's Mass (Roman Catholicism).[7] Quaintance has been involved in children's church activities since—at least—the 1970's (when Quaintance was in his 30's).[17]

Church Scandal

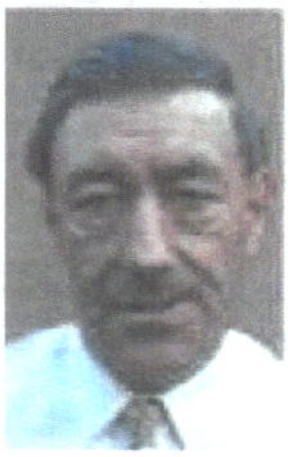

Vernon Quaintance (2007)[7]

In April of 2012—after learning of Quaintance's pedophilic nature—there was a mass walkout of the Order's governing council, which has its headquarters in St John's Wood, North London, from where it directs its charitable undertakings. Nine members, including Lord Guthrie, the former Chief of the Defence Staff, who is the vice-president, have resigned.[2]

Three members of the Order of Malta, known as knights, have been banned from entering the church of St John and Elizabeth in North London. Many resigned because they are unhappy to find that Vernon Quaintance is a pedophile; these include retail heir Mark Brenninkmeijer, City fund manager Stephen Mucklow-Smith, upmarket chocolate retailer Nick Crean, society party organiser Peregrine Armstrong-Jones' wife Caroline, publishing heir Adam Macmillan's ex-wife, Sarah, the Duke of Norfolk's cousin, Richard Fitzalan-Howard, financier Count Nicolas Reuttner and the organisation's former hospitaller Tim Orchard. One knight said "What we objected to was that the three members of the Order's senior body, the Grand Priory, who should have known about this man's background, did nothing."[11]

As a result, the Archbishop of Westminster, Vincent Nichols, the head of the Catholic Church in England, is considering banning the Order from using the church altogether.[2]

Photography Work

Some of Quaintance's photography can be viewed here (http://1.bp.blogspot.com/_KtGG618Wzx4/SF3dl-Y2xxI/AAAAAAAAADw/TrkAMrTn9To/s400/london.jpg) , from his own website.[34]

Quotes

Email

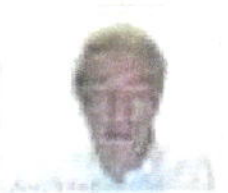

Photo of Quaintance from his photography website (http://www.traditions

Jake Waskett—the number one Wikipedia editor on all articles related to circumcision[25]—wrote a thank you letter to Quaintance in 2003 after obtaining his fantasy of becoming circumcised.[26] Waskett has said he is good friends with Quaintance.

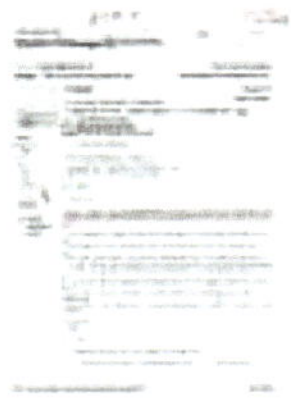

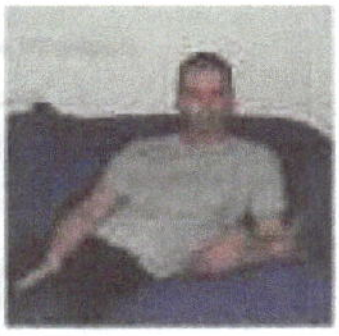

Jake Waskett, a close friend of Vernon Quaintance, and a fellow member of Circlist.

FROM: Jake H. Waskett

TO: Vernon Quaintance

SUBJECT: Circed At Last!

Hi Vernon

Thank you!

Yes, I recall our correspondence. I find it difficult to believe that I would regret something that I've regretted *not* having done since age 5!

I'm pleased to report that it's now day 9. I've taken all but one of the stitches out. The bruising has gone, and the skin has bonded well on the top and right sides. Dr. Zarifa warned me that the skin would open a little due to the tightness, and sure enough on the left and underside it has. He assured me that this would fill in and become a neat line, so I am trusting the mysterious processes of the human body to do this. I'm getting a couple of drops of blood from the frenulum area from nighttime erections. The swelling is slowly going down, though it has by no means gone.

Regards, Jake

– Yahoo Circlist Message #36133, 2003 July 30th (http://circleaks.org/images/b/bd/Waskett_2003-07-30.pdf) **More Here (http://circleaks.org/index.php?title=Jake_H._Waskett#2003_July_30th)**

Newsgroup

FROM: Vernon Quaintance <quainta...@oldpeter.agw.bt.co.uk>
SUBJECT: Circumcision as an aid to speed swimming

My nephew is 16 and a very good swimmer, representing his school and district in competitions. He keeps himself shaved for competitions to reduce the drag and now his coach has recommended that he get circumcised to further improve his performance. Jake is not averse to the idea of circumcision, but wonders how common this is as a speed aid. Does anyone have experience of swimming coaches advising circumcision? Anyone had it done to improve their own swimming? Does it work? Thanks. Date: 20 Nov 1995 1:00am

—rec.sport.swimming (13 Nov 1995 18:22:08 GMT)

FROM: Vernon Quaintance <quainta...@oldpeter.agw.bt.co.uk>
TO: Tina Johnson

Tina Johnson commented that her 7 month old son had been circumcised at birth but still had a lot of foreskin left [...] Irrespective of whether the arguments in favour of circumcision are really valid or not they _could_ only be valid in the case of a complete circumcision where the whole glans and coronal rim are permanently exposed. [...] If you leave it till later then it will be even more painful and embarrassing for the boy. [...] I know of several men who have chosen as adults to have a re-circumcision [...] the partial circumcision your son received will not do the job properly and you should seriously consider having it re-done properly

—misc.kids.health (Jul 1 1995, 3:00 am)
(http://webcache.googleusercontent.com/search?q=cache:Ja1[illegible].groups.google.sk/group/misc.kids.health/tree/browse_frm/month/1995-07/0a[illegible]%3Frnum%3D1%26_done%3D%252Fgroup%252Fmisc.kids.health%252Fbrowse_frm%252Fmonth%252F1995-07%253F[illegible]&ct=clnk&gl=sk&client=firefox-a)

Poetry

Vernon Quaintance Writes Poetry

Doctors

Some people claim that foreskins are fun
And keep the 'muzzle' on the gun
But many doctors do declare;
It's healthier with the glans laid bare
So, mum & dad, we say to you,
You must decide what's best to do,
Your son will benefit throughout his life,
As, incidentally, will his wife:
If you make the choice that's always wise
and do decide to circumcise

Quaintance. Quoted by (http://www.circumstitions.com/Schoens.html) Brian Morris. (2007, October). An old protector mandated Circumcision HPV Today pp 12-13 (http://www.circumstitions.com/Schoens.html)

Website

> Like the appendix, the foreskin is a remnant from our evolutionary past and now serves no essential purpose. Unlike the appendix, which is buried deep inside the abdomen, the foreskio is easily and safely removed as a preventative measure.
>
> — Quaintance, V. (2000). *Questions girls ask about male circumcision* (http://www.circinfo.com/questions/qga.html) Archive (http://circleaks.org/images/d/da/Quaintance_for_Girls.pdf)

> An additional hazard of having a redundant foreskin is the [illegible] with which it can get caught in a zipper. Many women complain of a lack of stimulation because a long or tight foreskin can stick to the walls of the vagina...
>
> — Quaintance, V. (2000). *Questions girls ask about male circumcision* (http://www.circinfo.com/questions/qga.html) Archive (http://circleaks.org/images/d/da/Quaintance_for_Girls.pdf)

See Also

- Discussion Page – See the talk page for more information about Quaintance that isn't yet added to this article.
- Circumfetish -- A description of the illness Quaintance suffers from.
- Brian J. Morris – A circumcision promoter that works with Quaintance to obtain circumcision propaganda pamphlets.
- Jake H. Waskett -- A friend of Quaintance who is the #1 Wikipedia editor on all circumcision articles.
- Gilgal Society – Quaintance's secret club.
- Circlist -- Quaintance is a moderator of this private circumfetish group that fantasizes about children.
- Cutting Club -- Quaintance is a member of this circumcision fetish group.
- Acorn Society – Quaintance is a member of this circumcision fetish group.
- Daniel T. Halperin -- A "Circumcision to prevent HIV" researcher that personally approved of Quaintance's materials.
- Edgar J. Schoen – A pro-circumcision doctor that personally approved of Quaintance's materials.
- Stephen Moses – A "Circumcision to prevent HIV" researcher that personally approved of Quaintance's materials.
- Bertran Auvert – A "Circumcison to prevent HIV" researcher that personally approved of Quaintance's materials.
- Robert C. Bailey – A "Circumcision to prevent HIV" researcher that personally approved of Quaintance's materials.
- Thomas E. Wiswell – A "Circumcision to prevent UTIs" researcher that personally approved of Quaintance's materials.

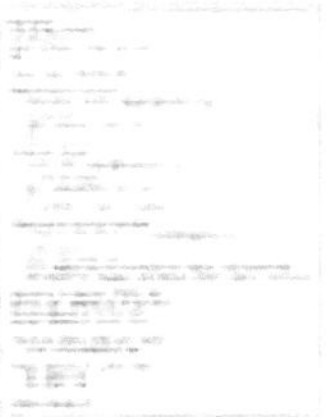

infocirc.com is also registered to Vernon Quaintance on behalf of The Gilgal Society. According to the main page "The International Circumcision Information Reference Centre is sponsored by The Gilgal Society"[47]

CircWatch

Posts about Vernon Quaintance on CircWatch (http://circwatch.org/tag/vernon-quaintance/)

External Links

- CIRCUMGATE (http://joseph4gi.blogspot.com/2012/04/circumgate-uk-circumfetish-czar-finally.html) – UK Circumfetish Czar Finally Caught Red-Handed
- GILGAL SOCIETY: Circumcision advocate, Vernon Quaintance, convicted of sex crime (http://www.circumcisionandhiv.com/2012/04/index.html) – Circumcision and HIV Weblog
- Photography by Vernon (http://www.traditionalcatholic.org.uk/Photography_by_Vernon.html) – A collection of Quaintance Photography.
- Q Audio-Visual (http://www.q-audio-visual.co.uk/vernon.html) – A self run business by Quaintance.
- Quaintance Family Gathering (http://replay.waybackmachine.org/20010813013123/http://www.martinq.dircon.co.uk/Qreunion/index.html) – Relatives (o)
- Two videos that mention Vernon Quaintance, here (http://youtu.be/gdGbXdFu93U) and here (http://youtu.be/vFH17Arkets)

References

Note: If a link is broken, you will find a PDF archive link directly behind it (under the same reference number).

1. ↑ "InCourts Daily" (http://incourts.co.uk/Daily/Monday/Southwark.html) . *InCourtsDaily*. 2012-04-16. http://incourts.co.uk/Daily/Monday/Southwark.html. Retrieved 2012-04-21 Archive (2012-04-21): http://circleaks.org/images/6/64/V-g-quaintance-incourt.pdf
2. ↑ [2.0 2.1 2.2 2.3 2.4 2.5 2.6] Kay, Richard (2012-04-25). "Sex scandal rocks Order of the Knights" (http://www.dailymail.co.uk/news/article-2134978/David-Cameron-son-PM-wife-Samantha-unveil-church-tribute-son-Ivan.html) . *MailOnline* (GlamEntertainment). http://www.dailymail.co.uk/news/article-2134978/David-Cameron-son-PM-wife-Samantha-unveil-church-tribute-son-Ivan.html. Retrieved 2012-04-26. Archive (2012-04-27): http://circleaks.org/images/6/66/Quaintance-disrupts-the-church%28malta%29.pdf
3. ↑ [3.00 3.01 3.02 3.03 3.04 3.05 3.06 3.07 3.08 3.09 3.10] "Croydon circumcision campaigner caught with child porn videos" (http://www.thisiscroydontoday.co.uk/Croydon-circumcision-campaigner-caught-child-porn/story-15866127-detail/story.html) . *Croydon Advertiser*. 2012-04-21. http://www.thisiscroydontoday.co.uk/Croydon-circumcision-campaigner-caught-child-porn/story-15866127-detail/story.html. Retrieved 2012-04-22. Archive 2012-04-21: http://circleaks.org/images/2/27/Www.thisiscroydontoday.co.uk-Croydon-circumcision-campaigner-caught-child-porn-s.pdf
4. ↑ [4.0 4.1] Harper. *Little Mikey H* (http://www.authonomy.com/books/20510/little-mickey-h-a-norbury-lad/read-book/?chapterid=194978) . http://www.authonomy.com/books/20510/little-mickey-h-a-norbury-lad/read-book/?chapterid=194978. Retrieved 2012-04-23. Archive (2012-04-21): http://circleaks.org/images/8/82/Little-mickey-h-a-norbury-lad-r.pdf
5. ↑ Vernon, Quaintance (2005-2007). "Photo Information" (http://www.traditionalcatholic.org.uk/2006RosaryCrusade/Photo_Information.html) . http://www.traditionalcatholic.org.uk/2006RosaryCrusade/Photo_Information.html. Retrieved 2011-03-13. Archive: http://circleaks.org/images/c/c6/VQ-Photo-Info.pdf
6. ↑ Circlist – See article for further evidence and citations
7. ↑ Gilgal Society – See article for further evidence and citations

8. † Quaintance, Vernon (Sep. 2001). "One Man's Account of His Adult Circumcision" (http://www.circinfo.com/an_account.html) . *Acorn Society Magazine*. Gilgal Society. http://www.circinfo.com/an_account.html. Retrieved 2011-04-27. *Archive* (2011-05-20): http://www.circleaks.org/images/2/2b/Acorn_Mag_-_Circ_Account.pdf
9. † [9.0 9.1] "Whois Record For InFocirc.com" (http://whois.domaintools.com/infocirc.com) . DomainTools. 2000-10-04. http://whois.domaintools.com/infocirc.com. Retrieved 2011-03-13.
10. † Archive (2011-05-20): http://www.circleaks.org/images/4/43/Who_is_infocirc.pdf "Whois Record For GilgalSoc.org" (http://whois.domaintools.com/gilgalsoc.org) . DomainTools. 2000-10-04. http://whois.domaintools.com/gilgalsoc.org. Retrieved 2011-03-13. Archive (2011-05-20):http://www.circleaks.org/images/2/2f/Who_is_gilgalso.pdf
11. † http://circleaks.org/index.php?title=Gilgal_Society#Gilgal_Porn
12. † Yahoo Circlist. Message #26333, 2003 July 30th
13. † [13.0 13.1] Morris, Brian (2007). Vernon Quaintance. ed. *Sex and circumcision: What every woman needs to know* (http://www.circinfo.net/pdfs/GFW-EN%200712-1.pdf) . London, England: Gilgal Society. http://www.circinfo.net/pdfs/GFW-EN%200712-1.pdf. Archive: File:Gilgal For Women leaflet.pdf
14. † [14.0 14.1] Morris, Brian; Quaintance, Vernon (2007). Vernon Quaintance. ed. *Circumcision: A guide for parents* (http://www.circinfo.net/pdfs/GFP-ENAU.pdf) . London, England: Gilgal Society. http://www.circinfo.net/pdfs/GFP-ENAU.pdf. Retrieved 2011-03-06. Archive: File:Gilgal Parents-Guide.pdf
15. † Christopher P Price. Male Non-therapeutic circumcision: The Legal and Ethical Issues. In Male and Female Circumcision, Medical, Legal, and Ethical Considerations in Pediatric Practice (Denniston GC, Hodges FM and Milos MF eds.) New York: Kluwer Academic/Plenum Publishers, 1999: 425-454. http://www.cirp.org/library/legal/price2/
16. † Quaintance, Vernon (1996). "One Man's Account of His Adult Circumcision" (http://www.circinfo.com/an_account.html) . Gilgal Society. http://www.circinfo.com/an_account.html. Retrieved 2011-05-22.
17. † Thomas, A. (2005). "Case histories and experiences of circumcision" (http://www.circleaks.org/images/d/d6/Gilgal_porn.pdf) . In Vernon Quaintance. *Circumcision: An Ethnomedical Study*. **Fourth Edition**. London, England: The Gilgal Society. pp. 191. EMS-EN 0304-2. http://www.circleaks.org/images/d/d6/Gilgal_porn.pdf.
18. † Christopher P Price. Male Non-therapeutic circumcision: The Legal and Ethical Issues. In Male and Female Circumcision, Medical, Legal, and Ethical Considerations in Pediatric Practice (Denniston GC, Hodges FM and Milos MF eds.) New York: Kluwer Academic/Plenum Publishers, 1999: 425-454. http://www.cirp.org/library/legal/price2/
19. † "WHOIS information for gilgalsoc.org" (http://www.whois.net/whois/gilgalsoc.org) . WhoIS.net. http://www.whois.net/whois/gilgalsoc.org. Retrieved 2011-04-27.
20. † "Gilgal" (http://en.wikipedia.org/wiki/Gilgal) . Wikipedia. http://en.wikipedia.org/wiki/Gilgal. Retrieved 2011-04-27.
21. † Christopher P Price. Male Non-therapeutic circumcision: The Legal and Ethical Issues. In Male and Female Circumcision, Medical, Legal, and Ethical Considerations in Pediatric Practice (Denniston GC, Hodges FM and Milos MF eds.) New York: Kluwer Academic/Plenum Publishers, 1999: 425-454. http://www.cirp.org/library/legal/price2/
22. † Morris, Brian (2007). Vernon Quaintance. ed. *Sex and circumcision: What every woman needs to know* (http://www.circinfo.net/pdfs/GFW-EN%200712-1.pdf) . London, England: Gilgal Society. http://www.circinfo.net/pdfs/GFW-EN%200712-1.pdf.
23. † Thomas, A. (2005). "Case histories and experiences of circumcision" (http://www.circleaks.org/images/d/d6/Gilgal_porn.pdf) . In Vernon Quaintance. *Circumcision: An Ethnomedical Study*. **Fourth Edition**. London, England: The Gilgal Society. pp. 191. EMS-EN 0304-2. http://www.circleaks.org/images/d/d6/Gilgal_porn.pdf.
24. † Shaw, Tony. "Circumcision, an ethnomedical study: A review by Tony Shaw" (http://www.gilgalsoc.org/b_reviews/ethnomed.html) . *Gilgal Society*. Gilgal Society. http://www.gilgalsoc.org/b_reviews/ethnomed.html. Retrieved 2011-02-28.
25. † [25.0 25.1] Quaintance, Vernon. "Adult Circumcision Video" (http://www.gilgalsoc.org/publications/acv.html) . Gilgal Society. http://www.gilgalsoc.org/publications/acv.html. Retrieved 2011-03-11. Archive: File:Gilgal Video.pdf
26. † "Croydon circumcision campaigner caught with child porn videos" (http://www.thisiscroydontoday.co.uk/Croydon-circumcision-campaigner-caught-child-porn/story-15866127-detail/story.html) . *Croydon Advertiser*. 2012-04-21. http://www.thisiscroydontoday.co.uk/Croydon-circumcision-campaigner-caught-child-porn/story-15866127-detail/story.html. Retrieved 2012-04-21. Archive (2012-04-21): http://circleaks.org/images/2/27/Www.thisiscroydontoday.co.uk-Croydon-circumcision-campaigner-caught-child-porn-s.pdf
27. † "Online Archive" (http://www.courtnewsuk.co.uk/online_archive/?courts=0&name=plied) . *Court News UK*. 2012-04-17. http://www.courtnewsuk.co.uk/online_archive/?courts=0&name=plied. Retrieved 2012-04-22.
28. † "Knights' former sacristan charged with abuse" (http://archive.thetablet.co.uk/article/12th-october-2013/30/knights-former-sacristan-charged-with-abuse) . *The Tablet: An International Catholic Weekly*.

http://archive.thetablet.co.uk/article/12th-october-2013/30/knights-former-sacristan-charged-with-abuse. Retrieved 2013-10-12.

29. ↑ "Former Knights of Malta member pleads guilty to abuse of young boys" (http://www.thetablet.co.uk/news/981/0/former-knights-of-malta-member-pleads-guilty-to-abuse-of-young-boys). *The Tablet: An International Catholic Weekly*. http://www.thetablet.co.uk/news/981/0/former-knights-of-malta-member-pleads-guilty-to-abuse-of-young-boys. Retrieved 2014-07-17.
30. ↑ "Upper Norwood circumcision fetishist jailed for asking schoolboys to show him their private parts" (http://www.croydonadvertiser.co.uk/Upper-Norwood-circumcision-fetishist-jailed/story-23040107-detail/story.html). *Croydon Advertiser*. http://www.croydonadvertiser.co.uk/Upper-Norwood-circumcision-fetishist-jailed/story-23040107-detail/story.html. Retrieved 2014-10-07.
31. ↑ Harper, Mike (2010-04-22). "12" (http://www.authonomy.com/books/20510/little-mickey-h-a-norbury-lad/read-book/?chapterid=194978). *Little Mikey H - A Norbury Lad*. England: Authonomy. http://www.authonomy.com/books/20510/little-mickey-h-a-norbury-lad/read-book/?chapterid=194978. Retrieved 2012-04-21. Archive (2012-04-21): http://circleaks.org/images/8/82/Little-mickey-h-a-norbury-lad-r.pdf
32. ↑ [32.0] [32.1] Quaintance, Vernon (2007-04-07). "Q Audio-Visual Computer Consultancy - The Proprietor" (http://www.q-audio-visual.co.uk/vernon.html). Q Audio-Visual. http://www.q-audio-visual.co.uk/vernon.html. Retrieved 2011-03-13. Archive (2011-05-20): http://www.circleaks.org/images/c/c2/Q_audio_visual.pdf
33. ↑ Harper, Mike (2010-04-22). "12" (http://www.authonomy.com/books/20510/little-mickey-h-a-norbury-lad/read-book/?chapterid=194978). *Little Mikey H - A Norbury Lad*. England: Authonomy. http://www.authonomy.com/books/20510/little-mickey-h-a-norbury-lad/read-book/?chapterid=194978. Retrieved 2012-04-21. Archive (2012-04-21): http://circleaks.org/images/8/82/Little-mickey-h-a-norbury-lad-r.pdf
34. ↑ "Photography by Vernon Quaintance" (http://www.traditionalcatholic.org.uk/Photography_by_Vernon.html). http://www.traditionalcatholic.org.uk/Photography_by_Vernon.html. Retrieved 2012-04-26.
35. ↑ "User contributions" (http://en.wikipedia.org/wiki/Special:Contributions/Jakew). Wikipedia. http://en.wikipedia.org/wiki/Special:Contributions/Jakew
36. ↑ Waskett, Jake H.; Vernon Quaintance (2003-07-30). "Circed at last" (http://circleaks.org/index.php?title=Jake_H._Waskett#2003_July_30th). Circlist. http://circleaks.org/index.php?title=Jake_H._Waskett#2003_July_30th
37. ↑ "Whois Record For InFocirc.com" (http://whois.domaintools.com/infocirc.com). Domain Tools. http://whois.domaintools.com/infocirc.com. Retrieved 2011-03-09.
38. ↑ Quaintance, Vernon (1998-10-03). "The Quaintance Family Gathering" (http://replay.waybackmachine.org/20010813013323/http://www.martinq.dircon.co.uk/Qreunion/index.html). http://replay.waybackmachine.org/20010813013323/http://www.martinq.dircon.co.uk/Qreunion/index.html. Retrieved 2011-03-13. Archive (2011-05-19): http://circleaks.org/index.php?title=File:Quaintance_Family_Gathering.pdf

Retrieved from "http://intactwiki.org/w/index.php?title=Vernon_G._Quaintance&oldid=1097"
Categories: People | CircLeaks

- This page was last modified on 8 May 2015, at 06:34.
- This page has been accessed 1,185 times.
- Content is available under Public Domain unless otherwise noted.

Howard J. Stang

From IntactWiki

In 1998, Howard J. Stang and Leonard W. Snellman co-authored "Circumcision Practice Patterns in the United States," an article promoting circumcision that was published in *Pediatrics*,[1] but he failed to mention his conflict of interest for a previous infant circumcision restraint patent he received in November 3, 1992.[2]

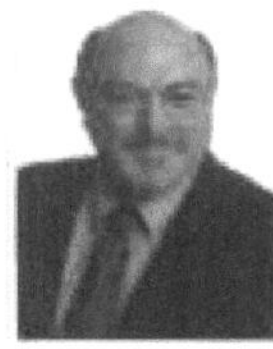

Howard J. Stang

Associates with:
Gilgal Society

References

1. ↑ Stang, Howard J.; Leonard W. Snellman (6 June 1998). "Circumcision Practice Patterns in the United States" (http://pediatrics.aappublications.org/cgi/content/full/101/6/e5) . *Pediatrics* **101** (6): e5. http://pediatrics.aappublications.org/cgi/content/full/101/6/e5. Retrieved 2011-05-02.
2. ↑ "United States Patent 5,160,185" (http://patft.uspto.gov/netacgi/nph-Parser?Sect1=PTO1&Sect2=HITOFF&d=PALL&p=1&u=%2Fnetahtml%2FPTO%2Fsrchnum.htm&r=1&f=G&l=50&s1=5160185.PN.&OS=PN/5160185&RS=PN/5160185) . November 3, 1992. http://patft.uspto.gov/netacgi/nph-Parser?Sect1=PTO1&Sect2=HITOFF&d=PALL&p=1&u=%2Fnetahtml%2FPTO%2Fsrchnum.htm&r=1&f=G&l=50&s1=5160185.PN.&OS=PN/5160185&RS=PN/5160185. Retrieved 2011-05-02. "Infant support and restraint system"

Retrieved from "http://intactwiki.org/w/index.php?title=Howard_J._Stang&oldid=291"
Categories: People CircLeaks

- This page was last modified on 23 April 2015, at 21:46.
- This page has been accessed 179 times.
- Content is available under Public Domain unless otherwise noted.

" If you're wearing a hat on the head of your penis. "

-- kunavu. (2001, May 25). Penn & teller on circumcision part 2. (http://youtu.be/jE3oa4Mx9hs?t=50s)

NOTE: The "*hat*" presumably referring to the visible glans.

Associates With

Circlist

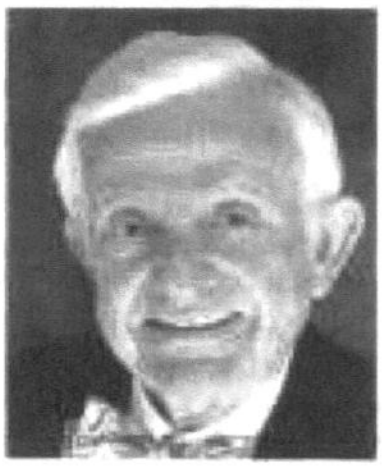

Schoen has been noted sending emails to and from the Circlist email list.[8] Circlist is a website and discussion group for men who sexually fantasize about performing and receiving circumcisions,[9] often on small children.[10]

Gilgal Society

Schoen is also listed as approving content for a Gilgal Society brochure.[11] Groups such as the Gilgal Society openly admit to a morbid fascination with circumcision to the point of sado-masochistic fetish. These groups advertise that doctors are among their members. There are those on the Internet who discuss the erotic stimulation they experience by watching other males being circumcised, swap fiction and about it, and trade in videotapes of actual circumcisions.[12]

Office

Schoen's office is in the Julia Morgan building on Broadway that houses Kaiser Permanente's genetics department in San Fransico. Only a few yards from the home office of Daniel Halperin, assistant professor of anthropology at UCSF's Center for AIDS Prevention Studies (CAPDS).[13]

Quote

Circumcision

" "It's like apple pie. It's part of being American." "

--Schoen. Prue. (2011-5-5). Both sides of the debate: Two Jewish doctors offer opinions on circumcision. J Weekly. (http://www.jweekly.com/article/full/61692/both-sides-of-the-debate-two-jewish-doctors-offer-opinions-on-circumcision/)

References

1. ↑ "UCSF On-line Campus Directory: People Search" (http://directory.ucsf.edu/people_detail.jsp?FNO=Edgar.Schoen@ucsf.edu&retLink=1&school_code=all&last_name=schoen&first_name=&offset=0) . http://directory.ucsf.edu/people_detail.jsp?

FNO=Edgar.Schoen@ucsf.edu&retLink=1&school_code=all&last_name=schoen&first_name=&offset=0. Retrieved 2011-05-27.
2. ↑ American Journal of Diseases in Children, Vol 141: 128. February 1987
3. ↑ Slack, Gordy (2000-05-19). "The Case For Circumcision" (http://circleaks.org/images/3/32/Edgar_Schoen_%26_Daniel_Halperin_%281999-2000%29.pdf) . *Express Online*. http://circleaks.org/images/3/32/Edgar_Schoen_%26_Daniel_Halperin_%281999-2000%29.pdf.
4. ↑ http://www.circinfo.net/pdfs/GFW-EN%200712-1.pdf
5. ↑ "Error: no |title= specified when using {{ (http://www.cirp.org/library/statements/aap/#a1989) Cite web}}". http://www.cirp.org/library/statements/aap/#a1989.
6. ↑ "Error: no |title= specified when using {{ (http://www.cirp.org/library/statements/aap1999/) Cite web}}". http://www.cirp.org/library/statements/aap1999/.
7. ↑ = "Penn & Teller on Circumcision" (http://youtu.be/vLGcqPE7xu0?t=7m50s) . *kunavu*. YouTube. 2011-05-25. http://youtu.be/vLGcqPE7xu0?t=7m50s. Retrieved 2011-09-25.
8. ↑ Schoen, E. (2006, April 22). *My recent circ pubs* [Online Forum Comment]. Retrieved from http://health.groups.yahoo.com/group/MCIRC/message/16 Archive: http://circleaks.org/images/1/1f/MCIRC_-_Msg_16.pdf
9. ↑ Ben Winkie. (2005, June) *International Circumsexual Symposium*, Washington, D.C. (http://www.circumstitions.com/Glossary2.html)
10. ↑ Thomas, A. (2005). "Case histories and experiences of circumcision" (http://www.circleaks.org/images/d/d6/Gilgal_porn.pdf) . In Vernon Quaintance. *Circumcision: An Ethnomedical Study*. **Fourth Edition**. London, England: The Gilgal Society. pp. 191. EMS-EN 0304-2. http://www.circleaks.org/images/d/d6/Gilgal_porn.pdf.
11. ↑ Morris, Brian (2007). Vernon Quaintance. ed. *Sex and circumcision: What every woman needs to know*. (http://www.circinfo.net/pdfs/GFW-EN%200712-1.pdf) . London, England: Gilgal Society. http://www.circinfo.net/pdfs/GFW-EN%200712-1.pdf.
12. ↑ Christopher P Price. Male Non-therapeutic circumcision: The Legal and Ethical Issues. In Male and Female Circumcision, Medical, Legal, and Ethical Considerations in Pediatric Practice (Denniston GC, Hodges FM and Milos MF eds.) New York: Kluwer Academic/Plenum Publishers, 1999: 425-454. http://www.cirp.org/library/legal/price2/
13. ↑ Slack, Gordy (2000-05-19). "The Case For Circumcision" (http://circleaks.org/images/3/32/Edgar_Schoen_%26_Daniel_Halperin_%281999-2000%29.pdf) . *Express Online*. http://circleaks.org/images/3/32/Edgar_Schoen_%26_Daniel_Halperin_%281999-2000%29.pdf.

Retrieved from "http://intactwiki.org/w/index.php?title=Edgar_J._Schoen&oldid=278"

Categories: Articles with incorrect citation syntax | People | Physicians | American Academy of Pediatrics Promoters | Jewish | CircLeaks

- This page was last modified on 23 April 2015, at 21:31.
- This page has been accessed 422 times.
- Content is available under Public Domain unless otherwise noted.

Daniel T. Halperin

From IntactWiki
(Redirected from Daniel Halperin)

Daniel Halperin has published several papers on circumcision for HIV prevention,[1] which are being used by the World Health Organization to endorse circumcision as an HIV prevention method. In November 1999, colleagues Daniel Halperin and Robert C. Bailey published an article in the Lancet criticizing the public-health community for not pushing circumcision. Today, Halperin is the Senior Research Scientist at the Harvard AIDS Prevention Research Project.[2]

Halperin is a member of Circlist,[3] and a proud promoter of the group.[4] Halperin's home office is only a stone's throw from the office of Edgar J. Schoen (leading pro-circumcision advocate).[5]

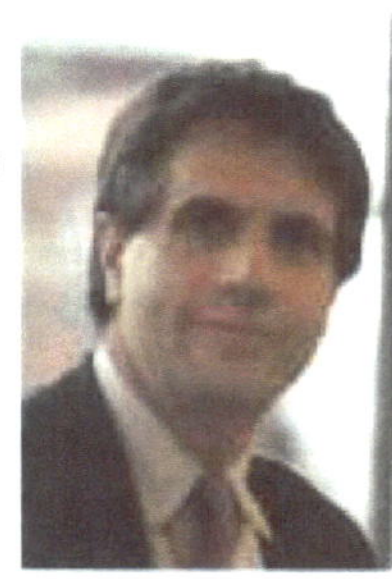

Associates With:

Circlist
Gilgal Society

Colleagues & Benefactors:

Robert C. Bailey
Edgar J. Schoen
Brian J. Morris
Thomas E. Wiswell
Jake H. Waskett

Contents

Religious & Cultural Bias

- His grandfhather was a Mohel, born in Russia, died in Chicago. "I don't have an agenda about foreskins" said Halperin in an interview for the Eastbay Express. When asked if being Jewish affects his pro-circumcision bias, he denied it, but said that his Judaism has "crept in now and then". He explains, "think of it as maybe a kind of health/cultural innovation ahead of it's time. So it's made me appreciate my own heritage more. And who knows, maybe finding out to my surprise that my own granddad was a Mohel was a weird kind of confirmation that I'm maybe in some small way 'destined' to help pass along this health benefit to people in parts of the world where it could really make a difference and perhaps save many lives." [5]

Halperin Cites Vernon Quaintance, Brian Morris and Circlist

In an interview, Daniel Halperin cites Vernon Quaintance, Brian Morris and Circlist as credible resources in favor of circumcision.[6] It is important to note that Quaintance and Morris are both proud members and promoters of Gilgal Society and Circlist, which openly admit to a morbid fascination with circumcision to the point of sado-masochistic fetish. Morris has included CircList as a resource in a recent paper,[7] and Quaintance is both the head of Gilgal Society, and head moderator at Circlist. Vernon Quaintance was recently arrested for child pornography.[8][9]

Interview with Daniel Halperin

> **Moderator** Obviously, when you do a web search for good info on circumcision, one generally comes up with a ton of anti-circ sites. Do you know of any pro-circumcision sites?
>
> **Dr. Halperin** I know of several:
>
> ```
> http://www.users.dircon.co.uk/~vernon/ICIRC/
> http://www-personal.usyd.edu.au/~bmorris/Circ
> http://www.circumcisioninfo.com
> http://www.circlist.org
> ```

– circumcisioninformation.com (http://www.circumcisioninformation.com/halperin_interview1.html)[10]

Moyels Without Borders

On May 28th 2010, at the UNC School of Medicine, Halperin lectured on "Moyels without Borders?: Barriers to Scale-up of Circumcision" [11]

Promoting Circumcision in Africa

Halperin and Bailey convinced eastern and south African "healers" to perform foreskin removal "as a way to alleviate chronic STD infection and prevent AIDS" in the 1990's. During the nineties alone, they convinced hundreds of South African men that circumcision would prevent HIV.[5]

HIV/AIDS

Daniel Halperin has said he believes circumcision will go further than any other intervention available in stopping the HIV, and that circumcision will prevent HIV among homosexual men.[5]

Quotes

. Halperin was asked by Gordy Slack of the East Bay Express if his being Jewish factored into his work on circumcision. Halperin replied:

> " No. At least it didn't during the first couple of years I was doing research. I didn't think about the Jewish part at all. I'd vaguely heard about a guy in Boston who does a non-cutting ritual bris, and maybe that would have appealed to me, if I had a boy someday. But in recent years the Judaism aspect has crept in now and then. Some [non-Jewish and typically uncircumcised] doctors, for example, an oncologist in northeastern Brazil who has to amputate cancerous penises every week, would tell me not knowing that I was Jewish, 'Those Jews were so smart; thousands of years ago they figured out this way to prevent health problems.' That was one of the things that began to spin my head around from thinking of this as a savage ritual from the dark past to thinking of it as maybe a kind of health/cultural innovation ahead of its time... So I guess it has made me appreciate my own heritage more. And who knows, maybe finding out to my surprise that my own granddad was an occasional mohel was a weird kind of confirmation that I'm maybe in some small way 'destined' to help pass along this health benefit to people in parts of the world where it could really make a difference and perhaps save many lives. "
>
> – Daniel Halperin [17]

Other quotes...

> " I'm from California - I believe in things being natural; I don't like surgical interventions. But now, yes, I would - although I'd have it done the Jewish way. "
>
> – Daniel Halperin [17]

> " Don't you dare write that I think foreskins cause AIDS epidemics, any more than mosquitoes cause malaria. Mosquitoes are necessary for malaria, but not sufficient. You need all these cofactors to get an explosive AIDS epidemic, including foreskins. "

> -- Daniel Halperin. Slack, G. (2000, November 16). The case for circumcision . *Express Online*, (http://circleaks.org/images/3/32/Edgar_Schoen_%26_Daniel_Halperin_%281999-2000%29.pdf)

> "Circumcision is too human, too 'soft.'"
>
> -- Daniel Halperin. Slack, G. (2000, November 16). The case for circumcision . *Express Online*, (http://circleaks.org/images/3/32/Edgar_Schoen_%26_Daniel_Halperin_%281999-2000%29.pdf)

> "It's as if you went to a lung-cancer resource center and they had nothing at all about cigarettes. What the hell is going on? Why is everyone ignoring the elephant-sized foreskin in the living room?"
>
> -- Daniel Halperin. Slack, G. (2000, November 16). The case for circumcision . *Express Online*, (http://circleaks.org/images/3/32/Edgar_Schoen_%26_Daniel_Halperin_%281999-2000%29.pdf) .

See Also

- Circlist -- Halperin endorses Circlist.
- Gilgal Society -- Halperin helped create a Gilgal brochure.
- Robert C. Bailey -- Colleague & Benefactor of Halperin.
- Edgar J. Schoen -- Colleague & Benefactor of Halperin.
- Brian J. Morris -- Colleague & Benefactor of Halperin.
- Thomas E. Wiswell -- Colleague & Benefactor of Halperin.
- Jake H. Waskett -- Benefactor of Halperin.
- World Health Organization -- The WHO endorses Halperin's *research*.
- Bias -- Read about circumcision bias.

External Links

- Halperin links to Circlist (http://www.circumcisioninformation.com/halperin_inverview1.htm) -- Endorsing Circlist and Vernon Quaintance's website.

References

1. ↑ "Daniel Halperin circumcision" (http://www.ncbi.nlm.nih.gov/pubmed?term=Daniel%20Halperin%20circumcision) . *NCBI*. PubMed. http://www.ncbi.nlm.nih.gov/pubmed?term=Daniel%20Halperin%20circumcision. Retrieved 2011-04-29.
2. ↑ Halperin, Daniel. "AIDS Prevntion Research Project" (http://www.newparadigmfund.org/daniel-halperin.html) . http://www.newparadigmfund.org/daniel-halperin.html.
3. ↑ Halperin, D. (2006, April 22). *RE: My recent circ pubs* [Online Forum Comment]. Retrieved from http://health.groups.yahoo.com/group/MCIRC/message/16 Archive: http://circleaks.org/images/1/1f/MCIRC_-_Msg_16.pdf
4. ↑ "The Great Circumcision Debate with Daniel Halperin, PhD" (http://www.circumcisioninformation.com/halperin_inverview1.htm) . *Chat Transcript*. http://www.circumcisioninformation.com/halperin_inverview1.htm. Retrieved 2011-05-07. "Do you know of any pro-circumcision sites? Dr. Halperin I know of several: [...]circlist"
5. ↑ 5.0 5.1 5.2 5.3 - {{cite journal - | title = The Case For Circumcision - | journal = Express Online - | date = 2000-05-19 - | first = Gordy - | last = Slack - | id = - | url = http://circleaks.org/images/3/32/Edgar_Schoen_%26_Daniel_Halperin_%281999-2000%29.pdf - }} -
6. ↑ "The Great Circumcision Debate with Daniel Halperin, PhD" (http://www.circumcisioninformation.com/halperin_inverview1.htm) . *Chat Transcript*. http://www.circumcisioninformation.com/halperin_inverview1.htm. Retrieved 2011-05-07. "Do you know of any pro-circumcision sites? Dr. Halperin I know of several: [...]circlist"
7. ↑ Morris, Brian J.; Chris Eley (2011-08). "Male Circumcision: An Appraisal of Current Instrumentation" (http://www.intechopen.com/articles/show/title/male-circumcision-an-appraisal-of-current-instrumentation) . *InTech*: 1-40. http://www.intechopen.com/articles/show/title/male-circumcision-an-appraisal-of-current-instrumentation. Retrieved 2011-09-17.
8. ↑ "Croydon circumcision campaigner caught with child porn videos" (http://www.thisiscroydontoday.co.uk/Croydon-circumcision-campaigner-caught-child-porn/story-15866127-detail/story.html) . *Croydon Advertiser*. 2012-04-21. http://www.thisiscroydontoday.co.uk/Croydon-circumcision-campaigner-caught-child-porn/story-15866127-detail/story.html. Retrieved 2012-04-22. Archive 2012-04-21: http://circleaks.org/images/2/27/Www.thisiscroydontoday.co.uk-Croydon-circumcision-campaigner-caught-child-porn-s.pdf
9. ↑ Kay, Richard (2012-04-25). "Sex scandal rocks Order of the Knights" (http://www.dailymail.co.uk/news/article-2134978/David-Cameron-son-PM-wife-Samantha-unveil-church-tribute-son-Ivan.html) . *MailOnline* (GlamEntertainment). http://www.dailymail.co.uk/news/article-2134978/David-Cameron-son-PM-wife-Samantha-unveil-church-tribute-son-Ivan.html. Retrieved 2012-04-26. Archive (2012-04-27): http://circleaks.org/images/6/66/Quaintance-disrupts-the-church%28malta%29.pdf
10. ↑ Slack, Gordy (2000-05-19). "The Case For Circumcision" (http://www.eastbayexpress.com/archive/051900/cover1_051900.html) . *The Guardian*. http://www.eastbayexpress.com/archive/051900/cover1_051900.html. Retrieved 2000-11-16. "I ask Halperin whether his being Jewish factors into his work on circumcision..."
11. ↑ Halperin, Daniel (2010-05-28). ""Moyels without Borders?: Barriers to Scale-up of Circumcision (and Some Reflections on the Track Record of Other HIV Prevention Approaches)"" (http://www.med.unc.edu/www/events/moyels-without-borders-barriers-to-scale-up-of-circumcision-and-some-reflections-on-the-track-record-of-other-hiv-prevention-approaches) . UNC School of Medicine. http://www.med.unc.edu/www/events/moyels-without-

borders-barriers-to-scale-up-of-circumcision-and-some-reflections-on-the-track-record-of-other-hiv-prevention-approaches. Retrieved 2011-03-11. Archive: File:Moyels Without Borders.pdf
12. ↑ Slack, Gordy (2000-05-19). "The Case For Circumcision" (http://www.eastbayexpress.com/archive/051900/cover1_051900.html) . *The Guardian*. http://www.eastbayexpress.com/archive/051900/cover1_051900.html. Retrieved 2000-11-16. "I ask Halperin whether his being Jewish factors into his work on circumcision..."
13. ↑ Renton, Alex (2009-07-05). "So, would you have your son circumcised?" (http://www.guardian.co.uk/lifeandstyle/2009/jul/05/circumcicision-health-children?intcmp=239) . *The Guardian*. http://www.guardian.co.uk/lifeandstyle/2009/jul/05/circumcicision-health-children?intcmp=239. Retrieved 2012-02-25. "I'm from California - I believe in things being natural..."

Retrieved from "http://intactwiki.org/w/index.php?title=Daniel_T._Halperin&oldid=268"
Categories: People | Circumcision in Africa | Researchers | Jewish | CircLeaks

- This page was last modified on 23 April 2015, at 20:30.
- This page has been accessed 449 times.
- Content is available under Public Domain unless otherwise noted.

Robert C. Bailey

From IntactWiki

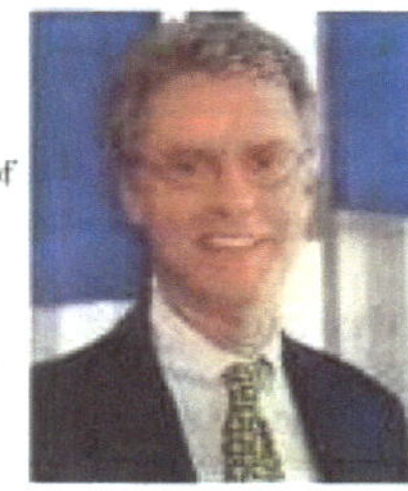

Associates with:
Gilgal Society
Colleagues & Benefactors:
Stephen Moses
Ronald H. Gray
Brian J. Morris
Bertran Auvert
Maria Wawer
Daniel T. Halperin

Robert C. Bailey is Professor of Epidemiology at the School of Public Health, University of Illinois at Chicago, and Research Associate at Field Museum in Chicago.[1] Bailey has been a circumcision proponent since at least 1998.[2] Bailey was responsible (along with Stephen Moses) for one of the three major African circumcision trials (funded by NIAID, the Canadian Institutes of Health Research, and the United States National Institutes of Health),[3][4][5] which are being used by the World Health Organization (under the guide of UNAIDS) to endorse circumcision as an HIV prevention method.[6] Bailey is associated with the Gilgal Society.[7]

Contents

- 1 Circumcision Research
- 2 Deceptive Tactics
- 3 Advocacy
- 4 Quote
- 5 References

Circumcision Research

Since 1995, Bailey has devoted most of his research activities to promoting male circumcision as a HIV prevention strategy.[8] He has conducted circumcision-related studies in varying communities in Uganda, Kenya, Malawi, Zambia, and the U.S. He has studied adverse events and conducted needs assessments associated with medical and traditional circumcisions in Kenya.

Bailey is the principal investigator of the randomized controlled trial of male circumcision to reduce HIV incidence in Kisumu, Kenya, and he has served as a consultant to WHO, UNAIDS, UNICEF, the World Bank, USAID, the CDC, and other national and international governmental and non-governmental agencies.[9]

In 2010, Bailey published a study with Brian J. Morris.[10]

Deceptive Tactics

In Bailey's trial, the circumcised group had specific instructions to abstain from sex and use condoms that the intact control group did not. Bailey has admitted that "repeated study visits and intensive behavioral counseling" of the circumcised men were needed to reduce risk behaviors.[11]

"Research" advocating infant circumcision has been published by the University of Illinois and the Nyanza Reproductive Health Society.[12] While it may appear as if two independent medical organizations are publishing research, Robert Bailey happens to be a Professor of Epidemiology and an adjunct professor of Anthropology in the University of Chicago at Illinois, as well as the Secretary of the Board of the Nyanza Reproductive Health Society.

Advocacy

Bailey is one of the primary modern day advocates for male circumcision. His research interest include "male circumcision as a strategy for HIV/STD prevention." He has written numerous articles advocating wholesale circumcision campaigns.[13] He is not a medical doctor or even a medical epidemiologist, but rather holds degrees in Anthropology and *behavioral epidemiology*.[14]" He has recently been described as "frustrated and impatient" with the alleged slowness to act on his research.[15]

Bailey and Daniel Halperin convinced eastern and south African "healers" to perform foreskin removal "as a way to alleviate chronic STD infection and prevent AIDS" in the 1990's. During the nineties alone, they convinced hundreds of South African men that circumcision would prevent HIV.[16]

Quote

Bailey says foreskin isn't pretty

" I know foreskin is not pretty, but these slides are pretty. "

--R. Bailey. Gajewski. (2008-05-02). The impacts of male circumcision in Africa. *The Lawrentian*. (http://www.lawrentian.com/features/the-impacts-of-male-circumcision-in-africa-1.1983582)

Bailey likes seeing men get circumcised

" "We're hacking away at it every month," Dr. Bailey said. "Those foreskins are flying." "

--R. Bailey. Pam Belluck. (2011-09-26). Obstacles Slow an Easy Way to Prevent H.I.V. in Men. *NY Times*. (http://www.nytimes.com/2011/09/27/health/27circumcision.html?pagewanted=all)

References

1. ↑ "Robert C. Bailey" (http://www.kaisernetwork.org/health_cast/uploaded_files/BAILEY_bio.pdf) (PDF). kaiser network. http://www.kaisernetwork.org/health_cast/uploaded_files/BAILEY_bio.pdf. Retrieved 2011-02-27.
2. ↑ Moses S, Bailey RC, Ronald AR. Male circumcision: assessment of health benefits and risks. Sex Transm Infect 1998;74(5):368-73.
3. ↑ "The Use of Male Circumcision to Prevent HIV Infection" (http://www.doctorsopposingcircumcision.org/info/HIVStatement.html) . Doctors Opposing Circumcision. 2008. Archived from the original (http://www.doctorsopposingcircumcision.org) on 2011-03-05. http://www.doctorsopposingcircumcision.org/info/HIVStatement.html. Retrieved 2011-03-05. "...funding from the United States National Institutes of Health to conduct randomized controlled trials (RCTs) in Africa."
4. ↑ Krieger JN, Bailey RC, Opeya J, *et al.* (November 2005). "Adult male circumcision: results of a standardized procedure in Kisumu District, Kenya". *BJU Int.* **96** (7): 1109–13. doi:10.1111/j.1464-410X.2005.05810.x (http://dx.doi.org/10.1111%2Fj.1464-410X.2005.05810.x) . PMID 16225538 (http://www.ncbi.nlm.nih.gov/pubmed/16225538) .
5. ↑ 12.Bailey RC, Moses S, Parker CB, et al. Male circumcision for HIV prevention in young men in Kisumu, Kenya: a randomised controlled trial. Lancet 2007;369:643-56
6. ↑ [Information Package on Male Circumcision and HIV Prevention "Information Package on Male Circumcision and HIV Prevention"] (PDF). *Info Pack.* World Health Organization. Information Package on Male Circumcision and HIV Prevention. Retrieved 2011-04-29
7. ↑ Morris, Brian; Vernon Quaintance (2007). "Sex and Circumcision What every Woman needs to know" (http://www.circinfo.net/pdfs/GFW-EN%200712-1.pdf) (PDF). The Gilgal Society. http://www.circinfo.net/pdfs/GFW-EN%200712-1.pdf. Retrieved 2011-02-27
8. ↑ "Pubmed Search: Robert C. Bailey" (http://www.ncbi.nlm.nih.gov/pubmed?term=Robert%20C.%20Bailey) . NIH. October 28, 2009. http://www.ncbi.nlm.nih.gov/pubmed?term=Robert%20C.%20Bailey. Retrieved 2011-02-27.
9. ↑ "Robert C. BAILEY" (http://www.kaisernetwork.org/health_cast/uploaded_files/BAILEY_bio.pdf) (PDF). kaiser network. http://www.kaisernetwork.org/health_cast/uploaded_files/BAILEY_bio.pdf. Retrieved 2011-02-27.
10. ↑ Gray RH, Bailey RC, Morris BJ (June 2010). "Keratinization of the adult male foreskin and implications for male circumcision". *AIDS* **24** (9): 1381; author reply 1381–2. doi:10.1097/QAD.0b013e3283392555 (http://dx.doi.org/10.1097%2FQAD.0b013e3283392555) . PMID 20559044 (http://www.ncbi.nlm.nih.gov/pubmed/20559044) .
11. ↑ "Circumcision Age-old surgery touted to reduce HIV" (http://www.circumstitions.com/news/News26.html#trinidad) . *Trinidad Express*. August 20, 2007. http://www.circumstitions.com/news/News26.html#trinidad. Retrieved 2011-02-27
12. ↑ Otieno, Samuel (2 July 2012). "Kenya: Nyanza Residents Warm Up to Infant Male Circumcision" (http://allafrica.com/stories/201207021653.html) . *All Africa*. http://allafrica.com/stories/201207021653.html. Retrieved 2012-07-06. ""The research, conducted

by the University of Illinois and the Nyanza Reproductive Health Society to assess the acceptability of infant male circumcision..."

13. ↑ "Pubmed Search: Robert C. Bailey" (http://www.ncbi.nlm.nih.gov/pubmed?term=Robert%20C.%20Bailey) . NIH. October 28, 2009. http://www.ncbi.nlm.nih.gov/pubmed?term=Robert%20C.%20Bailey. Retrieved 2011-02-27.
14. ↑ "Robert C. BAILEY" (http://www.kaisernetwork.org/health_cast/uploaded_files/BAILEY_bio.pdf) (PDF). kaiser network. http://www.kaisernetwork.org/health_cast/uploaded_files/BAILEY_bio.pdf. Retrieved 2011-02-27.
15. ↑ "GLOBAL: AIDS community moving too slowly on male circumcision" (http://www.plusnews.org/Report.aspx?ReportId=73388) . *Plus News* (IRIN). 24 July 2007. http://www.plusnews.org/Report.aspx?ReportId=73388. Retrieved 2011-02-27.
16. ↑ Slack, Gordy (2000-05-19). "The Case For Circumcision" (http://circleaks.org/images/3/32/Edgar_Schoen_%26_Daniel_Halperin_%281999-2000%29.pdf) . *Express Online*. http://circleaks.org/images/3/32/Edgar_Schoen_%26_Daniel_Halperin_%281999-2000%29.pdf.

Retrieved from "http://intactwiki.org/w/index.php?title=Robert_C._Bailey&oldid=343"
Categories: People | Researchers | Circumcision in Africa | CircLeaks

- This page was last modified on 25 April 2015, at 12:13.
- This page has been accessed 561 times.
- Content is available under Public Domain unless otherwise noted.

Ronald H. Gray

From IntactWiki

Ronald Gray is a North American circumcision proponent and biased researcher looking for justifications to roll-out mass circumcision programs around the world. He headed one of the three RCTs being used by the WHO to endorse circumcision as HIV prevention.[1] At their clinic, a music video promoting circumcision plays continuously.[2][3] He sometimes goes by the name Ron.[4]

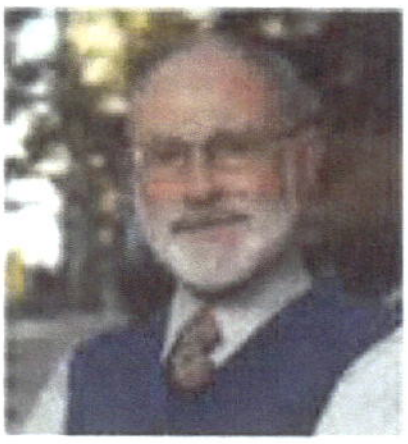

Married To:
Maria Wawer

Colleagues & Benefactors:
Maria Wawer
Robert C. Bailey
Bertran Auvert
Brian J. Morris
Aaron Tobian
Thomas Quinn

Funded By:
Bill and Melinda Gates Foundation
Johns Hopkins
National Institutes of Health

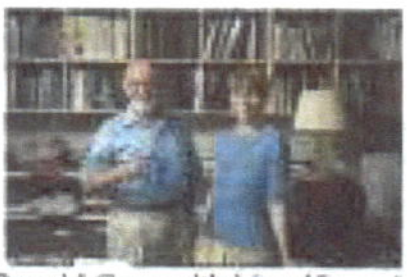

Ronald Gray with his wife, and colleague, Maria Wawer.

Ronald Gray's RCT

Of the three RCTs being used by the WHO to promote circumcision as HIV prevention, Gray supervised the RCT that was carried out in Uganda.[5] Two other RCTs were supervised by Robert C. Bailey and Bertran Auvert respectively. All three RCTs were funded by the American National Institutes of Health.[6]

In 2010,[7] and again in 2011,[4] Gray published studies with Brian J. Morris.

Quotes

> "We've never used surgery to prevent an infectious disease. It's a completely new concept, a new paradigm. How can we train all the surgeons to do this procedure and equip them."

--Ronald Gray. JohnsHopkinsSPH. (2009). *[illegible]* (http://www.youtube.com/watch?v=[illegible])

> "It's been hard to change policy, because this is a whole new paradigm. We've never used surgery to prevent an infectious disease. Policy makers have to really take some time to wrap their minds around it."

--Ronald Gray. JohnsHopkinsSPH. (2010). *Rakai project* (http://www.youtube.com/watch?v=[illegible])

" It's taken longer than I would like to see these programs emerge. "

–Ronald Gray. JohnsHopkinsSPH, (2010). *Rakai project.* (http://www.youtube.com/watch?v=1mXFdXJaG8k#t=7m39s)

The Latest Fight Over Foreskin

" If you were to ask me, should the U.S. be promoting circumcision, my answer would be, 'no,' What I do think ought to be the policy is that parents should be informed about the potential protective effects. "

–Ronald Gray. N.Y. Times, The Latest Fight Over Foreskin, (8/29/2009) (http://www.nytimes.com/2009/08/30/weekinreview/30rabin.html?_r=4)

References

1. ↑ "Information Package on Male Circumcision and HIV Prevention" (http://www.who.int/hiv/mediacentre/infopack_en_1.pdf) . World Health Organization. http://www.who.int/hiv/mediacentre/infopack_en_1.pdf. Retrieved 2011-05-07.
2. ↑ "Rakai Project" (http://www.youtube.com/watch?v=1mXFdXJaG8k#t=8m37s) . *JohnsHopkinsSPH*. YouTube. 2010-10-01. http://www.youtube.com/watch?v=1mXFdXJaG8k#t=8m37s. Retrieved 2011-04-10.
3. ↑ "Rakai Male Circumcision Video By Stephen Mugamba Feat Jemima Sanyu.mpg" (http://www.youtube.com/watch?v=0rtEdNI322Q) . *smugamba*. YouTube. 2010-06-06. http://www.youtube.com/watch?v=0rtEdNI322Q. Retrieved 2011-04-10.
4. ↑ [4.0] [4.1] Morris, Brian James; Ron Gray, Xavier Castellsagué, F. Xavier Bosch, Daniel T. Halperin, C. A. Hankins, and Jake H. Waskett (2011-03-09). "The Strong Protective Effect of Circumcision Against Cancer of the Penis" (http://www.hindawi.com/journals/au/aip/812368/) . *Advanced in Urology*. http://www.hindawi.com/journals/au/aip/812368/. Retrieved 2011-03-13.
5. ↑ Gray RH, Kigozi G, Serwadda D, et al. Male circumcision for HIV prevention in men in Rakai, Uganda: a randomised trial. Lancet 2007;369:557-66.
6. ↑ "The Use of Male Circumcision to Prevent HIV Infection" (http://www.doctorsopposingcircumcision.org/info/HIVStatement.html) . Doctors Opposing Circumcision. 2008. Archived from the original (http://www.doctorsopposingcircumcision.org) on 2011-03-05. http://www.doctorsopposingcircumcision.org/info/HIVStatement.html. Retrieved 2011-03-05. "...funding from the United States National Institutes of Health to conduct randomized controlled trials (RCTs) in Africa."
7. ↑ Gray RH, Bailey RC, Morris BJ (June 2010). "Keratinization of the adult male foreskin and implications for male circumcision". *AIDS* **24** (9): 1381; author reply 1381–2. doi:10.1097/QAD.0b013e3283392555 (http://dx.doi.org/10.1097%2FQAD.0b013e3283392555) . PMID 20559044 (http://www.ncbi.nlm.nih.gov/pubmed/20559044)

Retrieved from "http://intactwiki.org/w/index.php?title=Ronald_H._Gray&oldid=344"
Categories: People | Circumcision in Africa | Researchers | CircLeaks

- This page was last modified on 25 April 2015, at 12:14.
- This page has been accessed 334 times.
- Content is available under Public Domain unless otherwise noted.

Maria J. Wawer

From IntactWiki
(Redirected from Maria Wawer)

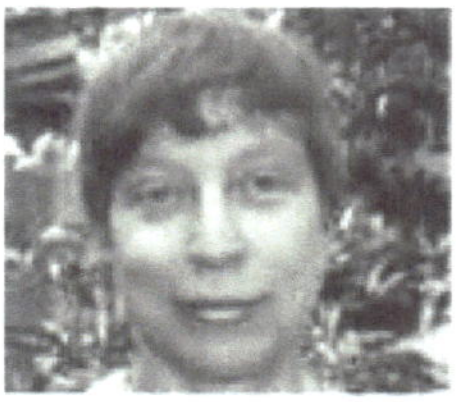

Married To:

Ronald Gray

Colleagues:

Ronald Gray
Bertran Auvert
Robert C. Bailey
Thomas Quinn

Funded By:

Johns Hopkins
NIH

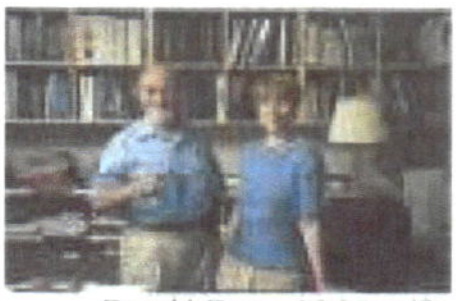

Ronald Gray with his wife, and colleague, Maria Wawer.

Maria J. Wawer is a biased pro-circumcision researcher [1] looking for justifications to roll-out mass circumcision programs around the world. Wawer is married to another biased pro-circumcision researcher Ronald Gray.[2] Her *research* has been funded by Johns Hopkins and the Bill and Melinda Gates Foundation.[2] In the waiting room at their clinic, a music video promoting circumcision plays continuously.[3][4]

Quotes

When Wawer found out she could push circumcision

" You almost feel like crying "

--M. Wawer, JohnsHopkinsSPH (2009, May 29) *Impact*

NOTE: *When she found a reason to push mass circumcision. How could she find joy in that?*

" Once circumcision programs become more widespread, more available, it's very likely that HIV positive men will also seek the procedure. Partly (because) you don't want to be the only guy on the block who hasn't been circumcised. "

--M. Wawer, MedPageToday (2008, February 08) *CROI: Circumcising HIV-Pos Men Doesn't Block Transmission*

NOTE: *This is the goal? To make men feel uncomfortable?*

> " We found a benefit to the (HIV) positive men of becoming circumcised. "
>
> --M. Wawer, MedPageToday. (2008, February 08). *CROI: Circumcising HIV-Pos Men Doesn't Block Transmission.*

NOTE: *They are already HIV positive. You'd think this was a joke.*

> " Where you don't have complete keratinization of the remaining mucosa, then that could in effect increase the transmission of (the) virus. "
>
> --M. Wawer, MedPageToday. (2008, February 08). *CROI: Circumcising HIV-Pos Men Doesn't Block Transmission.*

NOTE: *While pro-circ HIV "researchers" are claiming keratinization is a fact, pushers such as Brian J. Morris and Jake H. Waskett claim there is no keratinization. The keratinization reduces sensation.*

> " We are providing male circumcision as a service now to negative men, but also to positive men. Again, because we don't want them to become stigmatized if they refuse the service. "
>
> --M. Wawer, MedPageToday. (2008, February 08). *CROI: Circumcising HIV-Pos Men Doesn't Block Transmission.*

NOTE: *i.e., she promotes the cutting of anyone for any reason. No logic required.*

> " It's amazing, cultures do change once people see there's a real advantage of a certain action (circumcision) on their part. "
>
> --M. Wawer, JohnsHopkinsSPH. (2010, December 01). *Rakai project.*

NOTE: *You heard that right. She want's to make circumcision part of the culture. i.e., the norm.*

Contradictory Quotes

Male Circumcision does NOT protect women

" We haven't seen a benefit to women for the procedure. "

—M. Wawer, MedPageToday. (2008, February 08). *CROI: Circumcising HIV-Pos Men Doesn't Block Transmission*

NOTE: *In fact, she found that male circumcision increases risk of HIV transmission to women.*

Male Circumcision DOES protect women

" You asked yourself the question, 'If it reduces the risk of acquisition it presumably reduces the risk of transmission to female partners." (Maria nods in agreement) "

—Interviewer, MedPageToday. (2008, February 08). *CROI: Circumcising HIV-Pos Men Doesn't Block Transmission*

NOTE: *Ignoring her own findings when they don't support male circumcision.*

Male Circumcision does NOT protect women

" Disappointingly, when we looked at the women partners of the (HIV) positive men, who've been circumcised, compared to the partners who had not been circumcised, we actually found a slightly higher rate of transmission from the positive circumcised men than from positive uncircumcised men. "

—M. Wawer, MedPageToday. (2008, February 08). *CROI: Circumcising HIV-Pos Men Doesn't Block Transmission*

NOTE: *Interestingly, Maria has said on numerous occasions that circumcision will reduce the rate of transmission to female partners, even though her research doesn't support this. Here she contradicts herself, yet again.*

References

1. ↑ "Maria Wawer circumcision". *PubMed*. NCBI. http://www.ncbi.nlm.nih.gov/pubmed/?term=Maria%20Wawer%20circumcision. Retrieved 2011-04-24.

2. ↑ [2.0] [2.1] Willyard, Cassandra (2007). "Cutting the Risk". *Johns Hopkins Magazine*. http://www.jhu.edu/jhumag/0907web/cutting.html. Retrieved 2011-04-24.
3. ↑ "Rakai Project". *JohnsHopkinsSPH*. YouTube. 2010-10-01. http://www.youtube.com/watch?v=1mXFdXJaG8k#t=8m37s. Retrieved 2011-04-24.
4. ↑ "Rakai male circumcision video by Stephen Mugamba feat Jemima Sanyu". *smugamba*. YouTube. 2010-06-06. http://www.youtube.com/watch?v=0rtEdNl322Q. Retrieved 2011-04-24. "Rakai Health Sciences Program funded the production of an MC promotion song which was done by Stephen Mugamba and Jemima Sanyu. This was done under the supervision of one Uganda's best audio producers; Henry Kiwuuwa of Grayce Records."

Retrieved from "http://intactwiki.org/w/index.php?title=Maria_J._Wawer&oldid=308"
Categories: People | Circumcision in Africa | Researchers | CircLeaks

- This page was last modified on 24 April 2015, at 21:26.
- This page has been accessed 260 times.
- Content is available under Public Domain unless otherwise noted.

Stephen Moses

From IntactWiki

Professor, Depatrments of Medical Microbiology, Community Health Sciences and Medicine. Stephen Moses has been a circumcision proponent since at least 1994.[1] Moses (along with Robert C. Bailey) was responsible for one of the three major African circumcision trials (funded by NIAID and the Canadian Institutes of Health Research)[2] which are being used by the World Health Organization (under the guide of UNAIDS) to endorse circumcision as an HIV prevention method.[3]

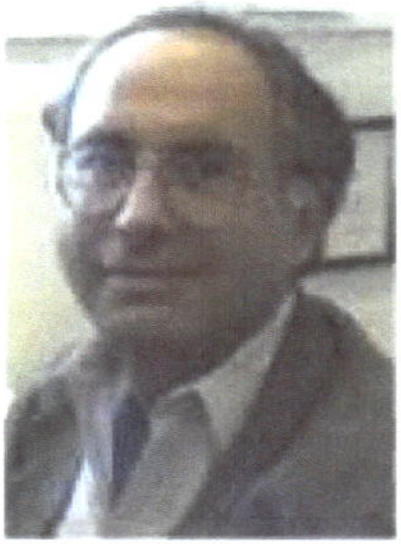

Associates With:

Gilgal Society
Circlist

Colleagues & Benefactors:

Daniel T. Halperin
Edgar J. Schoen
Robert C. Bailey
Bertran Auvert
Maria J. Wawer
Brian J. Morris

Avahan project

Funded by The World Bank

Contents

- 1 Interests
- 2 RCT in Kenya
- 3 Active Projects
- 4 Recent Publications
- 5 References

Interests

According to Stephen's bio, his interest is in biological and behavioural risk factors for STI/HIV transmission.[4] Moses has been an advocate of circumcision since at least 1994.[5]

RCT in Kenya

Of the three RCTs being used by the WHO to endorse circumcision as HIV prevention, Stephen Moses and Robert C. Bailey headed the RCT that was carried out in Kenya.[6] All three trials were funded by the American National Institutes of Health.[7]

Active Projects

- A randomized, controlled trial of male circumcision to reduce HIV incidence in Kisumu , Kenya.[4]

  National Institutes of Health

- Scaling up HIV prevention in Karnataka and southern Maharashtra , Phase II. [4]

  Bill & Melinda Gates Foundation

- Monitoring and evaluation of the Avahan project in India.[4]

  Bill & Melinda Gates Foundation.

- Technical assistance to improve maternal, neonatal & child health through National Rural Health Mission, India.[4]

  Bill & Melinda Gates Foundation

- Mapping key populations for HIV prevention in Sri Lanka.[4]

  World Bank.

Recent Publications

- Prevalence and risk factors for human papillomavirus infection by penile site in uncircumcised Kenyan men.[8]

  Smith JS, Hudgens MG, **Bailey RC**, Agot K, Ndinya-Achola JO, Moses S, et al. Int J Cancer 2010; 126: 572-7.

- Top Achievements in Health Research: Male circumcision: a new approach to reducing HIV transmission.[9]

  Moses S. CIHR/CMAJ 2009; 181: E134-5.

- Does sex in the early period after circumcision increase HIV-seroconversion risk? Pooled analysis of adult male circumcision clinical trials.[10]

  Mehta SD, **Gray RH, Auvert B**, Moses S , Kigozi G, Taljaard D, Puren A, Agot K, Serwadda D, Parker CB, **Wawer MJ, Bailey RC**. AIDS 2009; 23: 1557-64.

- Male circumcision for HIV prevention in young men in Kisumu , Kenya: a randomised controlled trial.[11]

  Bailey RC, Moses S , Parker CB, Agot K, Maclean I, Krieger JN, et al. Lancet 2007; 369: 643-56.

- Modelling the public health impact of male circumcision for HIV prevention in high prevalence areas in Africa.[12]

  Nagelkerke NJD, Moses S, de Vlas S, **Bailey RC**. BMC Infect Dis 2007; 7: 16.

- Adult male circumcision outcomes: experience in a developing country setting.[13]

  Krieger J, **Bailey RC**, Agot K, Parker C, Ndinya-Achola JO, Moses S, et al. Urol Int 2007; 78: 235-40

References

1. ↑ Moses S., Plummer FA, Bradley, JE, Ndinya-Achola, JO, Nagelkerke NJ, and Ronald AR. The association between lack of male circumcision and risk for HIV infection: a review of the epidemiological data. Sex Transm Dis 1994;21:201-10. 1.

2. ↑ Krieger JN, Bailey RC, Opeya J, *et al.* (November 2005). "Adult male circumcision: results of a standardized procedure in Kisumu District, Kenya". *BJU Int* **96** (7): 1109–13. doi:10.1111/j.1464-410X.2005.05810.x. PMID 16225538.
3. ↑ "WHO and UNAIDS announce recommendations from expert consultation on male circumcision for HIV prevention". World Health Organization. 2007-03-27. http://www.who.int/hiv/mediacentre/news68/en/index.html. Retrieved 2011-02-23
4. ↑ 4.0 4.1 4.2 4.3 4.4 4.5 Moses, Stephen. "Dr. Stephen Moses". University of Manitoba. http://umanitoba.ca/faculties/medicine/units/medical_microbiology/faculty/StephenMoses.html. Retrieved 2011-02-23.
5. ↑ Moses S., Plummer FA, Bradley, JE, Ndinya-Achola, JO, Nagelkerke NJ, and Ronald AR. The association between lack of male circumcision and risk for HIV infection: a review of the epidemiological data. Sex Transm Dis 1994;21:201-10.
6. ↑ Bailey RC, Moses S, Parker CB, et al. Male circumcision for HIV prevention in young men in Kisumu, Kenya: a randomised controlled trial. Lancet 2007;369:643-56. Abstract
7. ↑ "The Use of Male Circumcision to Prevent HIV Infection". Doctors Opposing Circumcision. 2008. Archived from the original on 2011-03-05. http://www.doctorsopposingcircumcision.org/info/HIVStatement.html. Retrieved 2011-03-05. "...funding from the United States National Institutes of Health to conduct randomized controlled trials (RCTs) in Africa."
8. ↑ Smith JS, Backes DM, Hudgens MG, *et al.* (January 2010). "Prevalence and risk factors of human papillomavirus infection by penile site in uncircumcised Kenyan men". *Int. J. Cancer* **126** (2): 572–7. doi:10.1002/ijc.24770. PMID 19626601.
9. ↑ Moses S (October 2009). "Male circumcision: a new approach to reducing HIV transmission". *CMAJ* **181** (8): E134–5. doi:10.1503/cmaj.090809. PMID 19786481.
10. ↑ Mehta SD, Gray RH, Auvert B, *et al.* (July 2009). "Does sex in the early period after circumcision increase HIV-seroconversion risk? Pooled analysis of adult male circumcision clinical trials". *AIDS* **23** (12): 1557–64. doi:10.1097/QAD.0b013e32832afe95. PMID 19571722.
11. ↑ Bailey RC, Moses S, Parker CB, *et al.* (February 2007). "Male circumcision for HIV prevention in young men in Kisumu, Kenya: a randomised controlled trial". *Lancet* **369** (9562): 643–56. doi:10.1016/S0140-6736(07)60312-2. PMID 17321310.
12. ↑ Nagelkerke NJ, Moses S, de Vlas SJ, Bailey RC (2007). "Modelling the public health impact of male circumcision for HIV prevention in high prevalence areas in Africa". *BMC Infect. Dis.* **7**: 16. doi:10.1186/1471-2334-7-16. PMID 17355625.
13. ↑ Krieger JN, Bailey RC, Opeyu JC, *et al.* (2007). "Adult male circumcision outcomes: experience in a developing country setting". *Urol. Int.* **78** (3): 235–40. doi:10.1159/000099344. PMID 17406133.

Retrieved from "http://intactwiki.org/w/index.php?title=Stephen_Moses&oldid=351"
Categories: People | Researchers | Circumcision in Africa | CircLeaks

- This page was last modified on 25 April 2015, at 12:18.
- This page has been accessed 176 times.
- Content is available under Public Domain unless otherwise noted.

- This page was last modified on 25 April 2015, at 12:18.
- This page has been accessed 170 times.
- Content is available under Public Domain unless otherwise noted.

Bertran Auvert

From IntactWiki

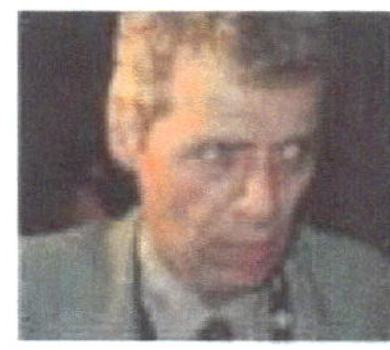

Associates with:
Gilgal Society
Member of:
Bill & Melinda Gates Foundation
Colleagues & Benefactors:
Ronald H. Gray
Stephen Moses
Robert C. Bailey
Brian J. Morris
Bill Gates

Bertran Auvert is a biased pro-circumcision researcher of French origin who has been a circumcision proponent since at least 2003.[1][2] Auvert was responsible for one of the three latest African circumcision trials,[3] which are being used by the World Health Organization to endorse circumcision as an HIV prevention method.[4] He associates with the Gilgal Society,[5] and is good friends with Bill Gates.[6]

Contents

- 1 Auvert's Circumcision Study
- 2 Bill Gates
- 3 See Also
- 4 External Links
- 5 References

Auvert's Circumcision Study

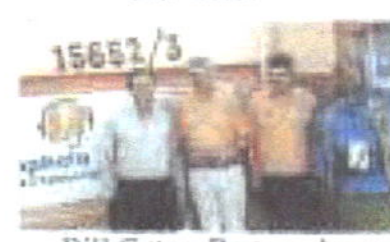

Bill Gates, Bertran Auvert, Dirk Taljaard, Cynthia Nhlapo

An RCT funded by the United States National Institutes of Health (NIH)[7] was carried out in Orange Farm, South Africa under the supervision of Bertran Auvert.[8] The British medical journal the Lancet decided against publishing Bertran's study. Lancet officials, following standard policy at the journal, refused to comment on why the study was turned down.[9]

In a Medscape interview, Bertran was asked, "in the group of men who were circumcised, I understand from the presentation that they were advised not to engage in sexual relations for approximately 5 weeks in order to recovery from the surgery. Is that correct?" Bertran replied, "Yes. We were very careful to recommend them to abstain from sex for 44 days, which is about 6 weeks after the surgical procedure, in order that they didn't have any risk of getting infected by HIV during this healing period."[10] Later in the interview he says "We also have 2 ongoing trials in Uganda and Kenya." (Notice the word "We")

Bill Gates

Bill Gates: Discussing Bertran's Circumcision *Studies*

> Bertran Auvert, is so modest about his work, but he has new theories that we're putting money behind and he is just making it work. "
>
> Lyons, D. (2010, January 25). Saving the world, 2.0. *Newsweek*. (http://www.newsweek.com/2010/01/24/saving-the-world-2-0.html)

"

See Also

- Gilgal Society -- Auvert associates with this circumfetish group.
- Bill & Melinda Gates Foundation -- Auvert is on the staff.
- Bill Gates -- Colleague & Benefactor of Auvert.
- Ronald H. Gray -- Colleague & Benefactor of Auvert.
- Stephen Moses -- Colleague & Benefactor of Auvert.
- Robert C. Bailey -- Colleague & Benefactor of Auvert.
- Brian J. Morris -- Colleague & Benefactor of Auvert.
- National Institutes of Health -- Funded Auvert's study.
- World Health Organization -- Endorces Auvert's study.

External Links

- Gilgal Society Association (http://www.circinfo.net/pdfs/GFW-EN%200712-1.pdf) -- Auvert contributed to a brochure created by Gilgal.

References

1. ↑ Rain-Taljaard RC, Lagarde E, Taljaard DJ, Campbell C, MacPhail C, Williams B, Auvert B. Potential for an intervention based on male circumcision in a South African town with high levels of HIV infection. Aids Care 2003;15(3):315-27
2. ↑ Rain-Taljaard RC, Lagarde E, Taljaard DJ, Campbell C, MacPhail C, Williams B, Auvert B. Potential for an intervention based on male circumcision in a South African town with high levels of HIV infection. Aids Care 2003;15(3):315-27. [PubMed]
3. ↑ Auvert, Bertran; Dirk Taljaard, Emmanuel Lagarde, Joëlle Sobngwi-Tambekou, Rémi Sitta, Adrian Puren (October 25, 2005). "Randomized, Controlled Intervention Trial of Male Circumcision for Reduction of HIV Infection Risk: The ANRS 1265 Trial" (http://www.plosmedicine.org/article/info:doi/10.1371/journal.pmed.0020298) . *PLoS Med* (November 2005). http://www.plosmedicine.org/article/info:doi/10.1371/journal.pmed.0020298. Retrieved 2011-03-03.
4. ↑ "WHO Male circumcision for HIV prevention" (http://www.who.int/hiv/topics/malecircumcision/en/index.html) . World Health Oranization. http://www.who.int/hiv/topics/malecircumcision/en/index.html. Retrieved 2011-03-03.
5. ↑ Morris, Brian; Vernon Quaintance (2007). "Sex and Circumcision What every Woman needs to know" (http://www.circinfo.net/pdfs/GFW-EN%200712-1.pdf) (PDF). The Gilgal Society. http://www.circinfo.net/pdfs/GFW-EN%200712-1.pdf. Retrieved 2011-02-27.

6. ↑ Lyons, Daniel (January 25, 2010). "Saving The World, 2.0" (http://www.newsweek.com/2010/01/24/saving-the-world-2-0.html) . *Newsweek* (Harman Newsweek LLC). http://www.newsweek.com/2010/01/24/saving-the-world-2-0.html. Retrieved 2011-03-03.
7. ↑ "The Use of Male Circumcision to Prevent HIV Infection" (http://www.doctorsopposingcircumcision.org/info/HIVStatement.html) . Doctors Opposing Circumcision. 2008. Archived from the original (http://www.doctorsopposingcircumcision.org) on 2011-03-05. http://www.doctorsopposingcircumcision.org/info/HIVStatement.html. Retrieved 2011-03-05. "...funding from the United States National Institutes of Health to conduct randomized controlled trials (RCTs) in Africa."
8. ↑ Auvert B, Taljaard D, Lagarde E, Sobngwi-Tambekou J, Sitta R, et al. (2005) Randomized, controlled intervention trial of male circumcision for reduction of HIV infection risk: The ANRS 1265 trial. PLoS Med 2:e298. Full Text (http://www.plosmedicine.org/article/info:doi/10.1371/journal.pmed.0020298)
9. ↑ Schoofs, M, Lueck, S, & Phillips, MM. (2005, July 05). Study says circumcision reduces AIDS risk by 70%. The Wall Street Journal, p. A1.
10. ↑ "Randomized Clinical Trial Shows Male Circumcision Has Great Potential to Curb HIV Infections in Africa" (http://www.medscape.org/viewarticle/509662) . Medscape. 07/29/2005. http://www.medscape.org/viewarticle/509662. Retrieved 2011-03-03

Retrieved from "http://intactwiki.org/w/index.php?title=Bertran_Auvert&oldid=242"
Categories: People | Researchers | Circumcision in Africa | CircLeaks

- This page was last modified on 22 April 2015, at 22:43.
- This page has been accessed 226 times.
- Content is available under Public Domain unless otherwise noted.

FALSE STUDIES

From Wiswell's UTI studies in which he is an advocate of early forced prepuce retraction, his practice increases what he statistically tests for and a cause of *Iatrogenic Pathophysiology*.

To Grey, Wawer and others who could not prove circumcision to reducing HIV/AIDS transmission in cohort studies the moved to Randomized Studies which Cooked the Book are, in part re: x

And Morris' citing wide ranges of statistical variations supporting his paraphilic erotic fetish. And so on with others involved: Demographic Choices: Testing Sites, Test Populations based on Religious and social practices, non- Muslin Socialized Multiple Concurrent Partners, Dry Sex. And, so on extending back beyond 170 years.

FALSE, FAKED, MEDICAL STUDIES: Net Search

Criminal Investigations > June 2, 2011: Physician, Researcher Charged with Falsifying Cl... Page 1 of 2

U.S. Food and Drug Administration
Protecting and Promoting Your Health

June 2, 2011: Physician, Researcher Charged with Falsifying Clinical Drug Trial

Food and Drug Administration
Office of Criminal Investigations

U.S. Department of Justice Press Release

For Immediate Release
June 2, 2011
United States Attorney
District of Kansas

TOPEKA, KAN. - A physician and a clinical research coordinator have been indicted on charges of falsifying study data in a clinical drug trial they were paid to conduct, U.S. Attorney Barry Grissom said today.

http://www.fda.gov/ICECI/CriminalInvestigations/ucm257769.htm 9/2/2015

Brian J. Morris

From IntactWiki

Notice: Brian Morris has been attempting to keep the information on this page from staying available to the public. On March 7th 2011, Morris attempted to remove this page; more on that here. On April 26th 2012, Morris removed information from his website and pamphlets due to information published on this page, information published about the Gilgal Society, and due to an arrest of Vernon Quaintance as a result of information on Quaintance's page. You can review this page, and the related pages, to see what Brian Morris doesn't want you to know

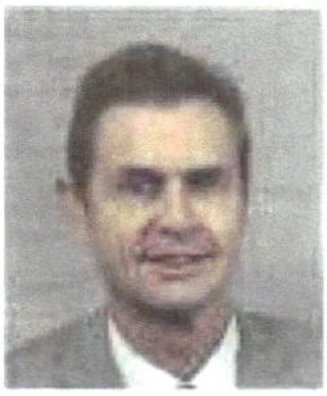

Member of:

Gilgal Society

Associates with:

Circlist

Cutting Club

Acorn Society

Colleagues & Benefactors:

Vernon Quaintance

Jake H. Waskett

Bertran Auvert

Robert C. Bailey

Daniel T. Halperin

Edgar J. Schoen

Stephen Moses

Thomas E. Wiswell

Gay Cox

Brian James Morris[1] is a molecular biologist and professor of molecular medical sciences at the University of Sydney, Australia.[2][3] He is an avid circumcision advocate,[4] who's never heard an argument for circumcision he didn't like.[5] He's the most vocal Australian circumcision promoter, stating that circumcision should be mandatory,[6] and uses regular scare tactics in an attempt to frighten parents into circumcising their children.[7]

Morris is also a member of the Gilgal Society,[8][9][10] who publishes circumcision propaganda, fetish stories of young boys being circumcised while others masturbate, and other materials. Gilgal Society has doctors and (circumcision to prevent HIV) researchers among their members.[11] Gilgal is headed by Vernon Quaintance, who was recently arrested for child pornography.[12][13]

Morris is in regular contact with Jake H. Waskett,[14] who is the number one Wikipedia editor of any articles on circumcision, or are even somewhat related to circumcision.[15]

Contents

Using Sydney University Prestige to Silence Dissent

Attempts to sack Dr. Karl S. Kruszelnicki

Brian Morris tried to use his status as a professor at the University of Sydney to pressure the university to sack Dr. Karl S. Kruszelnicki, from his position as Julius Sumner Miller Fellow in the School of Physics.[16] As a popular science writer, Dr. Kruszelnicki published an article in Sydney Morning Herald's Good Weekend" publication, titled "May the foreskin be with you."[17] prompting a fierce attack from Brian Morris. Firstly, Morris tried writing in response to the article. [18]

> **Good Weekend, 31 January 2004, Your Say**
>
> — Dr Karl Kruszelnicki ignores the massive scientific support for the benefits of circumcision (Weekender, January 10) and instead presents only extremist anti-circ nonsense from the likes of Paul Fleiss. Dr K fails to even mention that male circumcision prevents a raft of diseases in both sexes, as well as sexual problems in men. Bacteria abound under the foreskin,* accounting for 11-fold higher urinary tract infections. The foreskin is, moreover, an "HIV magnet". Its removal may reduce the risk of AIDS, penile cancer and cervical cancer.
>
> *Professor Brian Morris*
> *University of Sydney*
>
> – *Good Weekend, Your Say* (http://www.cirp.org/Dr_Karl.html)

In addition to writing a letter to the newspaper, and trying to get the University of Sydney to sack Dr Kruszelnicki from his position, Morris also filed a formal complaint of bias against the Sydney Morning Herald with the Australian Press Council.[19] These efforts were not successful, however, and the press council dismissed his complaint.[20]

Attempts to block a research paper from being published

In 2011, Morten Frisch, an MD, PhD and Doctor of Medicine, a professor of sexual health epidemiology at Statens Serum Institut in Copenhagen and at Aalborg University in Denmark, published a study, which showed an excess of orgasm difficulties in circumcised men, as well as significantly increased frequencies of orgasm difficulties, pain during intercourse and a sense of incomplete sexual needs fulfillment in women with circumcised spouses.[21]

This study was preceded by three other publications based on the same dataset, dealing with sexual dysfunctions in Danish men and women in relation to socioeconomic factors, health factors and lifestyle factors, respectively, which were swimmingly published without serious criticisms from peer reviewers in the two most prestigious US journals of sexual health, the Journal of Sexual Medicine and Archives of Sexual Behavior. After adding the variable of male circumcision status to the analysis, however, the study was met with extremely critical reviews of everything about the entire dataset.[22]

In particular, Brian Morris, along with Jake Waskett and Ronald Gray made extensive, obstructive peer-review comments in a review which included serious insinuations of racism and amateurism.[23] According to a letter of appreciation written by Morten Frisch to the editors of the International Journal of Epidemiology for the publication of his study, Frisch was informed by a colleague that Morris used his mailing list to enact a campaign to write critical letters to the editors of the International Journal of Epidemiology. [24]

> **To IJE Editors**
>
> I would like to thank the IJE editors for withstanding the pressure from one particularly discourteous and bullying reviewer who went to extremes to prevent our study from being published. After the paper's online publication, I have received emails from colleagues around the world who felt our contribution was useful and potentially important. One colleague

> informed me that the angry reviewer was the first author of the above letter to the editor. In an email, Morris had called people on his mailing list to arms against our study, openly admitting that he was the reviewer and that he had tried to get the paper rejected. To inspire his followers, Morris had attached his two exceedingly long and aggressive reviews of our paper (12858 words and 5293 words, respectively), calling for critical letters in abundance to the IJE editors. Breaking unwritten confidentiality and courtesy rules of the peer-review process, Morris distributed his slandering criticism of our study to people working for the same cause.

Morten Frisch: Author's Response to: Does sexual function survey in Denmark offer any support for male circumcision having an adverse effect? (http://ije.oxfordjournals.org/content/41/1/312.full)

Connection to the Gilgal Society

Morris hides his association with the 'Gilgal Society'

On the 26th of April, 2012, documents suddenly disappeared from Brian Morris's website.[7] The documents were his leaflets promoting circumcision, bearing the imprint of the Gilgal Society.[9][10] Recently, the head of the Gilgal Society, Vernon Quaintance, has been convicted of possessing child pornography.[12][13]

Until the 26th of April, 2012, Morris's leaflet, "Circumcision: A Guide For Parents", said it was published by Brian Morris & The Gilgal Society, with the society's address and logo.[10][7] As of the 26th of April, 2012, all reference to the society are gone, along with a reference to Morris's "interest in circumcision".

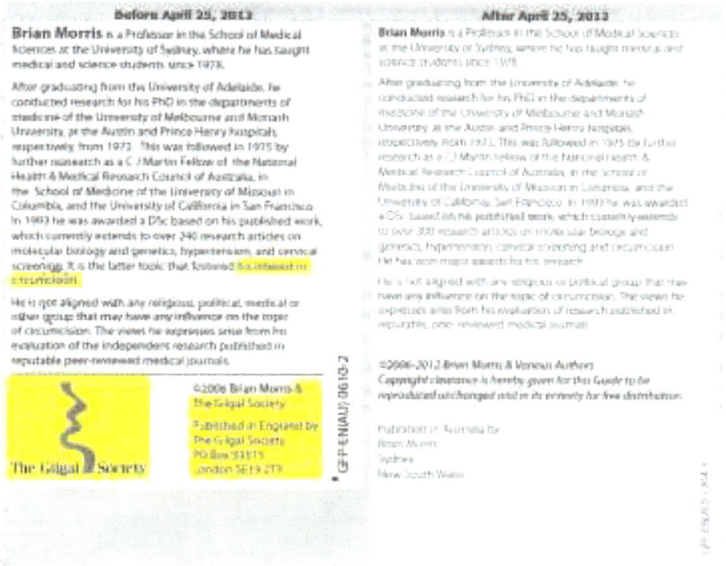

Before April 25, 2013

Brian Morris is a Professor in the School of Medical Sciences at the University of Sydney, where he has taught medical and science students since 1978.

After graduating from the University of Adelaide, he conducted research for his PhD in the departments of medicine of the University of Melbourne and Monash University, at the Austin and Prince Henry hospitals, respectively, from 1973. This was followed in 1975 by further research as a C J Martin Fellow of the National Health & Medical Research Council of Australia, in the School of Medicine of the University of Missouri in Columbia, and the University of California in San Francisco. In 1993 he was awarded a DSc based on his published work, which currently extends to over 240 research articles on molecular biology and genetics, hypertension, and cervical screening. It is the latter topic that fostered his interest in circumcision.

He is not aligned with any religious, political, medical or other group that may have any influence on the topic of circumcision. The views he expresses arise from his evaluation of the independent research published in reputable peer-reviewed medical journals.

The Gilgal Society

©2006 Brian Morris & The Gilgal Society

Published in England by The Gilgal Society PO Box [illegible] London SE19 2T[illegible]

GF-EN(AU) 0610-2

After April 25, 2013

Brian Morris is a Professor in the School of Medical Sciences at the University of Sydney, where he has taught medical and science students since 1978.

After graduating from the University of Adelaide, he conducted research for his PhD in the departments of medicine of the University of Melbourne and Monash University, at the Austin and Prince Henry hospitals, respectively, from 1973. This was followed in 1975 by further research as a CJ Martin Fellow of the National Health & Medical Research Council of Australia, in the School of Medicine of the University of Missouri in Columbia, and the University of California, San Francisco. In 1993 he was awarded a DSc based on his published work, which currently extends to over [illegible] research articles on molecular biology and genetics, hypertension, cervical screening and circumcision. He has won major awards for his research.

He is not aligned with any religious or political group that may have any influence on the topic of circumcision. The views he expresses arise from his evaluation of research published in reputable peer-reviewed medical journals.

©2006–2012 Brian Morris & Various Authors

Copyright clearance is hereby given for this Guide to be reproduced unchanged and in its entirety for free distribution.

Published in Australia by
Brian Morris
Sydney
New South Wales

Morris's leaflet for women, "Sex and Circumcision: What every woman needs to know", which boasted a long list of co-authors—a virtual roll-call of the pro-circumcision movement—was removed and later replaced by a black and white version (http://www.circinfo.net/pdfs/GFWomen-EN2012-b%26w.pdf) —again, with all reference to the Gilgal Society removed. Links to the Circumcision Foundation of Australia and the circumcision fetish site Circlist have been added.

Authors

The text of this brochure has received consensus support from the following circumcision experts (listed alphabetically), who contributed to its formulation:

Bertran Auvert, MD PhD (France)
Robert Bailey, PhD (Univ of Illinois, Chicago, USA)
Stefan Bailis, MA (Minnesota, USA)
Xavier Castellsague, MD PhD (Barcelona, Spain)
Mike Cormier (New Brunswick, Canada)
Guy Cox, DPhil (Univ of Sydney, Australia)
Rene Gelbaum, RN MOAM (Los Angeles, USA)
Daniel Halperin, PhD (Harvard, Boston, USA)
Dawn Harvey, MA(Hons) (Aberdeen, UK)
Sam Kunin, MD (Los Angeles, USA)
Edgar Schoen, MD (Oakland, USA)
Roger Short, AM FRS ScD (Univ of Melbourne, Australia)
Howard Stang, MD (Minnesota, USA)
Jake Waskett (Manchester, UK)
Helen Weiss, PhD (London Sch Hyg Trop Med, UK)
Robin Willcourt, MD (Newport Beach, USA & Adelaide, Aust)
Tom Wiswell, MD (Florida, USA)

Primary author: Brian Morris, DSc
Professor, School of Medical Sciences, University of Sydney, Australia

Further information

May be obtained from the following websites:

http://www.circinfo.net (Brian Morris, PhD DSc)
http://www.medicirc.com (Edgar Schoen, MD)
http://www.gilgalsoc.org (The Gilgal Society)
http://www.aboutcirc.info (Guy Cox, DPhil)
http://circumcision.com.au (Terry Russell, AOM, MB BS)
http://www.samkuninmd.com (Sam Kunin, MD)
http://circumcisioninfo.com (Pierre Lacock, PhD)
http://www.geocities.com/HotSprings/2754 (Mike Cormier)

A list of possible circumcisers in your region may be obtained from the Gilgal Society. See www.gilgalsoc.org for an order form, or www.circinfo.net for doctors in Australia and New Zealand.

Copyright clearance is hereby given for this Guide to be reproduced unchanged and in its entirety for free distribution. A pdf version can be downloaded for free from the Internet at www.circinfo.net for emailing to others and/or use to print unlimited copies.

© 2007 Brian Morris & The Gilgal Society
Published in England by The Gilgal Society
PO Box 59113, London, SE19 2TX

The Gilgal Society

Authors

The text of this brochure has received consensus support from the following circumcision experts (listed alphabetically), who contributed to its formulation:

Bertran Auvert, MD PhD (France)
Robert Bailey, PhD (Univ of Illinois, Chicago, USA)
Stefan Bailis, PsyD LP (Minnesota, USA)
Xavier Castellsague, MD MPH PhD (Barcelona, Spain)
Mike Cormier (New Brunswick, Canada)
Guy Cox, DPhil (Univ of Sydney, Australia)
Daniel Halperin, PhD (Univ of North Carolina, USA)
Dawn Harvey, MA(Hons) (Aberdeen, UK)
Sam Kunin, MD (Los Angeles, USA)
Edgar Schoen, MD (Oakland, USA)
Roger Short, AM FRS ScD (Univ of Melbourne, Australia)
Howard Stang, MD (Minnesota, USA)
Jake Waskett (Manchester, UK)
Helen Weiss, PhD (London Sch Hyg Trop Med, UK)
Robin Willcourt, MD (Queen Elizabeth Hospital, Australia)
Tom Wiswell, MD (Orlando, Florida, USA)

Primary author: Brian Morris, PhD DSc FAHA
Professor, School of Medical Sciences, Univ of Sydney, Australia

Further information

May be obtained from the following websites:

http://www.circinfo.net (Brian Morris, PhD DSc)
http://www.circumcisionaustralia.org (Circumcision Foundation of Australia)
http://www.medicirc.com (Edgar Schoen, MD)
http://www.circlist.com
http://www.aboutcirc.info
http://circumcision.com.au (Terry Russell, AO, MB BS)
http://www.samkuninmd.com (Sam Kunin, MD)

©2007–2012 Brian Morris & Various Authors
Copyright clearance is hereby given for this guide to be reproduced unchanged and in its entirety for free distribution. A pdf version can be downloaded for free from the Internet at www.circinfo.net for emailing to others and for use to print unlimited copies.

Published in Australia by
Brian Morris
Sydney
New South Wales

Since April 11th 2012 (the day Vernon Quaintance's court hearing was set, the Gilgal Society website has carried the message:
"We regret that as a result of major computer failure none of our publications are currently available to order from us." But Professor Morris's leaflets continue to be advertised on the site.

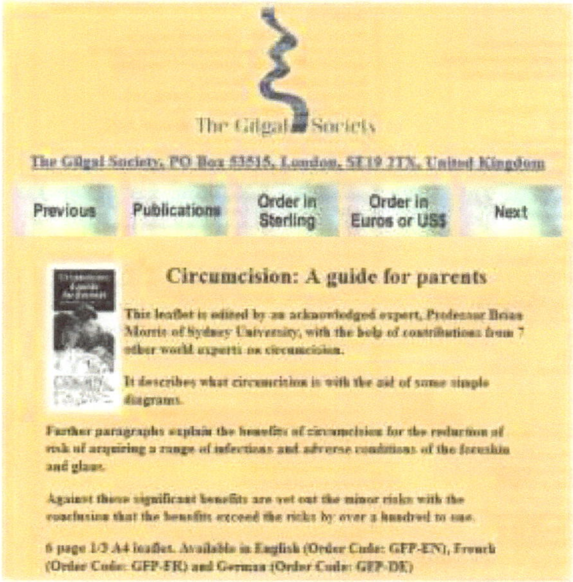

Morris's site continues to show a "circumcision humor" page, including a verse by Vernon Quaintance, directly under a picture of a baby with his foreskin trapped in a cellphone.[26]

Brian Morris' Websites

Original Website

Brian Morris ran a circumcision website hosted by the University of Sydney. While no longer on University of Sydney equipment, www.circinfo.net is again operational.[27] The University of Sydney asked Brian Morris not to associate his views on circumcision with his position at the university.

Recommended

Morris' website links to the following *recommended* websites and groups (8 of which are circumfetish sites, and 7 that sell devices to perform circumcisions):[28]

- The Gilgal Society[29]
- Circlist (German)[30]
- Circlist (Yahoo Asian)[31]
- Erotic Male Circumcision[31]
- Circumcised Kids[33]

- Circumcision Fetish[34]
- SCARandACORN[35]
- Teen Circ[36]
- Cutting Club[37]
- Beschnittene Gay Boys[38]
- Misc. Kids[39]
- Misc. Kids Health[40]
- Misc. Kids Pregnancy[41]
- A list of places to get circumcision devices[42][43][44][45][46][47][48]

Humor

Morris' website also has a circumcision humor section, which contains jokes about children, and even a video called "Don't cha wish your boyfriend was circumcized?"[49] It also contains a picture of a naked child, with a folding cellphone clamped onto his foreskin, dangling from the end of his penis, on the humor section of his website.[50] It appears as if an adult purposely put the cell phone there and took the picture.

Foreskin Fetish?

On several occasions Morris has called those against circumcision, foreskin fetishists. He sometimes cites a paper written in 1965 called "Foreskin fetishism and its relation to ego pathology in a male homosexual" (which links to Jake H. Waskett's website).[30][31] Waskett is homosexual.[32]

Allegations of a Homosexual Agenda Behind Intactivism

> " A subgroup of the gay community practise "docking", a sexual practice that requires the foreskin. Naturally such men would want to ensure that an adequate supply of boys with foreskins are coming up through the ranks, where a proportion will have an orientation towards males. Why don't those who wish to outlaw male circumcision be honest enough to admit the REAL reason for their campaign? And by the way, "docking" is regarded on gay health websites as unsafe sex, as it exposes the vulnerable mucosal inner lining of the foreskin to infection by HIV, to name just some of the medical hazards posed by the foreskin "
>
> — Brian J. Morris [illegible] 2011 at 12:33 am. Comment #38. Diary of a Wimpy Catholic (http://www.patheos.com/community/diaryofawimpycatholic/2011/[illegible]) [38]

Does it make sense to have a fetish about a genital organ?

> **fet·ish** [fet-ish, fee-tish]
> *Psychology.* Any object or nongenital part of the body that causes a habitual erotic response or fixation.[33]

Some of Brian Morris' Arguments for Circumcision

Mandatory

> " Circumcision should be made compulsory "
>
> Brian J. Morris. *Sunday Night* Circumcision (http://www.youtube.com/watch?v=[illegible])

Intact males are having sex

> "Because parents have been encouraged not to circumcise their kids, what we're now seeing is a big rise in number of uncircumcised males entering the sexually active community"
>
> —Brian J. Morris, *Sunday Night Circumcision* (http://www.youtube.com/watch?v=[illegible])

Bathroom Splatter

> "Boys and men who are not circumcised can be a source of irritation if they do not retract the foreskin when they urinate, as 'splatter' will occur."
>
> —Morris, B. (2010) *circinfo.net* (http://www.circinfo.net/physical_problems.html)

Zipper Injury

> "In uncircumcised boys the foreskin can become accidentally entrapped in zippers, resulting in pain, trauma, swelling and scarring of this appendage. Foreskin accidents in men can also occur."
>
> —Morris, B. (2010) *circinfo.net* (http://www.circinfo.net/physical_problems.html)

Saving lives?

> "Millions of lives will be saved by universal circumcision"
>
> —Brian J. Morris, *Sunday Night Circumcision* (http://www.youtube.com/watch?v=[illegible])

Women, be afraid!

> "Circumcision must be advocated for reducing AIDS, and the impact on cervical cancer and other conditions in women."
>
> —Brian J. Morris, *Sunday Night Circumcision* (http://www.youtube.com/watch?v=[illegible])

Intact penises kill people

> "The benefits exceed the risks by 100 to 1. One in three males—as a conservative estimate—will get a medical problem, many will die, if they're not circumcised. I'm being very serious about this."
>
> —Brian J. Morris, *Sunday Night Circumcision* (http://www.youtube.com/watch?v=[illegible])

A *Good Talking To*

> "For sure, there will be people who don't want it done, just as there are opponents of vaccination, but the benefits are so incredibly vast that any parent not wanting their child circumcised REALLY needs a good talking to."
>
> —Brian J. Morris, *Sunday Night Circumcision* (http://www.youtube.com/watch?v=[illegible])

Whose Responsibility?

> The greatest benefits accrue the earlier in life the procedure is performed. If left till later ages the individual has already been exposed to the risk of urinary tract infections, the physical problems and carries a residual risk of penile cancer. Moreover, it would take a very street-wise, outgoing, adolescent male to make this decision and undertake the process of ensuring that it was done. [...] many will suffer in silence rather than seek medical advice or treatment. Really though parental responsibility must over-ride arguments based on 'the rights of the child'

Morris, B. (2002, May 21). circinfo.net (http://web.archive.org/web/20020122071114/http://www.circinfo.net/Responsibility)

Published Work

In March of 2011, Morris published a paper in Am J Prev Med called "Circumcision denialism unfounded and unscientific." He had the paper co-authored by Daniel Halperin, Edgar J. Schoen, Stephen Moses, and others.[54]

In August of 2011, Morris published a paper called "Male Circumcision: An Appraisal of Current Instrumentation" with an editor of Circlist (a circumcision fetish group).[55]

Public Statements

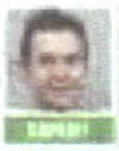

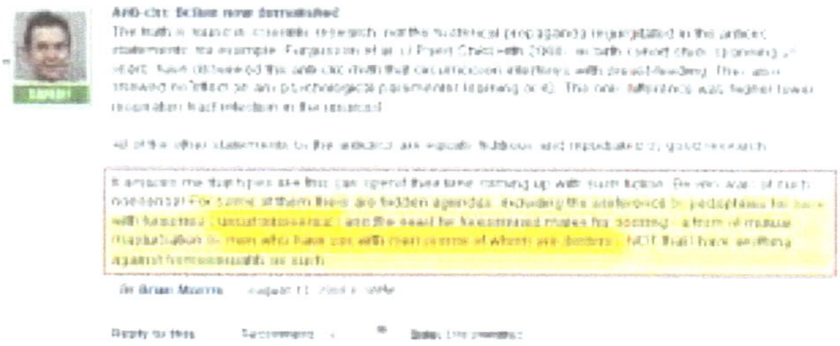

[illegible]

[56]

Private Statements

Female Circumcision

The following was an email response from Morris, to an email citing two studies that claim to show female circumcision does not reduce sexual pleasure.[57][58]

Re: [redacted]

From: [illegible]
To: [redacted]

Thank you [redacted]

Yes ... I am aware of the data on female sexual response after FGC.

The news media and medical profession are so 'politically correct' when it comes to reporting studies like this

I was not aware of the reduced incidence of HIV though

Best wishes

Brian

[illegible]

Mandatory Circumcision

Morris thinks circumcision should be required by law.[illegible]

Circumcision Tourism

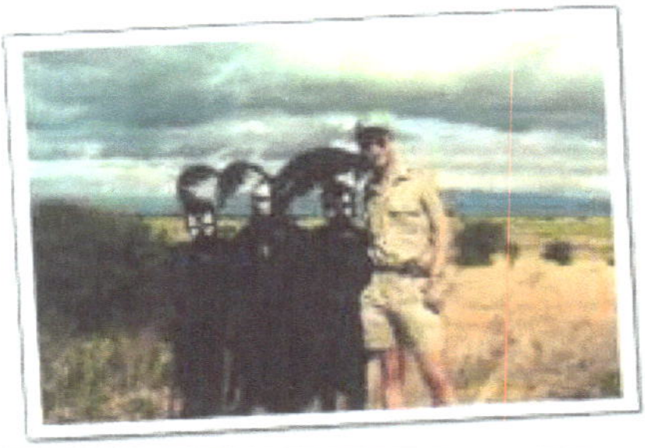

Brian Morris Watching Masai Boys During Circumcision Ritual in Kenya, 1989

> I have some wonderful photographs of a group of Masai boys in their early teens that I met in Kenya in 1989 dressed in their dark circumcision robes, with white feathers as headwear, and white painted facial decoration that stood out against their very black skin. Each wore a pendant that was the razor blade used for their own circumcisions. The ceremony that they had gone through is a special part of their tribal culture and was very important to these boys, who were proud to show that they were now 'men'. In other cultures it is associated with preparation for marriage and as a sign of entry into manhood.

— Brian Morris' personal website (archive) [illegible]

Circleaks Incident

On March 7th 2011, a new user account by the name of Brianm signed up for Circleaks,[60] attempted to blank this page,[61] then successfully blanked the page entirely.[62] A few minutes later Brianm added Brian Morris' website (circinfo.net) to the page,[63] then added and removed sda=brianm.[64][65] At this point an Administrator reverted the removal,[66] and locked the page due to repeated attempts of removal without discussion.[67] A message was then posted on Brianm's talkpage, notifying the user that their removals have been reverted, that if a statement is shown to be false it will be removed, and that registering simply to delete content that's incriminating to someone isn't compatible with Circleaks wiki policies.[68] A Circleaks administrator checked the IP address of brianm and found the user to be in Australia, New South Wales, Sydney, University of Sydney.[69] Soon after brianm's edits, Brian Morris sent an email to his mailing list regarding this page.

The following was an email response from Morris to his mailing list on March 7th 2011, several hours after User:Brianm made an account,[70] and blanked this page.[71]

Personal attacks on advocates of male circumcision

[illegible]

Dear all

There is now evidence that a growing proportion of opponents of male circumcision are starting to realize that they are losing the debate and that ad hominem attacks are all that's left for them.

In the past they have set up websites full of erroneous information about circumcision, and that promote foreskin mythology, and "restoration". As well this vocal minority orchestrate the bombardment of publishers and online news reports, using these as a platform to preach their fiction in the hope of perpetuating their fallacies.

But recently they have begun a campaign involving outrageous personal attacks on respected academics, clinicians and others worldwide (including Oprah Winfrey, Bill Gates, Bill Clinton, and the like) who have publicly supported male circumcision based on the considerable evidence now available.

Indeed, any intelligent analysis of the medical literature reveals male circumcision, especially when performed in infancy, provides a lifetime of benefits to public health and individual well-being, is very safe, and has no long-term adverse consequences [illegible]

The attacks are libelous and, as a consequence, the perpetrators have taken great care to hide their own identity.

Brian
-- Brian J. Morris, PhD DSc FAHA
Professor of Molecular Medical Sciences
Basic & Clinical Genomics Laboratory
School of Medical Sciences and Bosch Institute
Anderson Stuart Building (F13)
The University of Sydney
Sydney NSW 2006
Australia

On March 8th 2011, Morris posted an almost identical message on a science blog at Science 20.[77]

On accusations of libel:

CircLeaks prides itself on verifiable accuracy. Anyone may check the validity of any claim by checking the citations. If a claim is shown to be false, the claim will be altered or removed to reflect the new and more accurate information. If Morris finds anything on this page to be false, all he has to do is demonstrate the error, and said error will be removed or corrected. Blanking the entire page is not the way to resolve an error, and may instead appear to be an attempt to hide factual information. If you would like to challenge a claim on this page, please discuss it on the talk page.

See Also

- Circumfetish -- Traits consistent with Brian Morris' profile.
- Jake H. Waskett -- Morris uses Waskett to do his dirty work.
- Vernon Quaintance -- Morris uses Vernon to create his pro-circumcision brochures.
- Gilgal Society -- Morris is a member.
- Circlist -- Morris promotes and associates with Circlist.
- Cutting Club -- Morris promotes and associates with the Cutting Club.
- Acorn Society -- Morris promotes and associates with the Acorn Society.
- Daniel T. Halperin -- Coauthored a paper with Morris.
- Edgar J. Schoen -- Coauthored a paper with Morris.
- Stephen Moses -- Coauthored a paper with Morris.
- Bertran Auvert -- Colleague & Benefactor of Morris.
- Robert C. Bailey -- Colleague & Benefactor of Morris.
- Thomas E. Wiswell -- Colleague & Benefactor of Morris.

CircWatch

Posts about Brian Morris on CircWatch (http://circwatch.org/tag/brian-morris/)

External Links

- Crazy Man: Brian J. Morris (http://www.youtube.com/watch?v=gdGbXdEo93U) – Video
- Brian Morris' Biography (http://www.physiol.usyd.edu.au/~brianm/) – University of Sydney
- Brian Morris & His Circumfetish Push to Cut The World (http://www.drmomma.org/2009/11/brian-morris-his-circumfetish-push-to.html) – Analysis of Brian Morris

References

Note: If a link is broken, you will find a PDF archive link directly behind it (under the same reference number).

1. ↑ Morris, Brian James; Ron Gray, Xavier Castellsagué, F. Xavier Bosch, Daniel T. Halperin, C. A. Hankins, and Jake H. Waskett (2011-03-09). "The Strong Protective Effect of Circumcision Against Cancer of the Penis" (http://www.hindawi.com/journals/au/aip/812368/). *Advances in Urology*. http://www.hindawi.com/journals/au/aip/812368/. Retrieved 2011-03-13.
2. ↑ Morris, Brian J. (2010-03-04). "Professor Brian Morris" (http://sydney.edu.au/medicine/genetic/staff/profiles/bmorris.php). *The University of Sydney*. Head of Discipline. http://sydney.edu.au/medicine/genetic/staff/profiles/bmorris.php. Retrieved 2011-03-07.
3. ↑ Morris, Brian J. (2010). "About the Author - Professor Brian J. Morris" (http://www.circinfo.net/about_the_author_professor_brian_j_morris.html). circinfo.net. http://www.circinfo.net/about_the_author_professor_brian_j_morris.html. Retrieved 2011-03-07. Archive File:Circinfo about-the-author.pdf
4. ↑ Morris, Brian. *In favour of circumcision*. Sydney, NSW, Australia: University of New South Wales Press. ISBN 0-86840-537-X.
5. ↑ Morris, Brian J. (2010). "Circumcision - Physical Problems" (http://www.circinfo.net/physical_problems.html). circinfo.net. http://www.circinfo.net/physical_problems.html. Retrieved 2011-03-07. Archive: File:Circinfo physical-problems.pdf
6. ↑ [6.0 6.1] "Sunday Night Circumcision" (http://www.youtube.com/watch?v=7yDvL4hNny4#t=1m18s). http://www.youtube.com/watch?v=7yDvL4hNny4#t=1m18s. Retrieved 2011-03-06. Archive: http://www.youtube.com/watch?v=gdGbXdEo93U
7. ↑ Morris, Brian J. (2010). "Why Medical Bodies and Others Should Not Advise That Circumcision Should be Delayed Until the Boy Can Make the Decision for Himself" (http://www.circinfo.net/circumcision_why_you_should_not_delay.html). circinfo.net. http://www.circinfo.net/circumcision_why_you_should_not_delay.html. Retrieved 2011-03-07. Archive. File:Circinfo why-you-should-not-delay.pdf
8. ↑ [8.0 8.1] Morris, Brian (2007). Vernon Quaintance. ed. *Sex and circumcision. What every woman needs to know* (http://www.circinfo.net/pdfs/GFW-EN%200712-1.pdf). London, England: Gilgal Society. http://www.circinfo.net/pdfs/GFW-EN%200712-1.pdf. Archive: File:Gilgal For Women leaflet.pdf
9. ↑ [9.0 9.1 9.2] Morris, Brian; Quaintance, Vernon (2007). Vernon Quaintance. ed. *Circumcision: A guide for parents* (http://www.circinfo.net/pdfs/GFP-ENAU.pdf). London, England: Gilgal Society. http://www.circinfo.net/pdfs/GFP-ENAU.pdf. Retrieved 2011-03-06. Archive: File:Gilgal Parents-Guide.pdf
10. ↑ [10.0 10.1 10.2] "Guide For Women" (http://web.archive.org/web/20110518085430/http://www.circinfo.net/). http://web.archive.org/web/20110518085430/http://www.circinfo.net/. Retrieved 2011-05-81.
11. ↑ Gilgal Society - See article for citations
12. ↑ [12.0 12.1] "Croydon circumcision campaigner caught with child porn videos" (http://www.thisiscroydontoday.co.uk/Croydon-circumcision-campaigner-caught-child-porn/story-15866127-detail/story.html). *Croydon Advertiser*. 2012-04-21. http://www.thisiscroydontoday.co.uk/Croydon-circumcision-campaigner-caught-child-porn/story-15866127-detail/story.html. Retrieved 2012-04-22. Archive 2012-04-21. http://circleaks.org/images/2/27/Www.thisiscroydontoday.co.uk-Croydon-circumcision-campaigner-caught-child-porn-s.pdf
13. ↑ [13.0 13.1] Kay, Richard (2012-04-25). "Sex scandal rocks Order of the Knights" (http://www.dailymail.co.uk/news/article-2134978/David-Cameron-son-PM-wife-Samantha-unveil-church-tribute-son-Ivan.html). *MailOnline* (GlamEntertainment). http://www.dailymail.co.uk/news/article-

2134978/David-Cameron-son-PM-wife-Samantha-unveil-church-tribute-son-Ivan.html. Retrieved 2012-04-26. Archive (2012-04-27): http://circleaks.org/images/6/66/Quaintance-disrupts-the-church%28malta%29.pdf

14. † Waskett, Jake H.; Brian J. Morris (May 2007). "Fine touch pressure thresholds in the adult penis" (http://www3.interscience.wiley.com/cgi-bin/fulltext/118508593/HTMLSTART) . *BJU International* 99 (6): 1551–1552. doi:10.1111/j.1464-410X.2007.06970_6.x (http://dx.doi.org/10.1111%2Fj.1464-410X.2007.06970_6.x) . PMID 17537227 (http://www.ncbi.nlm.nih.gov/pubmed/17537227) . http://www3.interscience.wiley.com/cgi-bin/fulltext/118508593/HTMLSTART.
15. † Waskett, Jake H. "User contributions" (http://en.wikipedia.org/wiki/Special:Contributions/Jakew) . Wikipedia. http://en.wikipedia.org/wiki/Special:Contributions/Jakew. Retrieved 2011-03-08.
16. † "Dr Karl on the origins of circumcision" (http://www.circinfo.org/Dr_Karl.html) . *Circumcision Information Australia*. http://www.circinfo.org/Dr_Karl.html. Retrieved 2012-12-23. "Brian Morris tried to use his status as a professor at Sydney University to pressure the university to sack Dr Kruszelnicki from his position as Julius Sumner Miller Fellow in the School of Physics."
17. † Kruszelnicki, Karl S. (10 January 2004). "May the foreskin be with you". *Good Weekend*.
18. † "Dr Karl on the origins of circumcision" (http://www.circinfo.org/Dr_Karl.html) . *Circumcision Information Australia*. http://www.circinfo.org/Dr_Karl.html. Retrieved 2012-12-23. "Dr Karl Kruszelnicki ignores the massive scientific support for the benefits of circumcision (Weekender, January 10) and instead presents only extremist anti-circ nonsense from the likes of Paul Fleiss."
19. † "Dr Karl on the origins of circumcision" (http://www.circinfo.org/Dr_Karl.html) . *Circumcision Information Australia*. http://www.circinfo.org/Dr_Karl.html. Retrieved 2012-12-23. "Morris also filed a formal complaint of bias against the Sydney Morning Herald with the Australian Press Council."
20. † "May the foreskin be with you". *Sydney Morning Herald*. 13 April 2004. "The Australian Press Council has dismissed a complaint by Professor Brian Morris against the Good Weekend magazine, published by the Sydney Morning Herald, over a column by Dr Karl Kruszelnicki."
21. † Frisch M, Lindholm M, Grønbæk M. Male circumcision and sexual function in men and women: a survey-based, cross-sectional study in Denmark. Int J Epidemiol 2011 Oct;40(5):1367-81 [1] (http://www.ncbi.nlm.nih.gov/pubmed/21672947)
22. † "Circumcision and Sexual Function Difficulties" (https://www.youtube.com/watch?v=yfGkZZ-KzpU#t=01m34s) . YouTube. 2012-12-06. https://www.youtube.com/watch?v=yfGkZZ-KzpU#t=01m34s. Retrieved 2012-12-24.
23. † Morris BJ, Waskett JH, Gray RH. Does sexual function survey in Denmark offer any support for male circumcision having an adverse effect? Int J Epidemiol 2012 Feb;41(1):310-2 [2] (http://www.ncbi.nlm.nih.gov/pubmed/22422464)
24. † Frisch M. Author's Response to: Does sexual function survey in Denmark offer any support for male circumcision having an adverse effect? Int. J. Epidemiol. (2012) 41(1): 312-314 first published online November 28, 2011 [3] (http://ije.oxfordjournals.org/content/41/1/312.full)
25. † Young, Hugh. "Intactivism News" (http://www.circumstitions.com/news/news45.html#vernon2) . *Circumstitions*. http://www.circumstitions.com/news/news45.html#vernon2. Retrieved 2012-04-27.
26. † 26.0 26.1 Morris, Brian J.. "Circumcision Humor" (http://www.circinfo.net/circumcision_humor.html) . http://www.circinfo.net/circumcision_humor.html. Retrieved 2011-03-06. Archive: File:Circinfo-Humor.pdf
27. † Morris, Brian (2006-11-09). "Medical benefits from circumcision" (http://www-personal.usyd.edu.au/~bmorris/circumcision.shtml) . University of Sydney. http://www-personal.usyd.edu.au/~bmorris/circumcision.shtml. Retrieved 2011-09-17. Archive: http://wayback.archive.org/web/*/http://www-personal.usyd.edu.au/~bmorris/circumcision.shtml
28. † Morris, Brian J. (2007-08-29). "Circumcision Websites & Online Discussion Groups" (http://circleaks.org/images/3/31/Web.archive.org-web-20070829145507-circinfo.net-circumcision_websites_online_discussion_groups.html-1.pdf) . circinfo.net. http://circleaks.org/images/3/31/Web.archive.org-web-20070829145507-circinfo.net-circumcision_websites_online_discussion_groups.html-1.pdf. Retrieved 2011-03-06. Archive: http://web.archive.org/web/20070829145507/circinfo.net/circumcision_websites_online_discussion_groups.html
29. † Quaintance, Vernon. "The Gilgal Society" (http://www.gilgalsoc.org/) . The Gilgal Society. http://www.gilgalsoc.org/. Retrieved 2011-03-07. Archive: File:Gilgalsoc mainpage.pdf
30. † "Circlist" (http://www.circlist.hasibubu.de) . Circlist. http://www.circlist.hasibubu.de.
31. † "Asian-pro-circumcision" (http://groups.yahoo.com/group/asian_circlist/) . Yahoo. http://groups.yahoo.com/group/asian_circlist/.
32. † "Erotic Male Circumcision" (http://groups.yahoo.com/group/eroticmalecircumcision/) . Yahoo. http://groups.yahoo.com/group/eroticmalecircumcision/.
33. † http://groups.yahoo.com/group/circumcisedkids/
34. † Morris, Brian J. (2007-08-29). "Circumcision Websites & Online Discussion Groups" (http://circleaks.org/images/3/31/Web.archive.org-web-20070829145507-circinfo.net-

circumcision_websites_online_discussion_groups.html-1.pdf) . circinfo.net. http://circleaks.org/images/3/31/Web.archive.org-web-20070829145507-circinfo.net-circumcision_websites_online_discussion_groups.html-1.pdf. Retrieved 2011-03-06. Archive: http://web.archive.org/web/20070829145507/circinfo.net/circumcision_websites_online_discussion_groups.html

35. ↑ "SCARandACORN. Interested in the subject of circumcision, particularly those with personal experience. Against the tide of anti-circumcision." (http://groups.yahoo.com/group/SCARandACORN/) . Yahoo. http://groups.yahoo.com/group/SCARandACORN/.
36. ↑ "Teen Circumcision" (http://groups.yahoo.com/group/teen_circ_/) . Yahoo http://groups.yahoo.com/group/teen_circ_/.
37. ↑ "The Cutting Club" (http://www.eurocirc.org/cuttingclub) . EuroCirc. http://www.eurocirc.org/cuttingclub.
38. ↑ "BeschnitteneGayBoys - Circumcised guys do it better!!" (http://groups.yahoo.com/group/BeschnitteneGayBoys/) . Yahoo http://groups.yahoo.com/group/BeschnitteneGayBoys/.
39. ↑ "Usenet Newsgroup: misc.kids" (http://groups.google.com/group/misc.kids/topics?pli=1) http://groups.google.com/group/misc.kids/topics?pli=1.
40. ↑ "Usenet Newsgroup: misc.kids.health" (http://groups.google.com/group/misc.kids.health/topics?lnk=srg) http://groups.google.com/group/misc.kids.health/topics?lnk=srg.
41. ↑ "Usenet Newsgroup: misc.kids.pregnancy" (http://groups.google.com/group/misc.kids.pregnancy/topics?lnk=srg) . http://groups.google.com/group/misc.kids.pregnancy/topics?lnk=srg.
42. ↑ "Tara Klamp" (http://www.taraklamp.com/) . Tara Klamp. http://www.taraklamp.com/. Retrieved 2011-03-06.
43. ↑ "Find Supplies" (http://www.findsupplies.com/) . http://www.findsupplies.com/.
44. ↑ "Smart Klamp" (http://www.smartklamp.com/) . http://www.smartklamp.com/.
45. ↑ "Weihai Zhenxi Medical" (http://www.zhenxi-korea.com/) . http://www.zhenxi-korea.com/.
46. ↑ "Circ-Ring International" (http://www.zhenxi-europe.com/) . http://www.zhenxi-europe.com/.
47. ↑ "Cutting Ring" (http://www.cutting-ring.com/) . http://www.cutting-ring.com/.
48. ↑ "..." (http://gaja79.com/link/fow-mh1004.html) . http://gaja79.com/link/fow-mh1004.html.
49. ↑ Morris, Brian. "Circumcision Humor" (http://www.circinfo.net/circumcision_humor.html) . http://www.circinfo.net/circumcision_humor.html. Retrieved 2012-04-22. Archive (2012-04-21): http://circleaks.org/images/5/5a/Circinfo_humor.pdf
50. ↑ Morris, Brian J. (2010). "Anti - Circumcision Lobby Groups" (http://www.circinfo.net/anti_circumcision_lobby_groups.html) . circinfo.net. http://www.circinfo.net/anti_circumcision_lobby_groups.html. Retrieved 2011-03-09. Archive: File:B.Morris. Anti-Circ Lobby Groups.pdf
51. ↑ A-13. Khan MM. Foreskin fetishism and its relation to ego pathology in a male homosexual. Int J Psychoanal 1965; 46: 64-80. http://www.cirp.org/library/khan/
52. ↑ Waskett, Jake H.. "User:Jakew" (http://en.wikipedia.org/wiki/User:Jakew) . Wikipedia. http://en.wikipedia.org/wiki/User:Jakew. Retrieved 2011-03-08. Archive (2011-05-13): http://www.circleaks.org/index.php?title=File:En.wikipedia.org-wiki-User-Jakew.pdf
53. ↑ "Fetish" (http://dictionary.reference.com/browse/fetish) . Dictionary.com. http://dictionary.reference.com/browse/fetish. Retrieved 2012-04-27.
54. ↑ Banerjee J, Klausner JD, Halperin DT, *et al.* (March 2011). "Circumcision denialism unfounded and unscientific". *Am J Prev Med* **40** (3): e11–2. doi:10.1016/j.amepre.2010.12.005 (http://dx.doi.org/10.1016%2Fj.amepre.2010.12.005) . PMID 21335254 (http://www.ncbi.nlm.nih.gov/pubmed/21335254) .
55. ↑ Morris, Brian J., Chris Eley (2011-08). "Male Circumcision: An Appraisal of Current Instrumentation" (http://www.intechopen.com/articles/show/title/male-circumcision-an-appraisal-of-current-instrumentation) . *InTech*: 1-40. http://www.intechopen.com/articles/show/title/male-circumcision-an-appraisal-of-current-instrumentation. Retrieved 2011-09-17.
56. ↑ "Should boys be circumcised?" (http://www.opposingviews.com/questions/should-boys-be-circumcised/comments) . Opposing Views. 2008-08-13. http://www.opposingviews.com/questions/should-boys-be-circumcised/comments. Retrieved 2011-03-07. Archive: File:Should Boys be Circumcised.pdf
57. ↑ BJOG: An International Journal of Obstetrics and Gynaecology (vol 109, p 1089) http://www.newscientist.com/article/dn2837-female-circumcision-does-not-reduce-sexual-activity.html
58. ↑ Pleasure and Orgasm in Women with Female Genital Mutilation/Cutting (FGM/C). 1: J Sex Med. 2007 Nov;4(6):1666-78. http://www.ncbi.nlm.nih.gov/pubmed/17970975
59. ↑ Email from Brian Morris, submitted by *Anonymous*
60. ↑ Circleaks user creation log, 00:08 March 7th 2011 http://circleaks.org/index.php?title=Special%3ALog&type=newusers&user=Brianm&page=&year=&month=-1
61. ↑ Circleaks history log for Brian J. Morris, 00:15 March 7th 2011 http://circleaks.org/index.php?title=Brian_J._Morris&curid=28&diff=3112&oldid=2363

62. ↑ Circleaks history log for Brian J. Morris, 00:19 March 7th 2011 http://circleaks.org/index.php?title=Brian_J._Morris&curid=28&diff=3113&oldid=3112
63. ↑ Circleaks history log for Brian J. Morris, 00:24 March 7th 2011 http://circleaks.org/index.php?title=Brian_J._Morris&curid=28&diff=3114&oldid=3113
64. ↑ Circleaks history log for Brian J. Morris, 00:29 March 7th 2011 http://circleaks.org/index.php?title=Brian_J._Morris&curid=28&diff=3116&oldid=3114
65. ↑ Circleaks history log for Brian J. Morris, 00:29 March 7th 2011 http://circleaks.org/index.php?title=Brian_J._Morris&curid=28&diff=3117&oldid=3116
66. ↑ Circleaks history log for Brian J. Morris, 00:30 March 7th 2011 http://circleaks.org/index.php?title=Brian_J._Morris&curid=28&diff=3118&oldid=3117
67. ↑ Circleaks history log for Brian J. Morris, 00:31 March 7th 2011 http://circleaks.org/index.php?title=Special%3ALog&type=protect&user=&page=Brian+J.+Morris&year=&month=-1
68. ↑ Circleaks history log for User talk:Briamm, 19:02 March 7th 2011 http://circleaks.org/index.php?title=User_talk:Briamm
69. ↑ "IP Tracing and IP Tracking" (http://www.ip-adress.com/ip_tracer/129.78.32.22). IP-address.com. http://www.ip-adress.com/ip_tracer/129.78.32.22. Retrieved 2011-04-17.
70. ↑ Circleaks user creation log, 00:08 March 7th 2011 http://circleaks.org/index.php?title=Special%3ALog&type=newusers&user=Briamm&page=&year=&month=-1
71. ↑ Circleaks history log for Brian J. Morris, 00:19 March 7th 2011 http://circleaks.org/index.php?title=Brian_J._Morris&curid=28&diff=3113&oldid=3112
72. ↑ Campbell, Hank (2011-03-07). "Like AIDS? Then You Will Love The Anti-Circumcision Movement In San Francisco" (http://www.science20.com/cool-links/aids_then_you_will_love_anticircumcision_movement_san_francisco-76949). science20. http://www.science20.com/cool-links/aids_then_you_will_love_anticircumcision_movement_san_francisco-76949. Retrieved 2011-03-09. Archive: File:AIDS & Frisco.pdf

Mandated Report VA to CDC - Matteoli

Dr. Tom Freiden NY City Health under Bloomberg
Before becoming Director CDC

N.Y. / Region

New York City Plans to Promote Circumcision to Reduce Spread of AIDS

New York City's Department of Health and Mental Hygiene is planning a campaign to encourage men at high risk of AIDS to get circumcised in light of the World Health Organization's endorsement of the procedure as an effective way to prevent the disease.

While the Centers for Disease Control and Prevention in Atlanta is just beginning to convene meetings and design studies to help it formulate a national policy, New York City is moving ahead on its own.

In the United States, "New York City remains the epicenter of the AIDS epidemic," Dr. Thomas R. Frieden, the city's health commissioner, said in an interview. Referring to H.I.V., he said, "In some subpopulations, you have 10 to 20 percent prevalence rates, just as they do in parts of Africa."

His department has started asking some community groups and gay rights organizations to discuss circumcision with their members, and has asked the Health and Hospitals Corporation, which runs city hospitals and clinics, to perform the procedure at no charge for men without health insurance.

A spokeswoman for the corporation said it was "having conversations" with the health department but had not reached a decision.

"As you know, the research on this is pretty recent," the spokeswoman, Ana Marengo, said.

In three recent clinical trials in Africa, circumcision was shown to lower a man's risk of contracting the virus from heterosexual sex by about 60 percent. On March [illegible], the World Health Organization officially recommended that countries adopt the procedure as part of their AIDS prevention plans.

No spontaneous outcry for circumcision has arisen in New York, Dr. Frieden conceded.

"This is not something that has a lot of buzz," he said.

But he added that even 1,000 circumcisions in the right subgroups might slow the spread of AIDS.

For example, in Manhattan, [illegible] percent of all black men between 40 and 50 are infected with the virus that causes AIDS. About [illegible] percent of all gay men in the city are infected, and the rate rises to as high as 25 percent in the Chelsea neighborhood.

Dr. Frieden said black, Hispanic and foreign-born men were less likely to be circumcised than white Americans, and the percentage is smaller among men with lower incomes.

(About 65 percent of all male babies in the United States are circumcised, according to the National Center for Health Statistics, compared with about 30 percent of men worldwide, by W.H.O. estimates.)

Among men seeking treatment at the city's clinics for sexually transmitted diseases — another risk group for AIDS infection because of genital sores — a large proportion are uncircumcised, Dr. Frieden said.

There are clear limitations, however, on extrapolating data from Africa to New York.

The studies, done in Uganda, Kenya and South Africa, enrolled men who said they had sex with women, while New York's highest-risk groups are men who have sex with men, men who inject drugs and people who have sex with those men.

Nonetheless, Dr. Frieden said, it is logical to assume that circumcision would offer protection in some types of gay sex.

A man's risk from performing penetrative anal sex is about the same as his risk from vaginal sex, Dr. Frieden said, so circumcision would presumably confer the same protection as it did in the African trials.

The risk from receptive anal sex is five times higher, he said, and circumcision would obviously not protect those men. Oral sex is much less risky.

Also, cutting down infections among bisexual men — some of whom do not admit to female partners that they participate in gay sex — would protect women, he said.

Dr. Frieden said he thought health insurance companies might agree to pay for preventive circumcisions since they already covered them for infections and urinary blockage. City hospitals also offer the operation in those cases, Ms. Marengo said.

Peter Staley, a longtime AIDS activist and co-founder of ACT-UP New York, the Treatment Action Group and AIDSmeds.com, said he was "intrigued" by the idea of offering circumcisions but worried because those in the studies supporting it bore little relation to New York's risk groups.

"Should we proceed when we don't have hard data yet on the population here?" he asked. "On the other hand, if we wait the three years it would take to answer that question, how many will be infected in the meantime?"

Also, after reading many postings on gay Web sites about the Africa trials, he said he feared a backlash among black and Hispanic men to endorsements of circumcision from white public health officials or gay activists.

"I'm white, Frieden's white," he said. "It's going to sound like white guys telling black and Hispanic guys to do something that would affect their manhood."

Tokes Osubu, executive director of Gay Men of African Descent, a 20-year-old gay rights organization, agreed.

"There will always be conspiracy theorists," he said. "That's par for the course."

He also said he thought circumcision was "not the answer to our problems" and doubted that it would lower infection rates.

Many black men who have sex with men, he said, already face discrimination, stigma and an inability to talk about their sex lives with family members and sometimes even with doctors.

"No amount of circumcision is going to change that," he said.

Eric Bernas, manager of information and counseling for the Asian and Pacific Islander Coalition on H.I.V./AIDS, said his organization wanted to see studies done in the United States and among gay men before taking a position on the issue.

Circumcision is not common among Asian men, except those from Muslim countries and the Philippines, Mr. Bernas said, "and there might be cultural sensitivities around it."

More Articles in New York Region »

Tom Frieden

From Wikipedia, the free encyclopedia

Thomas R. Frieden has been since 2009 the Director of the U.S. Centers for Disease Control and Prevention (CDC) and Acting Administrator of the Agency for Toxic Substances and Disease Registry (ATSDR). He was appointed by President Barack Obama.[1] He served as Commissioner of the New York City Department of Health and Mental Hygiene from 2002 -09.

Tom Frieden

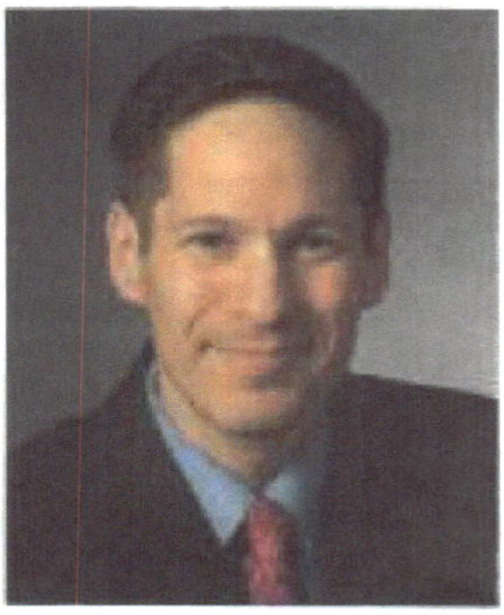

16th Director of the Centers for Disease Control and Prevention

Incumbent	
Assumed office June 8, 2009	
President	Barack Obama
Preceded by	Julie Gerberding
New York City Health Commissioner	
In office 2002–2009	
Mayor	Michael Bloomberg
Personal details	
Born	1960 (age 54–55)
Political party	Democratic
Education	Oberlin College Columbia University

Contents

Education

Frieden graduated from Oberlin College (BA, 1982), Columbia University College of Physicians and Surgeons (MD, 1986) and Columbia University Mailman School of Public Health (MPH, 1985). He completed training in internal medicine at Columbia-Presbyterian Medical Center and sub-specialty training in infectious diseases at Yale University.

Early career

Frieden's work on tuberculosis in New York fostered public awareness and helped improve public funding (city, state and federal) for TB control.[2][3] The epidemic was controlled rapidly, reducing overall incidence by nearly half and cutting multidrug-resistant tuberculosis by 80%.[4] The city's program became a model for tuberculosis control.[5][6]

From 1996 to 2002, Frieden was based in India, assisting with national tuberculosis control efforts. As a medical officer for the World Health Organization on loan from the CDC, he helped the government of India implement the Revised National Tuberculosis Control Program (RNTCP).[7][8][9][10] The 2008 RNTCP status report estimates the nationwide program resulted in 8 million treatments and 1.4 million saved lives.[11] While in India, Frieden worked to establish a network of Indian physicians to help India's state and local governments implement the program[12] and helped the Tuberculosis Research Center in Chennai, India, establish a program to monitor the impact of tuberculosis control services.[13][14]

Impact

Frieden served as head of the New York City DOHMH from 2002–2009. The agency employs more than 6,000 people[15] with an annual budget of $1.5 billion.[16][17]

Ebola outbreak

Frieden has been a prominent figure in the US and global response to the West African outbreak of Ebola. In a Congressional hearing on 10/16/2014, Frieden was questioned for his handling of the Ebola crisis following the spread of the disease to two nurses from the original patient in the US.[18] The previous day, the response of the CDC to the crisis led Rep. Tom Marino (R-PA) to call for Frieden's resignation.[19]

Tobacco control

Upon his appointment as Health Commissioner in January 2002, Frieden made tobacco control a priority [20] resulting in a rapid decline[21] after a decade of no change in smoking rates. Frieden established a system to monitor the city's smoking rate, and worked with New York City Mayor Michael R. Bloomberg to increase tobacco taxes,[22] ban smoking from workplaces including restaurants and bars, and run aggressive anti-tobacco ads and help smokers quit.[23] The program reduced smoking prevalence among New York City adults from 21.6% in 2002 to 16.9% in 2007 – a change that represents 300,000 fewer smokers and could prevent 100,000 premature deaths in future years.[21][24] Smoking prevalence among New York City teens declined even more sharply, from 17.6% in 2001 to 8.5% in 2007, and is now less than half the national rate.[25] The workplace smoking ban prompted spirited debate before it was passed by the New York City Council and signed into law by Mayor Bloomberg.[26] Over time, the measure has gained broad acceptance by the public and business community in New York City.[27][28] New York City's 2003 workplace smoking ban followed that of California in 1994. Frieden supports increased cigarette taxes as a means of forcing smokers to quit, saying "tobacco taxes are the most effective way to reduce tobacco use."[29] He supported the 62-cent Federal tax on each cigarette pack sol(in the United States, introduced in April 2009.[30] One side-effect of the increased taxes on tobacco in New York is a large increase in cigarette smuggling into the state from nearby states, such as Virginia, which has a much lower tobacco tax. The Tax Foundation estimates that "60.9% of cigarettes sold in Ne York State are smuggled in from other states".[31] In addition, some New Yorkers have begun to make their own cigarettes, and tobacco trucks have been hijacked. A 2009 Justice Department study found tha "The incentive to profit by evading payment of taxes rises with each tax rate hike imposed by federal, state, and local governments".[32]

Take Care New York

Frieden also introduced Take Care New York, the city's first comprehensive health policy. This program targeted ten leading causes of preventable illness and death for concerted public and personal action.[33][34] By 2006, New York City had made measurable progress in eight of the ten priority areas.[35]

HIV/AIDS

As Health Commissioner, Frieden sought to fight HIV/AIDS with public health principles used successfully to control other communicable diseases.[36] The most controversial aspect of this strategy was a proposal to eliminate separate written consent for HIV testing. He believes the measure would encourage physicians to offer HIV tests during routine medical care,[37] as the CDC recommends.[38] Some community and civil liberties advocates fought this legislation arguing it would undermine patient rights and lead eventually to forced HIV testing.[39][40] In 2010, New York State passed a new law that eased the requirement for separate written consent in some circumstances.[41] On 14 February 2007, the NYCDHMH introduced the NYC Condom,[42][43] prompting Catholic League president Bill Donohue to respond, "What's next? The city's own brand of clean syringes?"[44] More than 36 million condoms were given away by the program in 2007.[45]

Diabetes

Frieden worked to raise awareness about diabetes in New York City, particularly among pregnant women,[46] and established an involuntary, non-disclosed hemoglobin A1C diabetes registry that tracks patients' blood sugar control over several months and report that information to treating physicians in an effort to help them provide better care.[47][48]

The New York City Board of Health's decision to require laboratories to report A1C test results has generated a heated debate among civil libertarians, who view it as a violation of medical privacy and an intrusion into the doctor-patient relationship. Although patients may elect not to receive information fron the program, there is no provision enabling patients to opt out of having their glycemic control data entered in the database.[49][50] NPOV

Food policies

To combat cardiovascular disease, New York City has adopted regulations since 2006 to eliminate trans fat from all restaurants.[51][52][53] The restaurant industry and its political allies condemned the trans-fat measure as an assault on liberty by an overzealous "nanny state"[54][55] and the measure has inspired similar laws in several US cities and the state of California.[56] The Health Department also required chain restaurants to post calorie information to raise consumer awareness of fast food's caloric impact. The measure requires chains with 15 or more outlets to post calorie counts on menus and menu boards. It has prompted two lawsuits by the New York State Restaurant Association. In the first, New York State Restaurant Association v. New York City Board of Health, a U.S. District Court judge ruled that federal law pre-empted New York City's action and overturned it.[57] The NYC Board of Health then repealed and re-enacted the measure.[58] Most chains now post calorie information in their New York City outlets.[59][60] Section 4205 of the Patient Protection and Affordable Care Act, signed into law in 2010, requires menu labeling nationally, for restaurant chains, disclosing on the menu boards, calories, total calories, calories from fat, amounts of fat and saturated fat, cholesterol, sodium, total and complex carbohydrates, sugars, dietary fiber, and protein.[61]

Epidemiology

During Frieden's tenure as Commissioner, the Health Department expanded the collection and use of epidemiological data, launching an annual Community Health Survey[62] and the nation's first community-based Health and Nutrition Examination Survey.[63][64]

Electronic health records

To improve quality and efficiency of medical care, the agency launched a large community-based electronic health records project to improve preventive care for more than one million at-risk New Yorkers.[65]

Director of CDC and Administrator of ATSDR

On May 15, 2009 the White House and the Department of Health and Human Services named Dr. Frieden the 16th director of Centers for Disease Control and Prevention (CDC) and administrator of the Agency for Toxic Substances and Disease Registry (ATSDR); he assumed his position on June 8, 2009 from the acting head, Dr. Richard E. Besser.[66]

On announcing Frieden's appointment, President Obama said, "America relies on a strong public health system and the work at the Centers for Disease Control and Prevention is critical to our mission to preserve and protect the health and safety of our citizens".[67] Frieden had previously worked for the CDC from 1990 to 2002 as an Epidemic Intelligence Service Officer in New York City and then as part of CDC's tuberculosis control program.

Bloomberg philanthropies

Frieden also served as health advisor to New York City Mayor Bloomberg, supporting the Bloomberg Initiative to reduce tobacco use.[67]

Publications

- Frieden TR, Sterling T, Pablos-Mendez A, Kilburn JO, Cauthen GM, Dooley SW (February 1993). "The emergence of drug-resistant tuberculosis in New York City". *New England Journal of Medicine* **328** (8): 521–26. doi:10.1056/NEJM199302253280801 (https://dx.doi.org/10.1056%2FNEJM199302253280801). PMID 8381207 (https://www.ncbi.nlm.nih.gov/pubmed/8381207).
- Frieden TR, Fujiwara PI, Washko RM, Hamburg MA (July 1995). "Tuberculosis in New York City – Turning the Tide". *New England Journal of Medicine* **333** (4): 229–33. doi:10.1056/NEJM199507273330406 (https://dx.doi.org/10.1056%2FNEJM199507273330406). PMID 7791840 (https://www.ncbi.nlm.nih.gov/pubmed/7791840).
- Ounces of Prevention – The Public Policy Case for Taxes on Sugared Beverages (http://content.nejm.org/cgi/content/full/360/18/1805)

Awards

- Honorary degree, Doctor of Public Service, Tufts University (2011)
- Honorary degree, Doctor of Science, Oglethorpe University (2015)

References

1. "President Obama Appoints Dr. Thomas Frieden as CDC Director" (http://www.whitehouse.gov/the_press_office/President-Obama-Appoints-Dr-Thomas-Frieden-as-CDC-Director/). May 15, 2009.
2. Lobato MN, Wang YC, Becerra JE, Simone PM, Castro KG (2006). "Improved Program Activities Are Associated with Decreasing Tuberculosis Incidence in the United States" (https://www.ncbi.nlm.nih.gov/pmc/articles/PMC1525263). *Public Health Reports* **121** (2): 108–15. PMC 1525263 (https://www.ncbi.nlm.nih.gov/pmc/articles/PMC1525263). PMID 16528941 (https://www.ncbi.nlm.nih.gov/pubmed/16528941).
3. Leff DR, Leff AR (November 1, 1997). "Tuberculosis control policies in major metropolitan health departments in the United States. VI. Standard of practice in 1996" (http://ajrccm.atsjournals.org/cgi/pmidlookup?view=long&pmid=9372665). *American Journal of Respiratory and Critical Care Medicine* **156** (5): 1487–94. doi:10.1164/ajrccm.156.5.9704105 (https://dx.doi.org/10.1164%2Fajrccm.156.5.9704105). PMID 9372665 (https://www.ncbi.nlm.nih.gov/pubmed/9372665).
4. *TB Annual Summary, 2006* (http://www.nyc.gov/html/doh/downloads/pdf/tb/tb2006.pdf) (PDF). New York: New York City Department of Health and Mental Hygiene. 2008.
5. World Health Organization Tuberculosis Programme (1995). "New York City's Success Story". *Stop TB at th Source*. Geneva: World Health Organization. ISBN 978-0-11-951529-9. OCLC 181876135 (https://www.worldcat.org/oclc/181876135).
6. Steinhauer, Jennifer (February 14, 2004). "Gladly Taking The Blame For Health In the City" (http://www.nytimes.com/2004/02/14/nyregion/gladly-taking-the-blame-for-health-in-the-city.html). *The New York Times*. Retrieved July 8, 2009.

7. Drazen JM (October 2002). "A milestone in tuberculosis control". *New England Journal of Medicine* **347** (18): 1444. doi:10.1056/NEJMe020135 (https://dx.doi.org/10.1056%2FNEJMe020135). PMID 12409549 (https://www.ncbi.nlm.nih.gov/pubmed/12409549).
8. Khatri GR, Frieden TR (October 2002). "Controlling tuberculosis in India". *New England Journal of Medicine* **347** (18): 1420–25. doi:10.1056/NEJMsa020098 (https://dx.doi.org/10.1056%2FNEJMsa020098). PMID 12409545 (https://www.ncbi.nlm.nih.gov/pubmed/12409545).
9. Udwadia ZF, Pinto LM (2007). "Review series: the politics of TB: the politics, economics and impact of directly observed treatment (DOT) in India". *Chronic Respiratory Disease* 4 (2): 101–06. doi:10.1177/1479972307707929 (https://dx.doi.org/10.1177%2F1479972307707929). PMID 17621578 (https://www.ncbi.nlm.nih.gov/pubmed/17621578).
10. Chauhan LS, Tonsing J (2005). "Revised national TB control programme in India". *Tuberculosis* **85** (5–6): 271–76. doi:10.1016/j.tube.2005.08.003 (https://dx.doi.org/10.1016%2Fj.tube.2005.08.003). PMID 16253562 (https://www.ncbi.nlm.nih.gov/pubmed/16253562).
11. *TB India 2008: RNTCP Status Report: I am Stopping TB* (http://www.tbcindia.org/pdfs/TB%20India%202010.pdf) (PDF). New Delhi: Ministry of Health and Family Welfare. March 2008. p. 3. ISBN 81-902652-3-7. Retrieved July 8, 2009.
12. Frieden TR, Khatri GR (September 2003). "Impact of national consultants on successful expansion of effective tuberculosis control in India" (http://openurl.ingenta.com/content/nlm?genre=article&issn=1027-3719&volume=7&issue=9&spage=837&aulast=Frieden). *The International Journal of Tuberculosis and Lung Disease* 7 (9): 837–41. PMID 12971666 (https://www.ncbi.nlm.nih.gov/pubmed/12971666).
13. Subramani R, Radhakrishna S, Frieden TR et al. (August 2008). "Rapid decline in prevalence of pulmonary tuberculosis after DOTS implementation in a rural area of South India" (http://openurl.ingenta.com/content/nlm?genre=article&issn=1027-3719&volume=12&issue=8&spage=916&aulast=Subramani). *The International Journal of Tuberculosis and Lung Disease* **12** (8): 916–20. PMID 18647451 (https://www.ncbi.nlm.nih.gov/pubmed/18647451).
14. Narayanan PR, Garg R, Santha T, Kumaran PP (2003). "Shifting the focus of tuberculosis research in India". *Tuberculosis* **83** (1–3): 135–42. doi:10.1016/S1472-9792(02)00068-9 (https://dx.doi.org/10.1016%2FS1472-9792%2802%2900068-9). PMID 12758203 (https://www.ncbi.nlm.nih.gov/pubmed/12758203).
15. *Public Health in New York City, 2004–06* (http://www.nyc.gov/html/doh/downloads/pdf/public/triennial_report.pdf) (PDF). New York City Department of Health and Mental Hygiene. p. 3. Retrieved July 8, 2009.
16. *Public Health in New York City, 2004–06* (http://www.nyc.gov/html/doh/downloads/pdf/public/triennial_report.pdf) (PDF). New York City Department of Health and Mental Hygiene. p. 61. Retrieved July 8, 2009.
17. Frieden TR, Bassett MT, Thorpe LE, Farley TA (October 2008). "Public health in New York City, 2002–2007: confronting epidemics of the modern era". *International Journal of Epidemiology* **37** (5): 966–77. doi:10.1093/ije/dyn108 (https://dx.doi.org/10.1093%2Fije%2Fdyn108). PMID 18540026 (https://www.ncbi.nlm.nih.gov/pubmed/18540026).
18. Congress Scrutinizes Handling of Ebola Cases in Texas (http://www.nytimes.com/2014/10/17/us/ebola-dallas-texas-presbyterian-hospital-apology.html), nytimes.com, October 17, 2014.
19. "White House scrambles to ease concerns over Ebola, lawmakers demand changes: CDC" (http://www.foxnews.com/politics/2014/10/15/white-house-scrambles-to-ease-concerns-over-ebola-lawmakers-demand-changes/?utm_source=feedburner&utm_medium=feed&utm_campaign=Feed%3A+foxnews%2Fpolitics+(Internal+-+Politics+-+Text)). Fox News. October 15, 2014. Retrieved October 15, 2014.
20. Steinhauer, Jennifer (February 15, 2002). "Commissioner Calls Smoking Public Health Enemy No. 1 and Asks Drug Firms for Ammunition" (http://www.nytimes.com/2002/02/15/nyregion/commissioner-calls-smoking-public-health-enemy-no-1-asks-drug-firms-for.html). *The New York Times*. Retrieved July 8, 2009.
21. Centers for Disease Control and Prevention (CDC) (June 2007). "Decline in smoking prevalence – New York City, 2002–2006" (http://www.cdc.gov/mmwr/preview/mmwrhtml/mm5624a4.htm). *Morbidity and Mortality Weekly Report* **56** (24): 604–08. PMID 17585290 (https://www.ncbi.nlm.nih.gov/pubmed/17585290).
22. Altman, Alex (June 6, 2008). "When Are Cigarette Taxes Too High?" (http://www.time.com/time/nation/article/0,8599,1812426,00.html). *Time*. Retrieved July 8, 2009.

23. Frieden TR, Mostashari F, Kerker BD, Miller N, Hajat A, Frankel M (June 2005). "Adult Tobacco Use Levels After Intensive Tobacco Control Measures: New York City, 2002 –2003" (https://www.ncbi.nlm.nih.gov/pmc/articles/PMC1449302). *American Journal of Public Health* **95** (6): 1016–23. doi:10.2105/AJPH.2004.058164 (https://dx.doi.org/10.2105%2FAJPH.2004.058164). PMC 1449302 (https://www.ncbi.nlm.nih.gov/pmc/articles/PMC1449302). PMID 15914827 (https://www.ncbi.nlm.nih.gov/pubmed/15914827).
24. "Michael Bloomberg and Bill Gates Join to Combat Global Tobacco Epidemic" (http://www.gatesfoundation.org/press-releases/Pages/bloomberg-gates-tobacco-initiative-080723.aspx) (Press release). Bill & Melinda Gates Foundation. July 23, 2008. Retrieved July 8, 2009.
25. The Lancet (January 2008). "New York City's bold antitobacco programme". *Lancet* **371** (9607): 90. doi:10.1016/S0140-6736(08)60078-1 (https://dx.doi.org/10.1016%2FS0140-6736%2808%2960078-1). PMID 18191665 (https://www.ncbi.nlm.nih.gov/pubmed/18191665).
26. Chang C, Leighton J, Mostashari F, McCord C, Frieden TR (August 2004). "The New York City Smoke-Free Air Act: second-hand smoke as a worker health and safety issue". *American Journal of Industrial Medicine* **46** (2): 188–95. doi:10.1002/ajim.20030 (https://dx.doi.org/10.1002%2Fajim.20030). PMID 15273972 (https://www.ncbi.nlm.nih.gov/pubmed/15273972).
27. Cooper, Michael (October 23, 2003). "Poll Finds Smoking Ban Popular" (http://www.nytimes.com/2003/10/23/nyregion/metro-briefing-new-york-manhattan-poll-finds-smoking-ban-popular.html). *The New York Times*. Retrieved 8 July 2009.
28. Rutenberg, Jim; Lily Koppel (February 6, 2005). "In Barrooms, Smoking Ban Is Less Reviled" (http://www.nytimes.com/2005/02/06/nyregion/06xsmoke.html). *The New York Times*. Retrieved July 8, 2009.
29. Altman, Alex (June 6, 2008). "When Are Cigarette Taxes Too High?" (http://www.time.com/time/nation/article/0,8599,1812426,00.html). *Time*. Retrieved August 11, 2010.
30. Jonsson, Patrik (November 17, 2009). "Federal and state governments look to smokers for more tax revenue: Though they hit poor Americans hardest, stiff taxes on tobacco can reduce healthcare costs by billions" (http://www.csmonitor.com/USA/2009/0411/p90s01-usgn.html). *Christian Science Monitor*. Retrieved August 8, 2010.
31. Smith, Aaron (January 10, 2013). "60% of cigarettes sold in New York are smuggled: report" (http://money.cnn.com/2013/01/10/news/companies/cigarette-tax-new-york/). *CNN Money*. Retrieved December 4, 2014.
32. Mathias, Christopher (April 3, 2014). "Inside New York City's Dangerous, Multimillion-Dollar Cigarette Black Market" (http://www.huffingtonpost.com/2014/04/03/cigarette-smuggling-new-york-_n_5041823.html). *Huffington Post*. Retrieved December 4, 2014.
33. "Cause of Death or Illness, New York City, 2002, and Amenability to Intervention". *Take Care New York. A Policy for a Healthier New York City* (http://www.nyc.gov/html/doh/downloads/pdf/tcny/tcny-policy.pdf) (PDF). New York City Department of Health and Mental Hygiene. March 2004. pp. 57–61. Retrieved July 9, 2009.
34. Pérez-Peña, Richard (March 24, 2004). "City sets goals for the health of New Yorker" (http://www.nytimes.com/2004/03/24/nyregion/city-sets-goals-for-the-health-of-new-yorkers.html). *The New York Times*. Retrieved July 8, 2009.
35. *Take Care New York: A Policy for a Healthier New York City (Third Year Progress Report)* (http://www.nyc.gov/html/doh/downloads/pdf/tcny/tcny-report-2007.pdf) (PDF). New York City Department of Health and Mental Hygiene. August 2007. p. 2. Retrieved July 9, 2009.
36. Frieden TR, Das-Douglas M, Kellerman SE, Henning KJ (December 2005). "Applying public health principles to the HIV epidemic". *New England Journal of Medicine* **353** (22): 2397–402. doi:10.1056/NEJMsb053133 (https://dx.doi.org/10.1056%2FNEJMsb053133). PMID 16319391 (https://www.ncbi.nlm.nih.gov/pubmed/16319391).
37. Mandavilli, A (April 2006). "Profile: Thomas Frieden". *Nature Medicine* **12** (4): 378. doi:10.1038/nm0406-378 (https://dx.doi.org/10.1038%2Fnm0406-378). PMID 16598275 (https://www.ncbi.nlm.nih.gov/pubmed/16598275).
38. Branson BM, Handsfield HH, Lampe MA et al. (September 2006). "Revised recommendations for HIV testin of adults, adolescents, and pregnant women in health-care settings" (http://www.cdc.gov/mmwr/preview/mmwrhtml/rr5514a1.htm). *Morbidity and Mortality Weekly Report* **55** (RR–14): 1–17; quiz CE1–4. PMID 16988643 (https://www.ncbi.nlm.nih.gov/pubmed/16988643).

39. Chan, Sewell (December 25, 2006). "Rifts Emerge on Push to End Written Consent for H.I.V.Tests" (http://www.nytimes.com/2006/12/25/nyregion/25hiv.html). *The New York Times*. Retrieved July 9, 2009.
40. Fairchild AL, Alkon A (August 2007). "Back to the future? Diabetes, HIV, and the boundaries of public health". *Journal of Health Politics, Policy and Law* **32** (4): 561–93. doi:10.1215/03616878-2007-017 (https://dx.doi.org/10.1215%2F03616878-2007-017). PMID 17639012 (https://www.ncbi.nlm.nih.gov/pubmed/17639012).
41. "HIV Testing Is Now a Routine Part of Health Care in New York" (http://www.nyc.gov/html/doh/html/pr2010/pr043-10.shtml) (Press release). New York City Department of Health and Mental Hygiene. September 1, 2010. Retrieved February 8, 2011.
42. Chan, Sewell (February 15, 2007). "A New Condom in Town, This One Named 'NYC' " (http://www.nytimes.com/2007/02/15/nyregion/15condom.html). *The New York Times*. Retrieved July 8, 2009.
43. "Health department launches the nation's first official city condom" (http://www.nyc.gov/html/doh/html/pr2007/pr008-07.shtml) (Press release). New York City Department of Health and Mental Hygiene. February 14, 2007. Retrieved July 8, 2009.
44. "NYC-Branded Condoms Are a Big Apple First" (http://gothamist.com/2007/02/15/condoms_1.php). *Gothamist*. Retrieved October 13, 2014.
45. "Health department releases new NYC Condom wrapper" (http://www.nyc.gov/html/doh/html/pr2008/pr011-08.shtml) (Press release). New York City Department of Health and Mental Hygiene. February 13, 2008. Retrieved July 8, 2009.
46. Kleinfield, N.R. (February 22, 2006). "City to Warn New Mothers of Diabetes Risk" (http://www.nytimes.com/2006/02/22/nyregion/nyregionspecial5/22diabetes.html). *The New York Times*. Retrieved July 9, 2009.
47. Steinbrook R (February 2006). "Facing the diabetes epidemic – mandatory reporting of glycosylated hemoglobin values in New York City". *New England Journal of Medicine* **354** (6): 545–48. doi:10.1056/NEJMp068008 (https://dx.doi.org/10.1056%2FNEJMp068008). PMID 16467539 (https://www.ncbi.nlm.nih.gov/pubmed/16467539).
48. "The New York City A1C Registry" (http://home2.nyc.gov/html/doh/html/diabetes/diabetes-nycar.shtml). New York City Department of Health and Mental Hygiene. Retrieved July 9, 2009.
49. Goldman J, Kinnear S, Chung J, Rothman DJ. "New York City's Initiatives on Diabetes and HIV/AIDS: Implications for Patient Care, Public Health, and Medical Professionalism" (https://www.ncbi.nlm.nih.gov/pmc/articles/PMC2374815). *American Journal of Public Health* **98** (5): 807–13. doi:10.2105/AJPH.2007.121152 (https://dx.doi.org/10.2105%2FAJPH.2007.121152). PMC 2374815 (https://www.ncbi.nlm.nih.gov/pmc/articles/PMC2374815). PMID 18381989 (https://www.ncbi.nlm.nih.gov/pubmed/18381989). Retrieved October 16, 2014.
50. Frieden TR (September 2008). "New York City's Diabetes Reporting System Helps Patients And Physicians" (https://www.ncbi.nlm.nih.gov/pmc/articles/PMC2509589). *American Journal of Public Health* **98** (9): 1543–44; author reply 1544. doi:10.2105/AJPH.2008.142026 (https://dx.doi.org/10.2105%2FAJPH.2008.142026). PMC 2509589 (https://www.ncbi.nlm.nih.gov/pmc/articles/PMC2509589). PMID 18633070 (https://www.ncbi.nlm.nih.gov/pubmed/18633070).
51. "Healthy Heart – Avoid Trans Fat" (http://home2.nyc.gov/html/doh/html/cardio/cardio-transfat.shtml). New York City Department of Health and Mental Hygiene. Retrieved July 9, 2009.
52. Okie S (May 2007). "New York to trans fats: you're out!". *New England Journal of Medicine* **356** (20): 2017–21. doi:10.1056/NEJMp078058 (https://dx.doi.org/10.1056%2FNEJMp078058). PMID 17507699 (https://www.ncbi.nlm.nih.gov/pubmed/17507699).
53. "Calorie Posting" (http://nyc.gov/html/doh/html/cdp/cdp_pan-calorie.shtml). New York City Department of Health and Mental Hygiene. Retrieved July 9, 2009.
54. Lueck, Thomas J.; Kim Severson (December 6, 2006). "New York Bans Most Trans Fats in Restaurants" (http://www.nytimes.com/2006/12/06/nyregion/06fat.html). *The New York Times*. Retrieved July 9, 2009.
55. Halpern, Dan (December 17, 2006). "Dr. Do-Gooder" (http://nymag.com/health/features/25642). *New York*. Retrieved July 9, 2009.
56. Steinhauer, Jennifer (July 26, 2008). "California Bars Restaurant Use of Trans Fats" (http://www.nytimes.com/2008/07/26/us/26fats.html). *The New York Times*. Retrieved July 9, 2009.

57. Feuer, Alan (September 12, 2007). "Judge Throws Out New York Rule Requiring Restaurants to Post Calories" (http://www.nytimes.com/2007/09/12/nyregion/12calories.html). *The New York Times*. Retrieved July 9, 2009.
58. Rivera, Ray (October 25, 2007). "New York City Reintroduces Calorie Rule" (http://www.nytimes.com/2007/10/25/nyregion/25calories.html). *The New York Times*. Retrieved July 9, 2009.
59. Barron, James (July 19, 2008). "Restaurants That Lack Calorie Counts Now FaceFines" (http://www.nytimes.com/2008/07/19/nyregion/19calorie.html). *The New York Times*. Retrieved July 9, 2009.
60. Rabin, Roni Caryn (July 16, 2008). "New Yorkers try to swallow calorie sticker shock" (http://www.msnbc.msn.com/id/25464987). MSNBC. Retrieved July 9, 2009.
61. "Menu & Vending Machines Labeling Requirements" (http://www.fda.gov/Food/IngredientsPackagingLabeling/LabelingNutrition/ucm217762.htm). FDA. Retrieved October 16, 2014.
62. "Community Health Survey" (http://www.nyc.gov/html/doh/html/survey/survey.shtml). New York City Department of Health and Mental Hygiene. February 2009. Retrieved July 9, 2009.
63. "NYC HANES Datasets and Related Documentation" (http://www.nyc.gov/html/doh/html/hanes/datasets.shtml). New York City Department of Health and Mental Hygiene. Retrieved July 9, 2009.
64. Thorpe LE, Gwynn RC, Mandel-Ricci J et al. (July 2006). "Study Design and Participation Rates of the New York City Health and Nutrition Examination Survey, 2004" (http://www.cdc.gov/pcd/issues/2006/jul/05_0177.htm). *Preventing Chronic Disease* 3 (3): A94. PMC 1637802 (https://www.ncbi.nlm.nih.gov/pmc/articles/PMC1637802). PMID 16776895 (https://www.ncbi.nlm.nih.gov/pubmed/16776895).
65. "Primary Care Information Project" (http://www.nyc.gov/html/doh/html/pcip/pcip.shtml). New York City Department of Health and Mental Hygiene. Retrieved July 9, 2009.
66. Profile (http://www.foxbusiness.com/story/thomas-r-frieden-md-mph-begins-role-cdc-director-atsdr-administrator), foxbusiness.com; accessed October 16, 2014.
67. "President Obama Appoints Dr. Thomas Frieden as CDC Director" (http://www.whitehouse.gov/the_press_office/President-Obama-Appoints-Dr-Thomas-Frieden-as-CDC-Director/). The White House. May 15, 2009.

External links

- CDC Director Dr. Tom Frieden (http://www.cdc.gov/about/cdcdirector/)

Wikimedia Commons has media related to *Tom Frieden*.

Awards and achievements		
Preceded by **Neal L. Cohen**	**New York City Department of Health and Mental Hygiene Commissioner** 2002–2009	Succeeded by **Thomas A. Farley**
Preceded by **Monique Dixon** **Diana Reyes**	**NY1's New Yorker of the Year**	Succeeded by **Common Cents**

Retrieved from "https://en.wikipedia.org/w/index.php?title=Tom_Frieden&oldid=679102282"

Categories: 1960 births | Living people | American physicians | American Jews
| United States Department of Health and Human Services officials | Obama Administration personnel
| Commissioners in New York City | People in public health
| Columbia University Mailman School of Public Health alumni
| Columbia University College of Physicians and Surgeons alumni | Oberlin College alumni

- This page was last modified on 2 September 2015, at 13:12.
- Text is available under the Creative Commons Attribution-ShareAlike License; additional terms may apply. By using this site, you agree to the Terms of Use and Privacy Policy. Wikipedia® is a registered trademark of the Wikimedia Foundation, Inc., a non-profit organization.

The New York Times http://nyti.ms/WDKQ0e

N.Y. / REGION

$1.1 Billion in Thanks From Bloomberg to Johns Hopkins

By MICHAEL BARBARO JAN. 26, 2013

BALTIMORE — He arrived on campus a middling high school student from Medford, Mass., who had settled for C's and had confined his ambitions to the math club.

But by the time Michael R. Bloomberg left Johns Hopkins University, with a smattering of A's and a lust for leadership, he was a social and political star — the president of his fraternity, his senior class and the council overseeing Greek life. "An all-around big man on campus," as he puts it.

His gratitude toward the university, starting with a $5 donation the year after he graduated, has since taken on a supersize, Bloombergian scale.

On Sunday, as he makes a $350 million gift to his alma mater — by far the largest in its history — the New York City mayor, along with the president of the university, will disclose the staggering sum of his donations to Johns Hopkins over the past four decades: $1.1 billion.

That figure, kept quiet even as it transformed every corner of the university, makes Mr. Bloomberg the most generous living donor to any education institution in the United States, according to university officials and philanthropic tallies.

The timing of his latest donation, as the mayor's third term draws to a close, offers a glimpse of the sky-is-the-limit philanthropy that he and his aides say is likely to dominate his life after City Hall. The mayor, who is 70, has pledged to give away all of his $25 billion fortune before he dies, and he has built up **a foundation** on the Upper East Side of Manhattan to carry out the task.

At the same time, the donations highlight the unusually close relationship between Mr. Bloomberg and Johns Hopkins, which, interviews show, has played an unseen role in several of his biggest undertakings as mayor.

In an interview here, Mr. Bloomberg said he was making his donations public to encourage greater charitable giving toward education. He lamented, "In our society, we are defunding education."

The mayor, a member of the class of 1964, explained his fidelity to the university in deeply personal terms. Johns Hopkins, he said, was where he escaped the crushing boredom of **Medford High** and discovered an urban campus of stately Georgian buildings brimming with new people and ideas.

"I just thought I'd died and gone to heaven," he said.

"If I had been the son of academics," he added, "maybe I would have been on campuses and would never have been as impressed as I was when I was here, because it's the first time I really was walking among people who were world leaders, who were creating, inventing."

Johns Hopkins as it exists today is inconceivable without Mr. Bloomberg, whose giving has fueled major improvements in the university's reputation and rankings, its competitiveness for faculty and students, and the appearance of its campus.

His wealth — not to mention a small army of his favored architects, art consultants and landscape designers — has bankrolled and molded the handsome brick-and-marble walkways, lamps and benches that dot the campus; has constructed a **physics building**, a **school of public health**, a **children's hospital**, a stem-cell research institute, a malaria institute and a library wing; has commissioned giant art installations by **Kendall Buster**, **Mark Dion** and **Robert Israel**; and has financed 20 percent of all need-based financial aid grants to undergraduates over the past few years. (Even his ex-wife and in-laws make a campus cameo, on the dedication plaque for a science building he financed.)

Mandated Report VA to CDC - Matteoli

"The modern story of Hopkins is inextricably linked to him," said Ronald J. Daniels, the university's president, as he walked around the campus recently. "When you look at these great investments that have transformed American higher education, it's Rockefeller, it's Carnegie, it's Mellon, it's Stanford — and it's Bloomberg."

Hopkins, in return, has become something of a brain trust for Mr. Bloomberg, shaping his approach to issues like cigarette smoking, gun violence and obesity.

It was faculty members at Hopkins who introduced Mr. Bloomberg, as a donor and as a trustee, to a growing body of science linking behavior and disease.

"That is when he discovered public health," said Alfred Sommer, the dean of the Johns Hopkins Bloomberg School of Public Health from 1990 until 2005.

At times, Mr. Bloomberg, then a high-flying entrepreneur, was resistant to paying for such research, arguing that some of the most intractable health problems were best left to government. "That's policy; that's politics," Mr. Sommer recalled him saying.

But the underlying ideas stuck, and, as mayor, Mr. Bloomberg pressed the City Council to ban smoking in city parks, and the Board of Health to require fast-food chains to post caloric counts and restaurants to stop selling oversize sodas.

"He was in a position to act on things he had once told us we really shouldn't be bothered with," Mr. Sommer said. "He has been the public health mayor ever since."

Years before he would banish cars from parts of Times Square, Mr. Bloomberg removed them from the quads of Johns Hopkins as chairman of the board of trustees, arguing they were unsightly and impeded socializing. (To hide them, he paid for an underground parking garage.)

The relationship between Mr. Bloomberg and Hopkins is, much like the college admissions process, the product of happenstance.

In high school, Mr. Bloomberg worked at an electronics company whose owner happened to have a doctorate from the university. She urged him to apply, despite his mediocre transcript.

"Let's be serious — they took a chance on me," Mr. Bloomberg said.

At Hopkins, the boyish-looking Mr. Bloomberg, whose high school classmates branded him "argumentative" in a class book, blossomed into a charismatic figure, eager to organize those around him. An engineering major, he persuaded his fraternity brothers to pay for a chef to replace a chaotic dinnertime routine, and he doled out assignments to lab mates. "He was like the project manager, at 19 years old," Jim Kelly, a classmate, said.

On campus, Mr. Bloomberg discovered the addictive power of the limelight. When a local judge, tired of hearing cases involving misbehaving Hopkins fraternity brothers, called for an end to Greek life at the college, Mr. Bloomberg challenged him to an hourlong public debate. A healthy crowd showed up for the occasion.

"Mike not only held his own," Mr. Kelly recalled, "he beat him."

Mr. Bloomberg still relishes his star turn in campus governance. "It's the first time that I ever headed something," he said. "The first time I got a chance to pull people together."

These days, his status as the university's top donor has given him mayorlike sway at Hopkins: deans routinely travel to New York to pitch him new programs and research.

His latest passion: genetically engineering mosquitoes to prevent the transmission of malaria. "He always asks about the mosquitoes," said Dr. Peter Agre, a Nobel Prize-winning professor at the university, where Mr. Bloomberg has paid for a temperature-controlled center to cultivate the bugs. The mayor of New York City now speaks of "building a better mosquito."

Mr. Bloomberg tends to finance ideas that appeal to his contrarian style and corporate ethos. For years he has rotated top executives around his media company to encourage collaboration. In the hope of replicating that experience, most of his

Bloomberg to Johns Hopkins — $1.1 Billion Thanks - The New York Times Page 5 of 5

latest donation, about $250 million, will be used to hire 50 new faculty members who will hold appointments in two departments as they pursue research in areas like the global water supply and the future of American cities. (The remaining $100 million will be devoted to financial aid.)

His approach to philanthropy at the university is remarkably hands-on. A trusted mayoral architectural adviser, Allen Kolkowitz, and an art guru, Nancy Rosen, guided the construction of the new Charlotte R. Bloomberg children's hospital, named for the mayor's mother. The building's colorful exterior is a whimsical take on Monet's paintings at Giverny. "He got very involved in the design," said Dr. Edward D. Miller, the former chief executive of Hopkins Medicine.

Of course, certain courtesies are extended to a donor at Mr. Bloomberg's level. When Dr. Miller realized that the Charlotte R. Bloomberg Children's Center would be connected to a new tower named for Sheik Zayed bin Sultan al-Nahayan, the former president of the United Arab Emirates, he nervously called the mayor.

"Will you have a problem with this?" he asked Mr. Bloomberg.

The mayor thanked him for the call, but made clear he had no objection. "A Jew on one side, an Arab on the other," he told Dr. Miller. "That's what we should do in this world."

A version of this article appears in print on January 27, 2013, on page A1 of the New York edition with the headline: Bloomberg to Johns Hopkins: Thanks a Billion (Well, $1.1 Billion).

<u>BEFORE TO BLOOMBERG DONATION</u>

Appears: Changed from Cohort to Randomized Studies

Gray, RH, Wawer M, et al., "Probability of HIV-1 transmission per coital act in monogamous, heterosexual, HIV-1 discordant couples in Rakai, Uganda," *Lancet*, Vol. 357: pp. 1149-1153, 14 April 2001.

"The risk of transmission was not significantly affected by the circumcision status of HIV-1 positive male partners." p. 1151.

BEHAVIOR

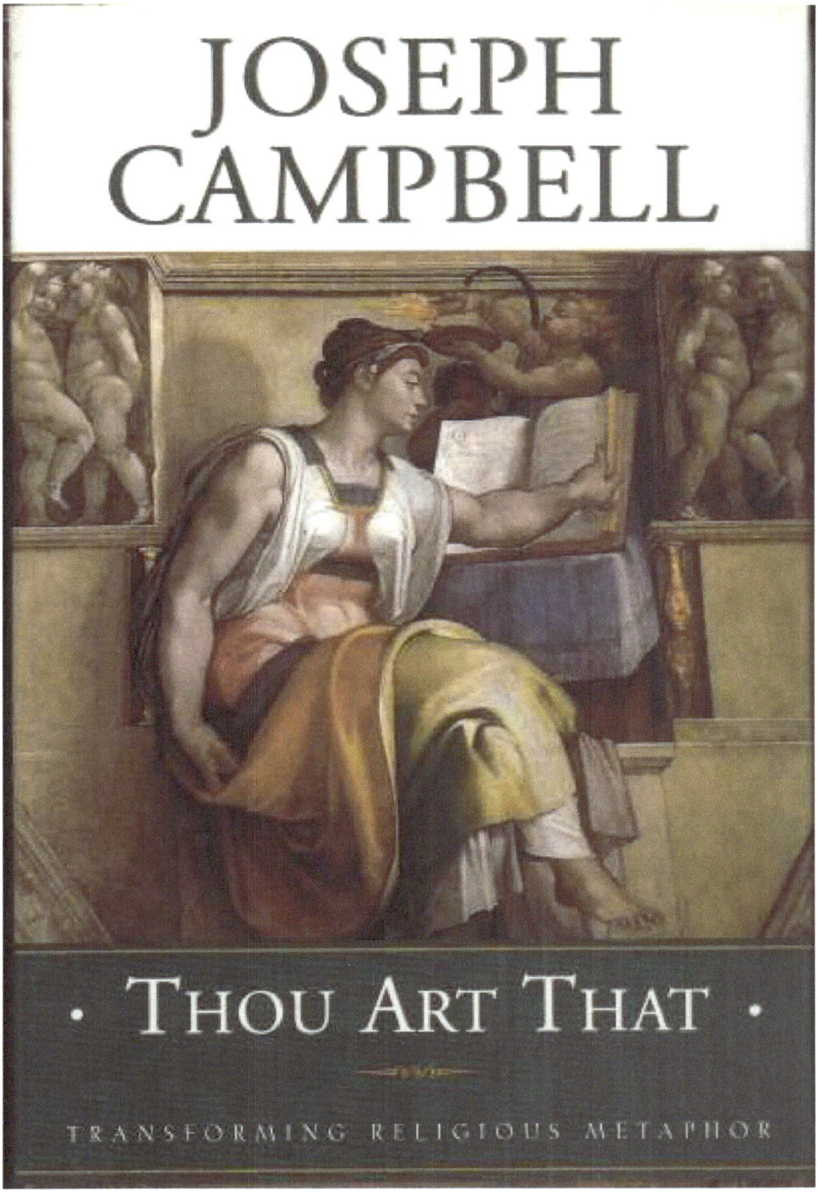
JOSEPH
CAMPBELL
· THOU ART THAT ·
TRANSFORMING RELIGIOUS METAPHOR

TO THE CONTRARY

US AIR FORCE, *JAMA*, 1970

Matriarchal Identity

THE CIRCUMCISION REFERENCE LIBRARY

JOURNAL OF THE AMERICAN MEDICAL ASSOCIATION, Volume 213, Number 11: Pages 1853-1858, September 14, 1970.

Whither the Foreskin?

A Consideration of Routine Neonatal Circumcision

CAPT E. Noel Preston, MC, USAF

Routine neonatal circumcision has been advocated as a means of preventing genitourinary diseases and genital cancers. However, the procedure has been found to have been of questionable benefit and to be associated with both immediate and delayed risks and complications. These in turn may produce undesirable psychologic, sexual, and medico-legal difficulties. Circumcision is considered with respect to carcinoma of the cervix, penis, and prostate; there is little evidence that circumcision of the newborn affords protection against subsequent development of these cancers in individuals who practice good personal hygiene.

[CIRP Note: This article is historic in nature. Preston's article along with that of Leitch, which was also published in 1970, disproved the false claim by Abraham Wolbarst that male circumcision could prevent penile cancer. Its publication influenced the American Academy of Pediatrics which issued a statement the following year that said "there are no valid medical indications for circumcision in the neonatal period."]

Circumcision of the newborn has been recommended to prevent the occurrence of various disorders such as phimosis, paraphimosis, and balanoposthitis,[1] venereal diseases including lymphogranuloma venereum, syphilitic chancres, and herpes progenitalis,[2] as well as carcinoma of the cervix[3,4] penis,[3,5] and prostate.[3,6] Routine circumcision of the newborn has been recommended to avoid emotional distress in the only uncircumcised boy in a high-school locker room or summer camp,[7] and to avoid psychologic, anesthetic, and surgical risks if it is performed at a later age.[10] Additionally circumcision has been advocated on the grounds that the circumcised phallus is cleaner,[2,8,11] that it provides greater pleasure during sexual intercourse,[12,13] and that it is more esthetic. Goodwin[13] has observed that, "circumcision is a beautification comparable to rhinoplasty, and a circumcised penis appears in its flaccid state as an erect uncircumcised organ - a beautiful instrument of precise intent."

Arguments against circumcision include the views that, like any other surgical operation, it is associated with certain infrequent but preventable hazards and complications and basically the operation is unnecessary.

Complications

Complications of circumcision may be regarded as immediate or delayed. The immediate complications fall into three categories: hemorrhage, infection, and surgical trauma.[14] Hemorrhage is the most common of these immediate complications. It may be caused by inadequate hemostasis, blood coagulapathies, or the existence of anomalous vessels.[14] Patel[15] studied 100 consecutive male infants who were circumcised at birth and who were reevaluated 6 to 18 months later. He found 35 instances of hemorrhage of which four required sutures.

Infection of the wound in circumcision is also a fairly common complication. It is manifested by local inflammatory changes, ulceration, and suppuration.[14] Occasionally infection may lead to more serious complications such as partial necrosis of the penis, or it may be a source of septicemia. Shulman et al[17] have recorded a case of staphylococcal septicemia giving rise to osteomyletis of the femur, and a fatal case of septicemia and pulmonary abscesses, both of which were ascribed to infection of circumcision wounds.

A common complication of circumcision is loss of penile skin. This can result from pulling too much of the skin from the shaft up over the glans during the operation. The remaining skin slides back, leaving a denuded penile shaft. Major losses of penile skin usually occur, however, because of a complicating infection, the use of the electocautery, or improper surgical technique. Van Duyn and Warr[11] reported a case of routine circumcision, performed by an experienced, competent pediatrician with use of a circumcision clamp, that resulted in wound dehiscence and required replacement by split skin grafting.

Additional complications include accidental lacerations of penile or scrotal skin, or both, incomplete circumcision with formation of adhesions and secondary penile deformity, and accidental amputation of the glans with secondary postoperative hemorrhage, and retraction of the penis into a subcutaneous position by contraction, healing, and fibrosis of the circular wound.[illegible]

Delayed complications of circumcision are related to the newly circumcised penis being in frequent and prolonged contact with feces and ammoniacal urine. One could logically expect the de-epitheialized, edematous, bleeding glans to become inflamed, bruised, or infected, with subsequent development of fibrosis and scarring.

Meatal stenosis, with its symptoms of dysuria, increased urinary frequency, and enuresis, is not related either to the method of circumcision or to the skill with which it is performed as it is a late complication.[1] The appearance of this condition indicates the fallacy of the argument that boys should be circumcised at birth so they will have "no trouble in later life." In Patel's series of 100 newborn circumcised boys who were examined 6 to 18 months later, 31 had developed meatal ulcers, 8 had meatal stenosis, 1 had phimosis ([1]) and 8 developed infections.

Delayed complications of circumcisions may not only be anatomic; they may also be psychologic. Settlage[illegible] has stated, "Concern for the psychologic development and future health of the child requires that events in the neonatal as well as any later stage of development be managed in such as a way as to keep tension in the child within tolerable limits." One cannot argue that structure and functions are intimately related, and at the same time shrug off with equanimity the fretful, circumcised newborn, his glans swollen and cyanotic for three to five days.

Is Circumcision Necessary?

It is interesting to note that all of the reasons advanced for routine circumcision have to do the prevention of certain conditions, not with the establishment of a condition such as strong teeth and bones or a normal cardiac reserve. Robertson[17] has stated: Avoidance of harm is not to be equated with provision of benefit; just because it doesn't kill, that doesn't mean it helps."

One of the reasons advanced for routine neonatal circumcision is the prevention of phimosis. Actually the presence of phimosis cannot be determined at birth because histologically the prepuce is still developing at this time and its separation is usually incomplete.[18,21] McKay[22] has observed: "The prepuce of the newborn infant is normally so tight and adherent that no information can be obtained as to later need for circumcision.

At birth only 4% of boys have a fully retractable foreskin; ; at 6 months of age, 15%; at one year of age 50%, and it is not until the age of 3 that 90% of boys have a completely retractable prepuce.[21] To diagnose phimosis one must find not only a nonretractable foreskin, but a small preputial opening. "Ballooning" of the prepuce occurs on micturation. **[CIRP Note: Ballooning is now regarded as a normal stage of development and not an indication of a need for circumcision.]**

Recurrent infection under a non-retractable foreskin in an older child seems a more legitimate reason for recommending operation to allow drainage. The fortunate rarity of this condition is possibly the result of the persisting attachment of the prepuce to the glans.[1]

Balanitis is uncommon in childhood when the prepuce is performing its protective function; in the circumcised penis the incidence of meatal ulcers is significantly increased precisely because the glans is deprived of the protection of the foreskin.[1,18,21,24] Most cases described as balanitis are nothing more than inflammation of the skin of the prepuce, which is usually due to ammonia dermititis from ammoniacal urine and circumcision is strongly contraindicated. In these cases the foreskin is carrying out its prime function of protecting the underlying glans;[1,12,18,21,24,25] if it is removed, a meatal ulcer due to the ammonia will almost certainly result.[25]

As to the argument that circumcision is of value in preventing the accumulation of venereal disease, Morgan[15] has observed:

> Venereal disease is more prevalent in the lower socioeconomic groups and these are the groups that are most likely to be uncircumcised. They are also the groups in which there is a poor standard of personal hygiene. The lower socioeconomic groups are also those with a higher incidence of tuberculosis but one could be excused for doubting that the retention of the prepuce renders one more susceptible to tuberculosis. Post hoc ergo propter hoc is invalid logic.

Herskowitz[21] has noted that Spock's[3] argument that circumcision helps a boy to feel "regular" is cultural, and wonders if Spock would favor circumcision of the clitoris in a society where that is the usual practice. It is the duty of the medical profession to lead rather than follow a community's standards of health care. **[CIRP note: Dr. Benjamin Spock later changed his mind and came to oppose circumcision.]**

Different opinions exist as to the importance of the foreskin in the act of coitus. On the one hand is Morgan's[13] assertion that coitus without a foreskin is comparable to viewing a Renoir while colorblind due to the prepuce lubricating the glans and permitting easier penetration. On the other is the statement that after circumcision the glans becomes less sensitive, resulting in a more delayed orgasm, and this a lessening of premature ejaculation. Goodwin[13] quoted a patient discussing delayed orgasm as prostatectomy as saying, "It takes about 15 minutes longer, doctor, but we don't begrudge a moment of it."

As to the argument that the circumcised penis is more esthetic, one is reminded that beauty is in the eye of the beholder, and that most Renaissance works of are show the male organ, if not with a fig leaf, at least with a foreskin. Morgan[12] noted:

> Perhaps why American mothers seem to endorse the operation with such enthusiasm is the fact that it is one way an intensely matriarchal society can permanently influence the physical characteristics of its males.

and concluded:

> the argument is also put forth that the circumcised organ is more hygienic for the prepuce collects nasty secretions. So does the ear, but the removal of this rather ugly appendage is frowned upon, and in one famous instance cutting it off lead to war - the so-called war of Captain Jenkin's ear. One can be grateful that this worthy mariner did not lose his prepuce under similar circumstances, for it is rather likely the battle would still be raging.[12]

[CIRP note: There now follows a discussion of cancer of the cervix. Later research has established the role of the human papillomavirus (HPV) and smoking in the etiology of cancer of the cervix. The foreskin is no longer believed to cause cancer.]

Circumcision and Cancer of the Cervix

Circumcision is only one of a large number of variables, many of them interrelated, which cannot be considered separately in epidemiologic studies of the etiology of cancer of the cervix. Factors known to be associated with a high degree of risk of developing cervical cancer include low socioeconomic status, early marriage, multiple marriages, extramarital relations, coitus at an early age, nonuse of contraceptives, syphilis, and multiparity.[15]

In 1932, Hanley[4] found only three cases of cancer among 90,000 Fijians who practice male circumcision at birth, but he found 26 cases among 70,000 Hindus who do not practice circumcision. The two populations live side by side but do not intermingle.

New data[22] from Fiji 25 years later, however indicated that natives of Fiji have a lower incidence of cancer in general, whereas the immigrant Hindus have a much higher incidence of cancer of all sorts. Also, while nearly 100% of the Fijians were circumcised in contrast to only 25% of the Hindus, there were 55 cases of the former with cancer of the cervix and only 101 of the latter, a ratio of 1:2 instead of the 1:9 of 25 years earlier. Perhaps this reflects improved methods on cancer detection developed over the intervening years, but in any case the data no longer retain their original significance.

Circumcision probably improves the hygienic status of the penis in circumstances where a low standard of hygiene would otherwise prevail. Kmet's[20] group studied circumcised orthodox Moslems, circumcised "emancipated" Moslems, and uncircumcised non-Moslems in Yugoslavia. They found premalignant lesions of the cervix to be 11 per 1,000 in the uncircumcised non-Moslems, 5.5 per 1,000 in the circumcised emancipated Moslems, and nil in the circumcised orthodox Moslems. This would indicate circumcision to be of questionable benefit in protecting women who live in cultures not adhering to religious rules regarding sexual hygiene, promiscuity, and genital cleanliness. A possible weakness in Kmet's study is that they were unable to obtain any data regarding the percent distribution of the circumcised males or the types of prepuces present in the uncircumcised.

Aitken-Swan and Baird's[21] group of 54 husbands whose wives had pre-clinical and clinical cancer of the cervix included 12 who were completely and 10 who were partly circumcised, compared with 56 husbands whose wives were in a control group, of whom 14 were completely and 14 partly circumcised. Thus complete circumcision was found about as frequently in husbands of patients with cancer as in husbands of controls.

Boyd and Doll[22] found the discovery rate for cancer of the cervix among non-Jewish women whose marital partners were circumcised to be no different from the rate among non-Jewish women with circumcised husbands. Jones et al[23] found the incidence of cancer of the cervix not to be related to the absence of circumcision in the spouse or other sexual partners. Circumcision was as common among the husbands of a group of women with certain cervical cancer as among husbands of a control group of women.

Khanolkar[24] found the cervix to be the site of origin of cancer more frequently in Moslem than in Parsee women with cancer, although the husbands of the former are circumcised and the those of the latter are not. The Parsees on the other hand, attach much greater importance to cleanliness. Additionally, Elliot[25] found English wives at the lower end of the socioeconomic scale to have a liability to cancer of the cervix more than ten times greater than those at the top.

Lack of circumcision supposedly leads to the accumulation of smegma beneath the prepuce[1,2] and smegma has been thought to be a carcinogenic substance.[3,4] If this were the case one would expect to find a difference in the rate of discovery of malignant and premalignant lesions of the cervix between groups not using such an obstructive form.

In support of such a theory, Boyd and Doll[12] found that fewer patients than controls had used obstructive methods of contraception, and Baird and Aitken-Swan[11] found that fewer patients than controls had "ever used" or "predominantly used" a sheath or cap contraceptive. Of 54 patients with cancer of the cervix, 13% had used an obstructive contraceptive as opposed to 43% of 56 controls. Stern and Nealy,[illegible] however discovered that the use of a sheath contraceptive by the marital partner was not to be associated with rate differences for cancer of the cervix between patient and control groups.

To determine whether smegma is indeed carcinogenic, Heins, in a study reported by Weiss,[illegible] inoculated monkeys through the vagina one to two times weekly for three years with raw human smegma and was unable to produce any cancers of the cervix or vagina. Additionally, Fishman's[illegible] group injected smegma from old men into the vaginas of mice two to three times weekly for 12 months and was unable to stimulate the production of genital cancers, although inoculation of similar animals with a known carcinogen regularly produced vaginal cancers.

Dodge's[illegible] investigations in Kenya have revealed not significant differences between the numbers of cervical cancer cases in women of tribe who men were or were not circumcised. He concluded: "The tribal distribution of cases does not seem in any way related to the practice of circumcision among the tribal males . . . thus it seems the role of smegma in the genesis of cervical cancer is of little importance."[illegible]

Lack of circumcision as a possible etiology for cancer of the cervix received attention from Gagnon's[illegible] being unable to find a single case of cervical carcinoma among 13,000 Catholic nuns over a 20-year period. This has lead to the idea that since Catholic nuns do not have intercourse with uncircumcised men, a lower rate of cervical cancer would obtain in those cultures where circumcision is performed.

Seemingly overlooked is the idea that Catholic nuns do not have intercourse with circumcised men either. It would appear that the decisive factor in the nuns' freedom from cervical cancer is related not to the presence or absence of the foreskin but to the absence of sexual relations.

In 1964, Reid[illegible] suggested that penetration of the epithelium by spermatozoa could initiate the process leading to cancer, and that an obstructive contraceptive would lessen the cancer risk by preventing spermatozoa from reaching the squamous epithelium. Boyd and Doll's[12] and Baird and Aitken-Swans[11] findings in this regard and Gagnon's[illegible] data from the Catholic nuns would seem to support this proposal.

[CIRP note: There now follows a discussion of carcinoma of the penis. Later research has established the role of the HPV virus and of smoking in the etiology of carcinoma of the penis.]

Circumcision and Carcinoma of the Penis

Lack of circumcision has been found to be associated with carcinoma of the penis. Many authors[2,3,5,7] have noted the rarity of penile cancers in circumcised men. Dodge and Kaviti[2] have stated that cancer of the penis occurs more frequently among European an Asian populations in the uncircumcised than among the circumcised. Others[21] have claimed that cancer of the penis has never been recorded in men circumcised at birth.

But, does the retention of the foreskin truly cause cancer of the penis? Is smegma actually carcinogenic? Or does the accumulation of smegma beneath the prepuce indicate a more basic problem, namely, that of poor genital hygiene? Proponents of circumcision have been unable to answer these questions with certainty.

In 1960, Apt[1] found only 15 cases of cancer of the penis, scrotum and other male genital organs (excluding cancer of the prostate and testis) in Sweden. Practically all of Sweden's 3.7 million males are not circumcised.

Anna-Munthrodo[11] recorded the incidence of carcinoma of the penis amongst Jamaicans and observed that 50% of them had gonococcal infection, 55% had positive blood Wassermann reactions, and 50% of them had positive complement-fixation tests for granuloma inguinale.

The Javanese, like the Jews, regularly perform ritual circumcision, but Sampoerno, in a study referred to by Herskowitz,[21] found seven carcinomas of the penis among 78 carcinomas of Javanese men.

Additionally, all 163 cases with cancer of the penis in Reddy's[6] series of Indian men belonged to the low-income group who are usually credited with low personal and genital hygiene. Dodge and Kaviti[2] found the rate of carcinoma of the penis among uncircumcised east African tribes to vary considerably and conceded that unexplored differences in personal hygiene or in dietary habits may be responsible. Lenowitz and Graham[12] found in 1946 that cancer of the penis was 5 times more common in American Negroes than in American whites, but skin cancer was seven times more common in whites.

The facts speak for themselves. Carcinoma of the penis is uncommon in uncircumcised men with a high standard of hygiene, as in Sweden, but circumcision affords little protection in populations where personal hygiene may be minimal. In cases of penile carcinoma, lack of hygiene is always striking.[22] If the uncircumcised man has a foreskin which he can retract and which he keeps clean, the risk of this cancer is removed.

Circumcision and Carcinoma of the Prostate

Some investigators[1,2] have attempted to show a correlation between uncircumcision and prostatic carcinoma.

Ravich[1] found that among his 1,275 Jewish private patients who underwent surgery for prostatic obstruction there were only 23 with cancer, an incidence of 1.8%. This compared with 35 cancers, or 19% in the 132 non-Jewish private patients, of whom he estimated "about" 5% were circumcised. Unfortunately, there are no data as to the age differences of his Jewish vs. non-Jewish patients. Since prostatic cancer is a disease associated with advanced age, the omission of this information renders his data inconclusive.

Interestingly, Ravich[2] also noted there was a 67% incidence of prior venereal infections in patients with cancer of the prostate as compared with 28% of the benign prostatic cases. He found that the incidence of cancer was significantly higher in both male Jews and non-Jews when gonorrhea had been present. This in turn would indicate a lower state of personal hygiene in prostatic cancer than in benign cases.

Apt[4] studied the cancer registers of Sweden and Israel for 1960 and found the number of prostatic cancers cases in Sweden to be 1,544 as opposed to 88 in Israel. This indicated the annual rate in Sweden to be 414 per million males in comparison to Israel's 88. Thus he concluded prostatic cancer to be 4.7 times more frequent in Sweden than in Israel. But, there were 3.7 million males in Sweden in 1960 and only 1.0 million males in Israel. Also, using Apt's own figures, 16% of the male population of Sweden was over 60 years old, as opposed to 8.3% of the Israeli male population being 60 or more years old. If one takes 16% of 3.7 million males, he finds that there were 0.592 million males over age 60 in Sweden. Taking 8.3% of 1.0 million males, one finds 0.083 million males over age 60 in Israel. There are thus seven times more men over age 60 in Sweden than in Israel, but prostatic cancer is only 4.7 times more frequent in Sweden. Would this mean that non-circumcision protects against prostatic cancer?

Comment

Circumcision is rarely performed or requested on the basis of its medical indications. Shaw and Robertson[5] interviewed 80 mothers of newborn male infants and found that 72% denied that a physician had ever discussed circumcision with them. The reasons for or against circumcision stated by 106 physicians questioned bore little of any resemblance to the reasons advanced by the 80 mothers. The results cast doubt on the belief that the decision to circumcise is reached in any scientific manner. Obviously, circumcision performed on the basis of religious beliefs is beyond the scope of this discussion.

Poor sexual hygiene, inadequate hygienic facilities, and venereal disease tend to increase the incidence of genitourinary cancers in ethnic groups or populations that do not practice circumcision. In these groups, then, circumcision would seem to be indicated.

However in groups where a high standard of cleanliness could reasonably be expected, circumcision at birth would not seem to be justified. Certainly phimosis, paraphimosis, balanoposthitis, and penile carcinoma are uncommon and could probably be prevented by adequate hygiene. It seems more likely that the presence of smegma in the uncircumcised is simply a sign of poor hygiene, and that this is the risk factor which increases the risk of both penile and cervical cancer.[19]

Proponents of circumcision will agree that in theory, personal hygiene may be as effective as circumcision in cancer prevention. The critical point however, is whether the necessary standards are, or can be achieved in practice. Newhill[13] has stated, "An uncircumcised boy has to be taught to keep his penis clean - which is likely to result in an undesirable concentration of attention on his penis every time he has a bath. A penis without a prepuce is permanently clean."

There is no question but that cleanliness must be taught. However, if a child can be taught to tie his shoes or brush his teeth or wash behind his ears, he can also be taught to wash beneath his foreskin. The foreskin is not fully retractable in 90% of males before age 3 anyway and not special attention is needed before this time. As to the boy paying an undesirable amount of attention to the genital area, most children in the genital stage of development will do exactly that. Children will play with themselves and with each other. Mere circumcision will not prevent such activity, nor is it supposed to.

In regard to the immediate surgical complications of circumcision, it is true that their incidence is small. They do however exist, and they are preventable. Such potential hazards as uncontrollable hemorrhage, lacerations, deformities, and amputations should be considered not only from the patient's and family's points of view but from a medico-legal one as well.Delayed complications of circumcision are more common, but less severe. Meatal ulcer, meatal stenosis, enuresis, and penile deformity secondary to scarring and fibrosis are potential sequelae of circumcision.

Justification of circumcision in order to save a boy later lockerroom embarrassment seems unrealistic. This is the latter half of the 20th century, a time supposedly to celebrate individuality and freedom of choice. One of the American ideals is independence and originality of expression. If being uncircumcised is embarrassing to a boy he can always be circumcised later. At any rate it will be his choice, and he will know why he chooses it.

Finally, to those physicians who would recommend the performance of untold numbers of circumcisions to prevent one case of cancer of the penis, there arises an interesting problem: The ultimate side effects and complications of the orally administered contraceptives have yet to be determined, but how many physicians who advocate circumcision as a cancer preventative continue to prescribe these anovulatory agents? How many of them still allow their patients, their wives or their children to smoke cigarettes, which are far more likely to be carcinogenic than is the foreskin?

Radiation of the thymus and routine tonsillectomy are no longer acceptable. This is because they have been found to be associated with certain dangers and to provide only questionable benefits. Perhaps routine neonatal circumcision will one day join these antiquated curiosities in medicine's attic.

Conclusion

Routine circumcision of the newborn is an unnecessary procedure. It provides questionable benefits and is associated with a small but definite incidence of complications and hazards. These risks are preventable if the operation is not performed unless truly medically indicated. Circumcision of the newborn is a procedure that should no longer be considered routine.

References

1. Wright JE: Non-therapeutic circumcision. *Med J Aust* 1:1083-1086, 1967.
2. Garvin CH, Persky L: Circumcision: is it justified in infancy? *J Nat Med Assoc* 58:233-238, 1966.
3. Ravich A: Role of circumcision in cancer prevention. *Acta Urol Jap* 11:79-86, 1965.
4. Handley WS: The prevention of cancer. *Lancet* 1:987, 1936.
5. Trainin N: Cervical carcinoma and circumcision. *Israel J Med Sci* 1:303-304, 1965.
6. Reddy DJ, Indira C: Some aspects of the pathology of carcinoma penis. *J Indian Med Assoc* 41:277-280, 1963.
7. Dodge OG, Kaviti JN: Male circumcision among the peoples of east Africa and the incidence of genital cancer. *E Afr Med J* 42:98-105, 1965.
8. Apt A: Circumcision and prostatic cancer. *Acta Med Scand* 178:493-504, 1965.
9. Spock B: *Baby and Child Care*. New York, Pocket Books, 1957, p 155.
10. Cansever G: Psychological effects of circumcision. *Brit J Med Psychol* 38:321-331, 1965.
11. Newill R: Circumcision. *Brit Med J* 2:419, 1965.
12. Bolande R: Ritualistic surgery: Circumcision and tonsillectomy. *New England J Med* 280:592-595, 1969.
13. Goodwin, quoted by Kaufman JJ: Should circumcision be done routinely? *Med Aspects Hum Sexual* 1:27-28, 1967.
14. Rosner F: Circumcision. *NY J Med* 66:2919-2922, 1966.
15. Shulman J, Ben-Hur N, Neuman Z: Surgical complications of circumcision. *Amer J Dis Child* 107:149-154, 1964.
16. Patel H: The problem of routine circumcision. *Canad Med Assoc J* 95:576-581, 1966.
17. Van Duyn J, Warr WS: Excessive penile skin loss from circumcision. *J Med Assoc Georgia* 51:394-396, 1962.
18. Morgan WKC: Penile plunder. *Med J Aust* 1:1102-1103, 1967.
19. Settlage CF: Psychologic development, in Nelson WE (ed): *Textbook of Pediatrics* ed 9. Philadelphia, WB Saunders, 1969, p 60.
20. Robertson WO: Should Circumcision be done routinely? *Med Aspects Hum Sexual* 1:27, 1967.
21. Herskowitz MS: The mechanistic distortion in treatment of infants and children. *J Amer Coll Neuropsych* 3:13-18, 1964.
22. McKay RJ: The newborn infant, in Nelson WE (ed): *Textbook of Pediatrics*, ed 9. Philadelphia, WB Saunders Co, 1969, p 357.
23. Gairdner D: The Fate of the Foreskin. *Brit Med J* 2:1433-1437, 1949.
24. St. John-Hunt D: Circumcision of the Newborn: Is it good preventive medicine? *Med J Aust* 1:1100-1101, 1967.

Mandated Report VA to CDC - Matteoli

25. Jolly, H: Circumcision. *Practitioner* 192:257, 1964
26. Morgan WKC: Re: The rape of the phallus. *JAMA* 194:309-311, 1965
27. Morgan WKC: The rape of the phallus. *JAMA* 193:223-224, 1965.
28. Circumcision and cervical cancer, editorial. *Brit Med J* 2:397-398, 1964.
29. Weiss C: Routine non-ritual circumcision in infancy. *Clin Pediatr* 3:560-563.
30. Kmet J Damjanovski L, Stucin M, et al: Circumcision and carcinoma colli uteri in Macedonia, Yugoslavia: I. Incidence of malignant and premalignant conditions. *Brit J Cancer* 19:217-227, 1965
31. Aitken-Swan J, Baird D: Circumcision and cancer of the cervix. *Brit J Cancer* 19:419-428, 1964.
32. Boyd JT, Doll R: Study of the aetiology of carcinoma of the cervix uteri. *Brit J Cancer* 18:419-428, 1964.
33. Jones EG, MacDonald I, Breslow L: Study of the epidemiologic factors in carcinoma of the uterine cervix. *Amer J Obstet Gynec* 76:1-10, 1958.
34. Khanolkar VR: Cancer in India. *Acta Un Int Cancer* 6:881-886, 1950.
35. Elliot RIK: On the prevention of carcinoma of the cervix. *Lancet* 1:232-232, 1964.
36. Stern E, Neely PM: Cancer of the cervix in reference to circumcision and marital history. *J Amer Med Wom Assoc* 17:739-740, 1962.
37. Fishman M, Shear MJ, Friedman HF, et al: Studies in carcinogenesis: local effect of repeated application of 3,4-benz-pyrene and of human smegma to vagina and cervix of mice. *J Nat Cancer Inst* 2:361-368, 1942.
38. Dodge OG, Linsell CA, Davies JNP: Circumcision and the incidence of carcinoma of the penis and cervix. *J Afr Med J* 40:440-444, 1963.
39. Gagnon F: Contribution to the study of the etiology and prevention of cancer of the cervix of the uterus. *Amer J Obstet Gynec* 60:516-522, 1950.
40. Reid BL: Circumcision and cancer of the cervix. *Lancet* 1:21, 1964.
41. Anna-Muntleodo H: Carcinoma of the penis. *J Int Coll Surg* 35:21-31, 1961
42. Lenowitz H, Graham HP: Carcinoma of the penis. *J Urol* 56:458-484, 1946.
43. Shaw RA, Robertson WO: Routine circumcision. *Amer J Dis Child* 106:216-217, 1963.

From the Pediatric Services, USAF Hospital, Vandenberg Air Force Base, California.
Opinions expressed in this paper are not necessarily those of the Department of Defense or the Department of the Air Force.
Reprint requests to 3644-E Chamblee-Tucker Road, Atlanta, GA 30341.

Correspondence in response to this article:

- Harnes J. The foreskin saga. *JAMA* 1971;217(9):1241-42.

Preston's reply:

- Preston EN. Letter. *JAMA* 1971;218(7):1051

Citation:

- Preston EN. Whither the foreskin. *JAMA* 1970; 213(11):1853-8.

(File revised 1 October 2006)

Return to CIRP library

http://www.cirp.org/library/general/preston/

Mandated Report VA to CDC - Matteoli

US NAVY – THAILAND, 2004
BUMED/FORCEMED
No AIDS Connection

U.S. Navy Finds That Circumcision Does Not Prevent HIV or STIs (http://www.thewholenetwork.org/twn-news/us-navy-finds-that-circumcision-does-not-prevent-hiv-or-stis)

10/25/2011

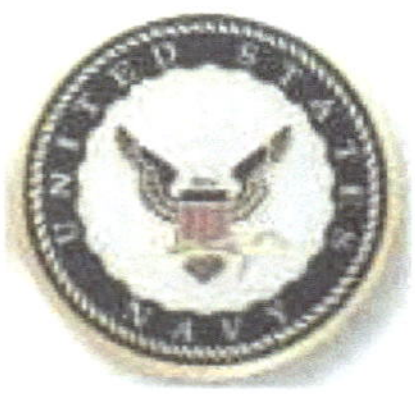

"Multiple logistic regressions were constructed separately to evaluate the role of circumcision in the acquisition of HIV and STI. Conclusions: [circumcision] is not associated with HIV or STI prevention in this U. S. military population."

Prevalence of male circumcision and its association with HIV and sexually transmitted infections in a U.S. navy population (http://www.dtic.mil/cgi-bin/GetTRDoc?AD=ADA458080)

Thomas AG, Bakhireva LN, Brodine SK, Shaffer RA. International Conference on AIDS (15th : 2004 : Bangkok, Thailand)

Int Conf AIDS. 2004 Jul 11-16; 15: abstract no. TuPeC4881. Naval Health Research Center, DHAPP, San Diego, CA, United States

Background: Lack of male circumcision has been found to be a risk factor for HIV and sexually transmitted infection (STI) in several studies performed in developing countries. However, the few studies conducted in developed nations have yielded inconsistent results. Policy regarding circumcision of male infants as a prevention measure against HIV/STI remains a controversial topic. This study describes the prevalence of circumcision and its association with HIV and STI in a U. S. military population.

Methods: This is a case-control study of male HIV infected U. S. military personnel (n=232) recruited from 7 military medical centers and male U. S. Navy controls (n=516) from a general aircraft carrier population. Cases and controls completed similar self-administered HIV behavioral risk surveys. Case circumcision status was abstracted from medical charts while control status was reported on the survey. Cases and controls were frequency matched on age. Multiple logistic regressions were constructed separately to evaluate the role of circumcision in the acquisition of HIV and STI.

Results: The proportion of circumcised men did not significantly differ between cases (84.9%) and controls (81.8%). Prevalence of circumcision among men born in the U. S. was higher (85.0%) than those born elsewhere (58.1%). After adjustment for demographic and behavioral risk factors lack of circumcision was not found to be a risk factor for HIV (OR = 0.9, 95% CI: 0.51, 1.7) or STI (OR = 1.08; 95% CI 0.52, 2.26). The odds of HIV infection were 2.6 higher for irregular condom users, 5 times as high for those reporting STI, 6.2 times higher for those reporting anal sex, 2.8-3.2 times higher for those with 2-7+ partners, nearly 3 times higher for Blacks, and 3.5 times as high for

facebook (https://www.facebook.com/WholeNetwork)

Search Our Site

Recent Articles:

ROYAL AUSTRALIAN ARMY

PRESENT

Personal Researcher Page for Gregory J. Boyle

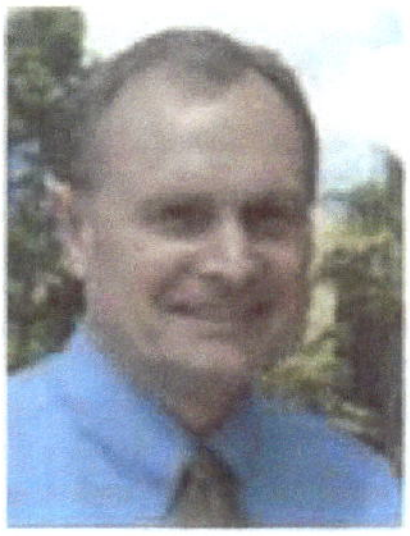

GREGORY J. BOYLE

Bond University

- Professor of Psychology

EXPERTISE

- Personality and Individual Differences
- Health Psychology

HONORS & AWARDS

- Vice-Chancellor's Research Grant, Bond University
- Canadian Donner Foundation Grant
- Buros Institute of Mental Measurements Distinguished Reviewer Award
- Elected Fellow, Australian Psychological Society
- Elected Fellow American Psychological Association
- Appointed LCOL, Australian Army Psychology Corps
- Awarded prestigious Doctor of Science Degree (UQ)

G+

BSc (Hons), MEd, PhD (Melbourne)

MA, PhD (Delaware)

DSc (Queensland)

Professor Boyle has spent over three decades undertaking quantitative research in the field of psychometrics, as related to the measurement of individual differences in personality, intelligence, and motivation, as well as undertaking studies within the fields of neuropsychology, clinical psychology, and educational psychology.

In more recent years, he has applied his extensive research skills to studies within the broad fields of medical/health psychology, and has undertaken many studies within the area of women's health. Lately, he has focused his attention more on research topics pertaining to men's health.

ARTICLES

Factor analyses of the McGill Pain Questionnaire (MPQ) in acute and chronic pain patients (with Bard H Boerresen and Deannah Jang), *Psychological Reports* (2015)

Empathy towards individuals of the same and different ethnicity when depicted in negative and positive contexts (with David Neumann and Raymond C.K. Chan), *Personality and Individual Differences* (2013)

Circumcision-generated emotions bias medical literature (with George Hill), *BJU International* (2012)

The case for boosting infant male circumcision in the face of rising heterosexual transmission of HIV... and now the case against (with George Hill), *Medical Journal of Australia* (2011)

Sub-Saharan African randomised clinical trials into male circumcision and HIV transmission: Methodological, ethical and legal concerns (with George Hill), *Journal of Law and Medicine* (2011)

BOOKS

Measures of personality and social psychological constructs (with Donald H. Saklofske and Gerald Matthews), *Measures of personality and social psychological constructs* (2015)

BOOK CHAPTERS

Criteria for selection and evaluation of scales and measures (with Donald H. Saklofske and Gerald Matthews), *Measures of personality and social psychological constructs* (2015)

Measures of affect dimensions (with Edward Helmes, Gerald Matthews, and Carroll E. Izard), *Measures of personality and social psychological constructs* (2015)

Measures of anger and hostility in adults (with Ephrem Fernandez and Andrew Day), *Measures of personality and social psychological constructs* (2015)

Measures of empathy: Self-report, behavioral, and neuroscientific approaches (with David Neumann, Raymond C.K. Chan, Yi Wang, and H. Rae Westbury), *Measures of personality and social psychological constructs* (2015)

Method of test administration as a factor in test validity: The use of a personality questionnaire in the prediction of cancer and coronary heart disease (with R. Grossarth-Maticek and H. J. Eysenck), *Psychological Assessment vol 1- 4* (2012)

CONFERENCE PAPERS

Ending forced genital cutting of children and violation of their human rights: ethical, psychological and legal considerations. 6th *International Symposium on Genital Integrity: Safeguarding fundamental human rights in the 21st century* (2000)

Meta-analytic procedure and interpretation of treatment outcome and test validity for the practitioner psychologist (with Ephrem Fernandez), *International Review of Professional Issues in Selection and Assessment* (1996)

Intelligence and personality measurement within the Cattellian psychometric model, *Personality Psychology in Europe* (1983)

OTHER

Review of the Personality Self-Portrait (Revised), *Humanities & Social Sciences papers* (2007)

Review of the International Personality Disorder Examination, *Humanities & Social Sciences papers* (2007)

Review of the Taylor-Johnson Temperament Analysis (2002 Edition), *Humanities & Social Sciences papers* (2007)

Review of the Trauma Symptom Checklist for Children, *Humanities & Social Sciences papers* (2007)

Editors' introduction: Contemporary perspectives on the psychology of individual differences. (with Donald H. Saklofske), *Humanities & Social Sciences papers* (2004) e-publications@bond

BOND UNIVERSITY

Gregory J. Boyle

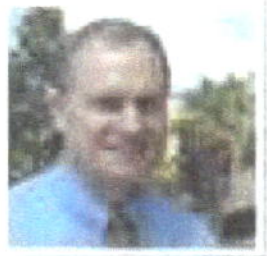

Professor of Psychology
Associate Dean (Research)

[illegible]

Fellow, Australian Psychological Society
Fellow, Association for Psychological Science

[illegible]

Documents by Subject Area

No subject area

- [illegible]
- Adverse Sexual and Psychological Effects of Male Infant Circumcision
- [illegible]

Gregory J. Boyle

Professor of Psychology
Associate Dean (Research)

Bond University

[illegible]

- Review of R. B. Cattell's (1983) Structured personality-learning theory: A wholistic multivariate research approach.
- Review of the (1985) Standards for educational and psychological testing: AERA, APA and NCME.
- Review of the International Personality Disorder Examination
- Review of the Personality Self-Portrait (Revised)
- Review of the Taylor-Johnson Temperament Analysis (2002 Edition)
- Review of the Trauma Symptom Checklist for Children
- Ritual and Medical Circumcision among Filipino boys: Evidence of Post-traumatic Stress Disorder
- Schizotypal Personality Traits: An Extension of Previous Psychometric Investigations
- Self-report measures of depression: Some psychometric considerations.
- Shortened halstead category test
- The enriched behavioral prediction equation and its impact on structured learning and the dynamic calculus
- The factor structure of "schizotypal" traits: A large replication study.
- The interaction of psychosocial and physical risk factors in the causation of mammary cancer, and its prevention through psychological methods of treatment.

CHEMICAL AXIOM LIKE DISSOLVES LIKE

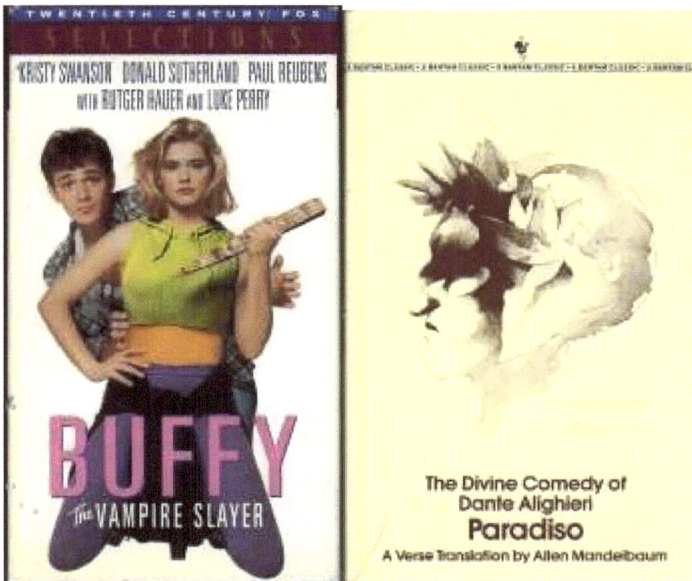

THE CIRCLE IS NOW COMPLETE

MOTHER'S MITOCHONDRIAL RUTHLESS/PROSOCIAL GENE
V.
FATHER'S WARRIOR GENE INACTIVE UNTIL RESURRECTED BY AND FOR THE SOCIAL

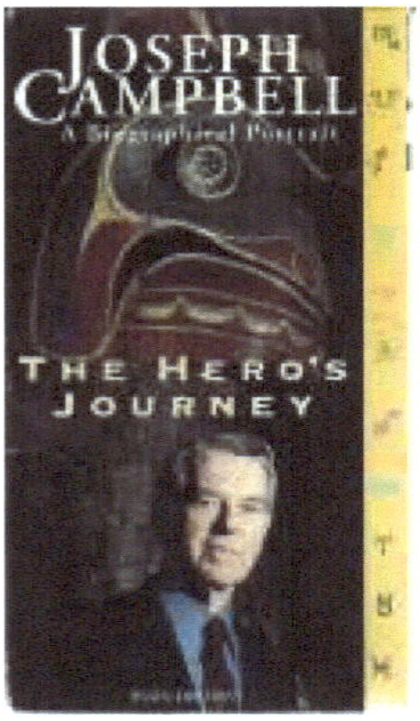

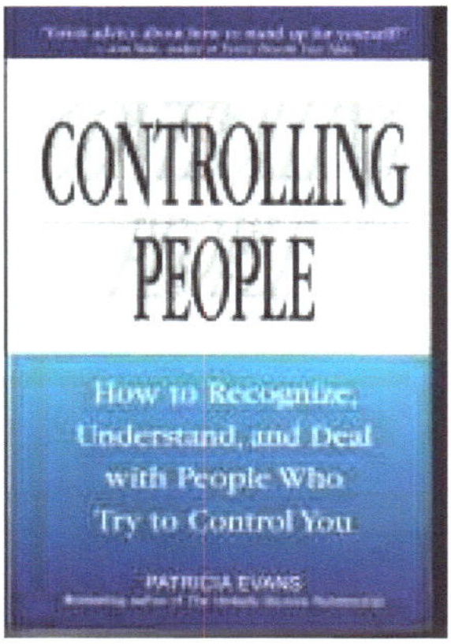

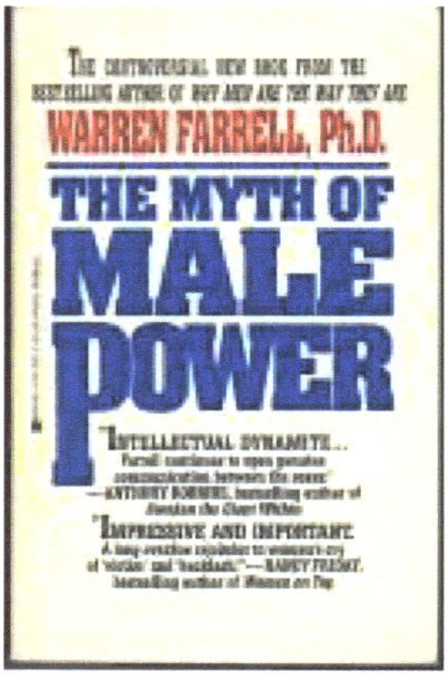

HERACLES

THE FATED MALE

RICHARD L. MATTEOLI

Mandated Report VA to CDC - Matteoli

OMINOUS FUTURE

GENETIC TESTING FOR PSYCHOPATHIC AND HOMICIDAL TENDENCIES BEYOND NONVIOLENT NORMAL FREUDIAN THANTOS

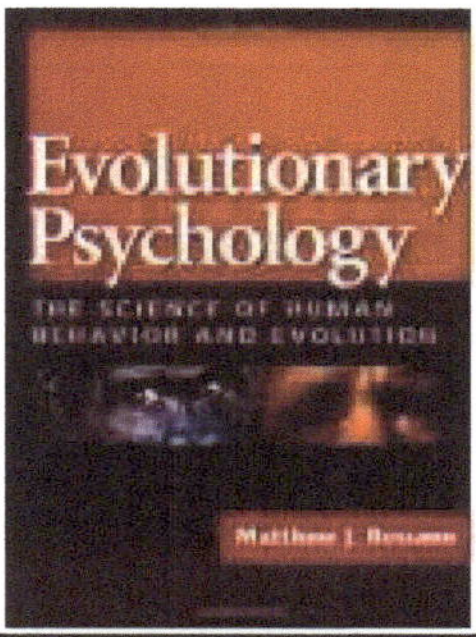

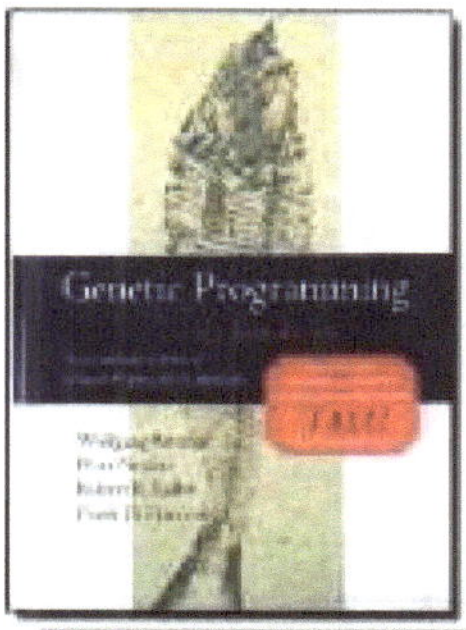

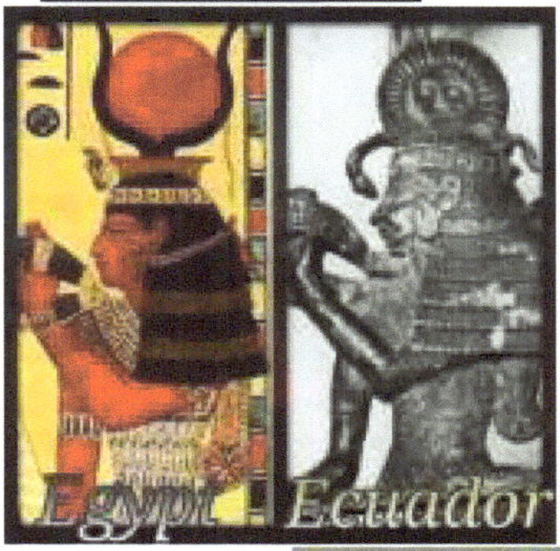

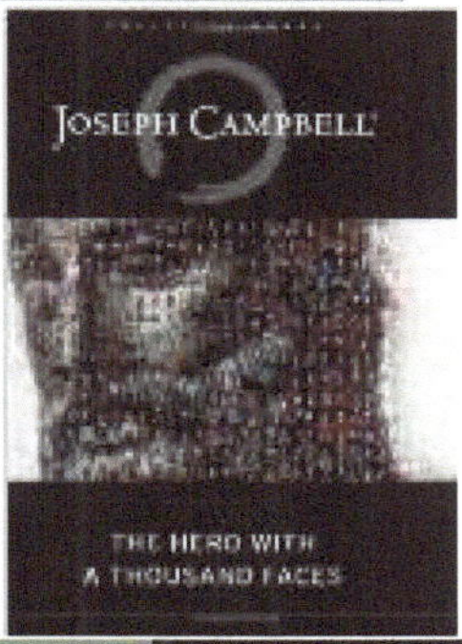

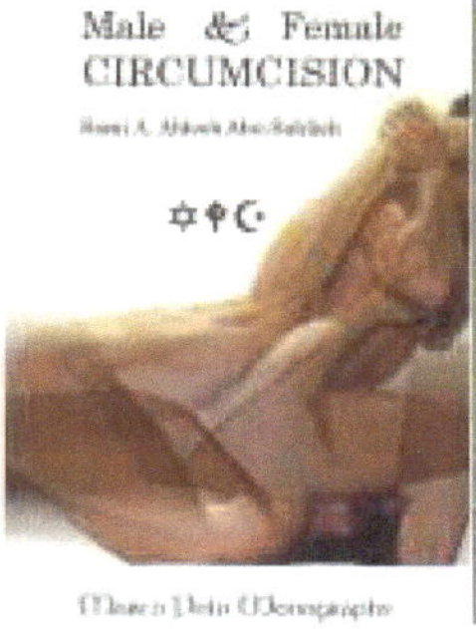

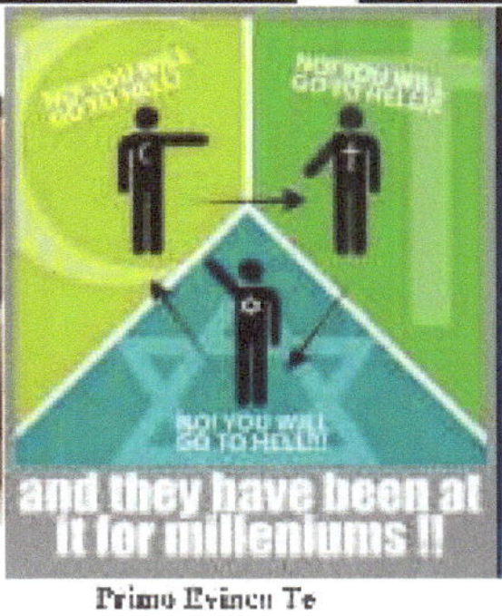

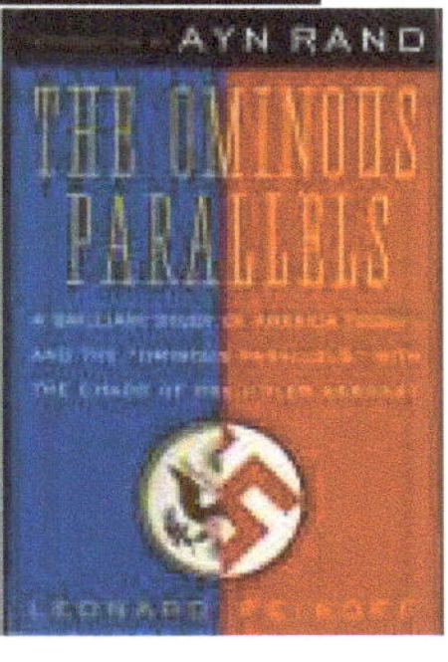

Primo Evincu Te
First Conquer Thyself:
Nemean Press
Monterey, CA 93940
USA
Richard L. Matteoli
with John J. Whitworth

www.ingramcontent.com/pod-product-compliance
Lightning Source LLC
Chambersburg PA
CBHW041303210326
41598CB00005B/8
* 9 7 8 1 9 4 3 3 4 7 1 4 8 *